D1728285

The Child in His Family

CHILDREN AND THEIR PARENTS IN A CHANGING WORLD

VOLUME 5

*YEARBOOK OF THE INTERNATIONAL ASSOCIATION
FOR CHILD PSYCHIATRY AND ALLIED PROFESSIONS*

EDITOR-IN-CHIEF—E. JAMES ANTHONY, M.D. (U.S.A.)

CO-EDITORS—CYRILLE KOUPERNIK, M.D. (FRANCE)

COLETTE CHILAND, M.D., Ph.D. (FRANCE)

Volume 1 **The Child in His Family**

E. James Anthony and Cyrille Koupernik, Editors

Volume 2 **The Child in His Family:
The Impact of Disease and Death**

E. James Anthony and Cyrille Koupernik, Editors

Volume 3 **The Child in His Family:
Children at Psychiatric Risk**

E. James Anthony and Cyrille Koupernik, Editors

Volume 4 **The Child in His Family:
Vulnerable Children**

E. James Anthony, Cyrille Koupernik, and Colette Chiland, Editors

Volume 5 **The Child in His Family:
Children and Their Parents in a Changing World**

E. James Anthony and Colette Chiland, Editors

The Child in His Family

CHILDREN AND THEIR PARENTS IN A CHANGING WORLD

VOLUME 5

Edited by

E. JAMES ANTHONY, M.D.
St. Louis, Missouri, U.S.A.

and

COLETTE CHILAND, M.D., PH. D.
Paris, France

Foreword by

ERIK H. ERIKSON

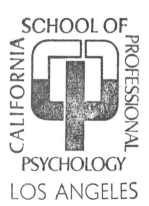

CALIFORNIA SCHOOL OF PROFESSIONAL PSYCHOLOGY LOS ANGELES

A WILEY-INTERSCIENCE PUBLICATION

JOHN WILEY & SONS, New York • Chichester • Brisbane • Toronto

Library of Congress Catalog Card Number: 78-120701

ISBN 0-471-04432-6

Printed in the United States of America

10 9 8 7 6 5 4 3 2 1

To *ERIK HOMBURGER ERIKSON,* who enabled us to look at the good, constructive, and helpful facets of evolving life (as well as what is negative) with an inquiring gentleness of spirit

Contributors

E. James Anthony (M.D.), Blanche F. Ittleson Professor of Child Psychiatry, and Director, Division of Child Psychiatry, Washington University School of Medicine, St. Louis, Missouri, U.S.A.

Helen Antonovsky (Ph.D.), Ben Gurion University, Beer Sheva, Israel.

D. M. Bassa (M.B., D.P.M., M.R.C.Psych.), Consultant Psychiatrist, Norfolk Area Health Authority, Bethel Hospital, Norwich, England.

Christopher C. Benninger (Ph.D.), Professor and Director, Centre for Development Studies and Activities, Poona, India.

Judith Blanc (M.A.), Ben Gurion University, Beer Sheva, Israel.

Gerald Caplan (M.D.), Professor of Psychiatry, Harvard Medical School, Boston, Massachusetts, U.S.A.; Visiting Professor of Psychiatry, Hebrew University of Jerusalem, Israel; Chairman, Department of Child Psychiatry, Hadassah University Hospital, Jerusalem, Israel.

G. Morris Carstairs (M.D.), Professor and Vice-Chencellor, University of York, York, England.

Colette Chiland (M.D., Ph.D.), Professor de Psychologie Clinique à l'Université René Descartes de Paris (Sorbonne), Paris, France.

Reuven Feuerstein (Ph.D.), Director, Hadassah-Wizo-Canada Research Institute, Jerusalem, Israel.

M. S. Gore (Ph.D.), Professor, Tata Institute of Social Sciences, Bombay, India.

Stephen P. Hersh (M.D.), Assitant Director, National Institute of Mental Health, Rockville, Maryland; Consultant, Pediatric Oncology Branch, National Cancer Institute, Bethesda, Maryland, U.S.A.

Erna Hoch (Ph.D.), Professor of Psychiatry, Medical College, Srinagar, India.

Mordecai Kaffman (M.D.), Medical Director, Kibbutz Child and Family Clinic, Tel Aviv, Israel.

Sudhir Kakar (Ph.D.), Visiting Professor of Behavioral Science, McGill University, Montreal, Canada.

David Kasilowsky (Ph.D.), Hadassah-Wizo-Canada Research Institute, Jerusalem, Israel.

Jon Lange (M.D.), Director, Child Psychiatry Clinic, Ulleval Hospital, Oslo, Norway.

Serge Lebovici (M.D.), Professeur Associé de Psychiatrie de l'Enfant à l'Université de Paris (Sorbonne), and Directeur, Centre Alfred Benet, Paris, France.

David J. de Levita (M.D.), Professor and Head of the Department of Child Psychiatry, University of Amsterdam, Amsterdam, The Netherlands.

Michaela Lifshitz (Ph.D.), University of Haifa, Haifa, Israel.

Reginald S. Lourie (M.D.), Professor Emeritus, George Washington School of Medicine, and Senior Consultant for the Psychiatric Institute, Washington, D.C.; and Senior Research Scioentist, Mental Health Study Center, National Institute of Mental Health, Adelphi, Maryland, U.S.A.

Kiyoshi Makita (M.D.), Professor and Chairman, Department of Psychiatry and Behavioral Science, Tokai University School of Medicine, Bohseidai, Isehara, Japan.

Mahmoud Meari (M.A.), Ben Gurion University, Beer Sheva, Israel.

Karen Moses (B.S.W.), Social Work Consultant to the Ministry of Defense of Israel, and affiliated with Paul Baerwald, School of Social Work, Hebrew University, Jerusalem, Israel.

Rafael Moses (M.D.), Clinical Director, Jerusalem Mental Health Center, Jerusalem, Israel; Professor of Psychiatry, Hebrew University, Jerusalem, Israel.

Peter B. Neubauer (M.D.), Director, Child Development Center; and Department of Child Psychoanalysis, Downstate Medical Center, NeNew York, New York, U.S.A.

Joseph Noshpitz (M.D.), Clinical Professor of Psychiatry, George Washington University School of Medicine, and Director of Training and Education, Children's Hospital, Washington, D.C., U.S.A.

Daniel Offer (M.D.), Chairman, Department of Psychiatry, Michael Reese Hospital and Medical Center; Professor, Department of Psychiatry, University of Chicago, Chicago, Illinois, U.S.A.

Phyllis Palgi (Ph.D.), Chief Anthropologist, Ministry of Health, Tel Aviv, Israel.

Ramlal Parikh (Ph.D.), B.M. Institute of Mental Health, Ahmedabad, India.

Anna Potamianou (Ph.D.), in private practice; formerly the Scientific Director of the Center for Mental Health and Research (1957-1968), Athens, Greece.

Luis E. Prego-Silva (M.D.), Professor of Child Psychiatry, University of Montevideo, Montevideo, Uruguay.

B. K. Ramanujam (M.D.), B.M. Institute of Mental Health, Ahmedabad, India.

Yaacov Rand (Ph.D.), Hadassah-Wizo-Canada Research Institute, Jerusalem, Israel.

Winston S. Rickards (M.D.), Department of Psychiatry, Royal Children's Hospital, Parkville, Victoria, Australia.

Alan Roland (Ph.D.), Psychoanalyst, New York, New York, U.S.A.; and Senior Research Fellow, American Institute of Indian Studies, Bombay, India.

Manoj Shah (Ph.D.), B.M. Institute of Mental Health, Ahmedabad, India.

Albert J. Solnit (M.D.), Professor, Departments of Pediatrics and Psychiatry, and Director, Child Study Center, Yale University School of Medicine, New Haven, Connecticut, U.S.A.

E. F. Thebaud (M.D.), John F. Kennedy Medical Center, Monrovia, Liberia.

James B. Welsh (Ph.D.), Research Fellow in Adolescence, Committee on Human Development, University of Chicago Department of Psychiatry, Michael Reese Hospital and Medical Center, Chicago, Illinois, U.S.A.

Sidney Werkman (M.D.), University of Colorado Medical Center, Denver, Colorado, U.S.A.

Edward Zigler (Ph.D.), Department of Psychology, Yale University, New Haven, Connecticut, U.S.A.

Foreword —
Reflections on Historical Change

IT FEELS SOMEWHAT PRESUMPTUOUS TO WRITE AN INTRODUCTORY foreword for a volume that promises to be in itself an introduction, rich in data, to a new phase in the alliance of the clinical and behavioral observation of childhood and in its relation to ongoing history. But since, over the years, I have helped to conduct seminars in two of the countries prominent in the reports collected here, namely, Israel and India, I may not be out of order in reflecting generally on the changes that are taking place in our very conception of historical change itself, as over the decades our attention has moved irresistibly from the case history to the human life cycle and on to the generational cycle and its historical setting.

HISTORY, OF COURSE, AS THE WORD CONNOTES, IS THE TRADITIONAL field of knowledge which reveals some logic in events that are sufficiently concluded that their completed story can be told and they can be compared and panoramically stored in some grand order classifying significant people, areas, and epochs. Historians can then take their time determining, in tune with the changing philosophies of their day, what men and what movements really made a difference in the way things inexorably turned out.

Up to a point, our case histories, singly and in comparative clusters, are historical in this sense, often too much so when they lead us to all too finite closures of diagnosis and induce us to see the developing present mostly in terms of the determining past. And yet, what we have learned about our role in the case history, from the moment we begin to record it, has led us to take a point of view more concerned with ongoing history than with history concluded—as is attested to by the existence of this volume.

The clinical and behavioral observation I am familiar with begins with Freud. In the psychoanalytic method he created an essentially life-historical approach which elicited from the patient data leading to a reconstruction of his repressed or unremembered past and a recognition of the origin of his symptoms in some stage of early history. But the patient can do so only by "transferring" some of his past into the treatment situation and thus reliving it; while the practitioner, in principle, must have learned to recognize in his own life the potentially pathogenic repressions and rationalizations that are apt to cloud man's memory. Moreover, the practitioner must be ready to recognize systematically the specific irrational responses evoked in him by a given patient's history. This, it must be realized, is a significant extension of the Hippocratic obligation. It also represents, in its ethical implications, a new and special form of age-old Caritas based on the acknowledgement of shared and universal human conflict. And finally, since in this kind of work the therapeutic process is also the method of observation, it also harbors a new attitude toward the life history—and toward history itself.

When I first became aware of this, I found myself allied to a philosophy of history that was formulated most memorably by R. G. Collingwood (*The Idea of History,* Oxford University Press, 1946) who concluded that "history is the life of mind itself which is not mind except so far as it both lives in the historical process and knows itself as so living." This statement to me connoted what I called the "systematic subjectivity" governing the clinical as well as the historical observer's objectivity.

If, by implication, I here seem to connect the historian's involvement and the clinician's Hippocratic task, I do not apologize: for as we approach a conjunction of the fields of history and of clinical and behavioral science we may well find that certain Hippocratic obligations extend to all dealings with ongoing history. To begin with, then: we certainly influence our patients' histories by the way we explore them; to this degree, at any rate, to *take* history means to *make* history.

BUT WHERE CAN HISTORICAL CHANGE ITSELF BE SEEN TO BE TAKING hold of our methods and insights? One of the (often apocryphal) stories that impressed us during our training in Vienna told of Freud's being accosted after a lecture by a listener who exclaimed, "But, Herr Professor, ten years ago you said exactly the opposite!" and reported Freud's answer: "Yes, that was right, then." In other words, a clinical method undergoes significant and continuous changes in the theories that emerge from it and, in turn, inform it.

We have also had to learn to understand historically that an overall concept such as the libido theory owed its original form to last century's scientific and economic preoccupation with energies and quantities meticulously to be accounted for in their transformations—and thus in all changes, for the better and for the worse: to find in all endeavours an "energy of equal dignity" to the energies that could be measured was the ethos of the science of that day. Nor do we have a right later to judge a theory wrong which, rooted in the spirit of its time, has established a firm first step essential to all later theories, attuned as they may be to their time and its dominant or contending world images. And as to the life histories of conceptual founders, we can discern in the correspondence between Freud and Jung how the two men, who agreed so creatively in certain basic clinical and theoretical matters—including the self-analytical approach—could not, at the end, agree on the overall world image to which these revolutionary observations belonged, and this clearly on the basis of their respective historical (ethnic and religious) backgrounds. They tried to understand this and to be honest about it; but whereas in our day our gradual attunement to modern science can make us understand a certain difference in standpoint as a true function of historical relativity, such an attempt at understanding would have appeared to be too relativistic for the founders' job-at-hand. And, indeed, to Freud's great persistence in letting each original observation and its theoretical implications "lead him as far as it would," step for step rather than in premature foreclosure, must be credited the fact that psychoanalysis survived the gigantic changes of World War I and emerged as an international movement, as it was then called, which was eventually to help revolutionize man's relation to his own history.

A formulation of special historical significance is a passage in Freud's *New Introductory Lectures on Psychoanalysis,* in a chapter determinedly called "Dissection of the Psychic Personality," where he locates some aspects of the historical process in the *super-ego.* As the *super* suggests, this is the inner agency of unremitting moralistic repression, which therefore must be a main focus in all attempts to free man from *inner suppression:*

As a rule parents and authorities analogous to them follow the precepts of their own super-egos in educating children. . . . They have forgotten the difficulties of their own childhoods and they are glad to be able now to identify themselves fully with their own parents who in the past laid such severe restrictions upon them. Thus a child's super-ego is in fact constructed on the model not of its parents but of its parents' super-ego; the contents which fill it are the same and it becomes the vehicle of tradition and of all the time-resisting judgments of value which have propagated themselves in this manner from generation to generation.

Then Freud, for once, briefly spars with Marxism—the contemporaneous world movement that made it its business to transcend all history as we know it by the revolutionary liquidation of *social oppression.*

It seems likely that what are known as the materialistic views of history sin in underestimating this factor. They brush it aside with the remark that human "ideologies" are nothing other than the product and superstructure of their contemporary economic conditions. That is true, but very probably not the whole truth. Mankind never lives entirely in the present. The past, the tradition of the race and of the people, lives on in the ideologies of the super-ego, and yields only slowly to the influences of the present and to new changes; and so long as it operates through the super-ego it plays a powerful part in human life, independently of economic conditions. (*Complete Psychological Works of Freud,* XXII, p. 67).

Accepting, for the moment, Freud's linkage of ideology and super-ego, we note, first of all, that with these formulations Freud indicated clearly that any true psychoanalytic procedure included, in principle, a study of the place of tradition in a patient's inner conflicts. He implies, furthermore, that the super-ego, the mainstay of moralistic conscience, is the inner agency that resists historical change—and thus all forms of liberationg8and can only be fought with the non-violent persuasion of psychoanalytic insight. From this original location of an archaic conscience both in the structure of the psyche and in an early period of the life cycle, there are, then, only a few steps to a corresponding assignment of other historical attitudes to other stages of the individual's developing psychic personality. There is, for example, the ripening of man's ego-identity in adolescence, a stage of life acutely responsive, both cognitively and emotionally, to the contemporary ideological changes of varying intensity and velocity. We will come back to that. Nevertheless, the psychoanalytic treatment of adults first became the method of choice in opening up the repressed past, whether in the form of childhood stages never before charted or in the form of reactionary moralities never before made responsible for mental suffering. Thus, even a culturally significant epidemiological item (such as hysteria at the turn of the century) was studied (and treated) by clarifying the role of the infantile super-ego in the repression of infantile drives; this became the first model for clinical description and analysis. The acute identity conflicts of hysterical patients at the time of the outbreak of the symptoms were not given the attention we would insist on today. Nor was the adult culture, characterized as it was by the double standards separating classes and sexes, spelled out as a historical phenomenon with a special pathogenic impact. It is, of course, characteristic of Freud's own case histories (as it is of his dream reports) that his description and discussion provide most telling hints for the study of other life stages and of corresponding historical conditions.

IN THE DAYS OF MY TRAINING IT WAS IMPRESSIVE TO BEHOLD HOW the psychoanalysis of children, while confirming many of the retrospective reconstructions of childhood by "adult" analysts, at the same time revealed developmental resources—for example, in the child patient's playful imagination and the searching verbalization that could be used directly in alleviating an all too stringent super-ego pressure. At the same time, Anna Freud's and August Aichhorn's work, in accounting for a child's acute life conflicts, also opened up for exploration and discussion the ongoing changes in the conditions of school life that were prone to occur in an education-conscious city such as Vienna. Later, of course, after her own exile, Anna Freud and her coworkers systematically studied the influence of war conditions on English children and the traumatic impact of concentration camp life on refugee children. However, these were primarily traumatic events, that is, radical upsets in what were then still considered to be regular conditions in the life of the generations, which at least in stable countries were expected to be restored post-traumatically both in their normality and in their foreseeable risks.

Since then, the world wars and world revolutions as well as worldwide industrialization have made historical change unilinear, irreversible, and permanent. As for its impact on the generational cycle, we must agree with Margaret Mead that today

Young people everywhere share a kind of experience that none of the elders ever have had or will have. Conversely, the older generation will never see repeated in the lives of young people their own unprecedented experience of subsequently emerging change. This break between generations is wholly new; it is planetary and universal. (*N. Y. Times Magazine,* April 26, 1970.)

BUT WHAT IMPRESSES AS A RADICAL CHANGE OF GENERATIONAL perspectives, wherever it becomes unpredictable in velocity and intensity, at least in the United States and in some other countries founded by immigrants, rather clearly corresponds to a traditional trend, which from the beginning made out of generational change itself a determined tradition cultivating the continuous emergence of a New Man, whether characterized primarily by a national, political, economic, or technological type—or all of these. True, the history of only a few countries (as different in their historical beginnings as the United States, Australia, Israel) has also offered to the "new man" a new territory, claimed on the basis of historical, if not divine, predestination. This permitted the development of a new native identity hospitable to a wide variety of eager immigrants and ingathered seekers of a homeland. Otherwise, in most countries, what for brevity's sake we may call the *modernization of identity* has to accommodate or be accommodated to the assumption that successive generations of children, youths, and adults will share essential experiences similar enough to attest to a world image confirmed by tradition and sealed by shared ritual.

How a variety of transitional conditions deal with this particular confrontation of old and new, and especially what specific psychopathology reflects the degree and kind of the resulting historical traumatization—this is a subject dominant in this volume. In this context it seems particularly important to discern in the material presented how historical change reaches into each stage of life and what each stage has to contribute to or is apt to lose from it. While, as indicated, Freud's formulation of "ideologies of the super-ego" primarily emphasizes the undue pressure of conscience and tradition on early life, one may well also ponder the normative need—in whatever system—for a stable orientation in the upbringing of children, that is, a firm and affirmative (rather than guilt-ridden) set of values that can later be mobilized for the aims of the society and against certain specified evils. Here, I will take the liberty of quoting myself:

In youth, the life history intersects with history; here individuals are confirmed in their identities and societies regenerated in their life style. But this process also implies a fateful survival of adolescent modes of thinking and of juvenile enthusiasm in man's historical and ideological perspectives, and a split between adult reason and idealistic conviction which is only too obvious in oratory, both political and clerical. (*Identity, Youth and Crisis.* New York, 1968. p. 257.)

This last "dig" obviously was meant to underline the necessity for giving serious attention to the function of the major age divisions (and each of their subdivisions) in historical change, and essentially also for a more informed assumption of adult responsibility. For if, indeed, adolescence is the hub of the wheel of generational turnover, and the imagination of adolescence is ready to experimentally endow many kinds of ideology with totalistic fervor, a whole young generation will not develop the true and healthy fidelity on which society depends without a convincing ideological link between past and future. Our problem is to know what combinations of old and new can convince youth that they have an active part in change—that is, whether change calls only for continuous readjustment or invites a live adaptation to institutions which, in turn, remain adaptable to inner as well as outer necessities.

All the more it is important for us even as we study children and youth to delineate what adulthood is and must become in an era marked by historical change. For recent events in a number of countries, and especially in the United States, have clearly shown that adult society can be all too ready to abandon the responsibility for rejuvenating change to ideologically inclined and yet inexperienced youth.

WE MUST NOW HASTEN TO ADMIT THAT WE HAVE MADE TOO MUCH OF Freud's use of the word *ideologies,* which in the context quoted was meant strictly for a comparison with the Marxian counterpoint. The proper designation for the social trend supported primarily by the super-ego is, of course, *moralities.* This would permit us to speak, in turn, of the *ideologies of the youthful ego-identity,* and, finally, of the *communal ethics of the mature ego.* Here I must hasten to underscore, however, that such an assignment of the rudiments of moralities to childhood and those of ideologies to youth does not make the first childish and the second juvenile—or not, at any rate, in a viable culture. As I have often explained, these are "epigenetic" matters—meaning that, while we develop the rudiments of our social personalities in successive pre-adult phases, every earlier gain is, in principle, renewed, transformed, and integrated in all subsequent ones, if, indeed, such development is facilitated by inner and outer conditions. Otherwise, they will, it is true, always invite regression. They must, therefore, be negotiated by the adult capacity to integrate past and foreseeable future and to counteract with an ever more inclusive communal ethics the adult tendency to reject other "species" of men.

And here it is not enough to say that ego strength means "adjustment to reality." In fact, as historically conscious observers we must consider how the connotations of such words change with the times—and in translation. For example, whether *ego* stands for the German *Ich,* or *reality* for *Wirklichkeit,* translations are always prone to rob matters of important philosophical connotations. I have therefore suggested that we must differentiate three functions of a viable living in reality: a maximum acceptance of *factuality*—that is, of what can be verified by the senses and by the existing methods of inquiry; a sense of *reality,* such as is conveyed only by shared world views assigning all facts to some intuitively convincing order; and, finally, a sense of *actuality*—that is, of a mutual actualization of all who share such world views. This suggests that there can be no inner-personal integration (or *ego*) which is not tuned to the *ethos* of an organized communality—and no ethos that does not have the support of the prevalent modes of ego-synthesis. In other words, ego and ethos complement each other.

I HAVE NOW ARRIVED AT SOME PRETTY LOFTY REQUIREMENTS OF what may be demanded of a healthy historical situation. As with all health, one can only hope that one has approached what in the nature of things seems to make for the optimum that is unrealized in ill-health. At any rate, the ego-synthesis that holds together a person passing through the human life cycle, and the generational synthesis that holds a social organization together seem to be all set to strive for such a mutually invigorating interplay. It is not my intention to claim, however, that we, with our clinical observations and developmental theories, can set out to plan such an optimum; health is always so much more than the sum of all observable, explainable, and manageable functioning. But insight and health, as gifts, are no strangers to each other. And even as medical men and women in the past could base their intercultural work on the knowledge of the workings of the all-human body, workers in clinical and behavioral science can, on the basis of their insights into the interplay of life cycle and generational cycle, become agents as well as observers of historical change.

To return to our Hippocratic discussion: such cultural interpenetration, as we said, commits the observer to some insight into the relativity of his own functioning within contending world views, including what he may consider scientificially most obvious. This, in turn, calls for special dialogues between observers who, in order to agree on aims of mental health and symptoms of mental ill-health, may have to make conscious, for themselves and their counterplayers, how culture-bound some of their habitual designations and theoretical preoccupations are. Well-known is our easy assumption of unconscious guilt; Eastern and Western discussants may want to clarify the different meanings of this word and its relation to a sense of shame or pollution—for example, in the context of the Judaeo-Christian and the Hindu traditions. What counts here is some agreement in regard to a developmental and social framework that will make it possible to pursue such matters through the various life stages and their relation to historical change.

BY THE SAME TOKEN WE MUST FIND WAYS OF COUNTERPOINTING OUR various means of systematic self-inspection. I, for one, would not hesitate to claim that psychoanalysis, in its use of the special state of attention called "free association," is a Western form of meditation designed to extend consciousness to inner areas obscured by defences and yet expressed in indirect, symbolic form. True, in its professional and historical setting this method became specialized as a means to the end of a cure or, at any rate, better adjustment, and at the same time as a means to the end of a scientistic theory explaining inner life in a quantitative and causal manner. Yet, psychoanalytic enlightenment touched on all forms of human endeavor and has by now become part and parcel of modern consciousness, wherever it spreads. At the same time, Eastern meditation, which in so many highly implicit and yet decisive ways dominates the thinking of Asian cultures, is attracting many adherents in the West. I cannot see how such Eastern and Western means of expanding human consciousness can fail to inform together an all-human historical awareness to which this volume contributes, I think, one specific tool. (As to a comparison of psychoanalytic and Hindu forms of thought I would point to the work of Professor Sudhir Kakar, who chaired with me a recent exploratory meeting convoked by the Indian Social Research Council in Delhi, *The Inner World, A Psychoanalytic Study of Hindu Childhood and Society*, New Delhi and New York: Oxford University Press, 1977; and for a report of our meetings, see Sudhir Kakar, Editor, *Identity and Adulthood in India*, New Delhi and New York: Oxford University Press [in press].)

IN CONCLUSION, AN ALLIANCE BETWEEN CLINICAL AND BEHAVIORAL observations can register and study the different forms taken by the human core disturbances under changing conditions—certainly one method of taking the pulse of changing history. Reflecting on their own function in worldwide communication, such observers will be aware of the necessity of studying not only the traditional and now disintegrating but also the emerging generational and historical consciousness on the part of adults all over the world. This, in turn, will impose new Hippocratic responsibilities on those who analyze and report historical change, whatever their method and approach; for, indeed, in today's world of communication, to report history is to make history. Note that clinical and behavioral theory can offer more than a powerful corrective; there can hardly be an all-inclusive therapeutic ideology. I am, in fact, reminded here that in some metropolitan areas the unavoidable and essential recognition of mental ill-health can become a substitute rather than a support for communal concerns; and we see young people for whom their own overdiagnosed case histories have become the only tangible identities they can envisage, and the interview the only setting where they feel they can find appreciation.

Our observations, then, must become part of a world image in which the community's responsibility for the verified resources of human growth is the dominant concern—and joy. This can, I think, be most significantly supported by students of childhood and youth. I do not think that I am stretching the utopian license of a foreword if I conclude by saying that nothing can reveal the evidence for one all-human species-hood (and the energies waiting for its universal recognition) as can the endeavor to look concernedly at each others' children, their suffering, and their miraculous readiness for full human development.

ERIK H. ERIKSON

Preface

In these brief prefatory remarks, the Editors would like to draw attention to the various steps in the making of this international, interdisciplinary series: *The Child in His Family.* At the beginning of every quadrennium immediately following the International Congress in Child Psychiatry and Allied Profession, the new International Executive chooses a theme that is felt to be innovative, widely ranging in its appeal to behavioral scientists, and potentially promising to clinicians although as yet untapped by them in the course of their everyday work. This theme is then investigated in detail and depth over the subsequent four years by an International Study Group of experts drawn from different disciplines, who visit countries that offer a sharp contrast with respect to the theme and collaborate with local specialists in examining the cultural and clinical variations imposed by local conditions. Thus, in the 1974–1978 period, the theme selected was that of change, and the International Study Group set about exploring the differences between rapidly developing societies, like Israel, and slowly developing societies, like India. In time, both countries became the locus of mini-conferences that involved, in addition to the interchanges with native-born colleagues, the arrangement of a series of supervised and reported site visits. The foreign experts understandably brought with them preconceived notions based on the training and experience in their own countries and were often compelled to develop new sets of theories and constructions to fit in with their observations. Our visitors found, as anthropologists have found for many years, that it is not easy to penetrate cultures rapidly and to empathize with alien visions of the world; but, with the help of colleagues born and bred in the tradition, they found themselves resonating to notions completely dystonic to them.

That they often left this *terra incognita* with more questions than answers and shorn of some the stereotypes that they brought with them was itself an indication of the way in which the investigating team was caught up in the process of change. The trend of these international, interdisciplinary discussions, as readers will find out for themselves, was toward an increasing convergence and synthesis of structural and functional aspects of change without an overreliance on Western theory. At times, during the exchanges, *structure* would become the predominant issue as reflected in efforts to classify and categorize observed and experienced phenomena; on other occasions, *process* would come to the forefront, as evident in dynamic descriptions of evolutions, developments, and transactions over time; and sometimes it was *content* that held the center of the stage, with "stories" of primitive behavior, ritualism, witchcraft, and bizarre symptomatology. To put all these features together in a single volume is by no means an easy task; besides which, the Editors have felt that in order to give something of the flavor of the Study Group, it was better not to edit the life out of the spontaneous and stimulating discussions.

Readers who have followed the series from the first to the present fifth volume will detect an overall logic that has also determined the progression of topics from one volume to the next. For example, in Volume 1, the family, across the world and down the centuries, was looked at for commonalities and divergences both in its nuclear and in its extended forms; in Volume 2, the response of the family and its membership to the natural disasters of disease and death were studied against the background of new and complex models of family life; in Volume 3, the risks were extended to include a wide spectrum of hazards and vicissitudes, with a special focus on coping and mastery; in Volume 4, it was recognized that some children confronted with these risks succumbed to them, whereas others proved extraordinarily resilient, and elements of both vulnerability and invulnerability were examined as they developed over the years; and now, in Volume 5, the theme of vulnerability is carried a step further in relation to the susceptibility or resistance to change, both internal and external, both developmental and environmental, and both historical and contemporary. Whether a new sub-science of "metabletics" will emerge in nonclinical and clinical forms remains to be seen, but it does represent an important field for the clinician to explore further.

Our thanks as usual go to Doris Diephouse, Martha Kniepkamp, and Sally Clayburgh for the excellent job that they have done in reducing some of the chaos and diversity of international contributions to sizable and manageable proportions within the theme of the book. The speed with which this particular volume has been produced reflects in part their skills as well as the experience and capacity of our publishers.

One must add the important comment that without the assistance of the William T. Grant Foundation and its sensitive and sympathetic president, Philip Sapir, there would be no meetings of the International Study Group and, consequently, no possibility of breaking ground in this new clinical area. We are deeply indebted to the Foundation for helping us in this way.

E. JAMES ANTHONY, M.D.
COLETTE CHILAND, M.D., PH.D.

St. Louis, Missouri, U.S.A.
Paris, France
May, 1978

Contents

The Child in His Family

CHILDREN AND THEIR PARENTS IN A CHANGING WORLD

VOLUME 5

GENERAL ASPECTS

An Introduction to the Psychology and Psychopathology of Change

E. James Anthony, M.D. (U.S.A.)

Ripening and rotting from hour to hour, as Shakespeare grimly reminded us, is the biological story of our lives: we seem inextricably caught up in anabolic-catabolic cycles, in circaddian rhythms, and in the menstrual ebb and flow. Change is also of the essence in our social and psychological lives, as pointed out by that evolutionary philosopher, Samuel Butler:

All our lives long, every day and every hour, we are engaged in the process of accommodating our changed and unchanged selves to changed and unchanged surroundings; living, in fact, is nothing else than this process of accommodation; when we fail in it a little we are stupid, when we fail flagrantly we are mad, when we suspend it temporarily, we sleep, when we give up the attempt altogether, we die.

What Butler is telling us here is that if we have to live our lives with change, we must learn how to cope with change and adjust to it, because unless we do, change inevitably will render us obsolete and sweep us under the carpet. There was never any place for stagnation, even in the hidden wards of insane asylums, but as the pace of life accelerated, the world was becoming increasingly intolerant of stasis.

Not the least of the many difficulties introduced by change is the paradoxical mode in which it presents itself to human percipients:

3

the more things seem to change, the more they appear to remain the same. All change inherently carries with it the notion of constancy and stability. Without this concomitant, it is doubtful whether we could ever be or feel ourselves for even a moment of time—to develop recognizable personalities, to forge enduring identities, one requires some underlying process of conservation to counteract the Protean mechanisms of change. The relationship between stability and change is by no means a fixed ratio; there are times, in the course of historical development, when one or the other is predominant in the foreground while the other remains unobtrusively in the background.

The ancients themselves were puzzled by the changing appearance of change: the Heraclitean model envisioned, like its modern Bergsonian counterpart, a state of flux—never stepping into the same stream of consciousness a second time, whereas the Parmenedean model is one of changelessness, with all change being an illusion. It would seem that human beings, in presumably different states of consciousness, experience change constantly or not at all, and one of the things that one needs to consider within a psychology of change is whether such vast discrepancies in awareness are functions of individual personalities, varying levels of threshold, or subtle physiological shifts. There is no doubt that there is often a striking difference in perspective. Some persons are constantly confronted and affronted by the rapidly changing world in which they live and by the swirl of political and social events about them and recognize that these leave their imprint on the social and personal scene. For others, the more introversive ones, external changes remain shadowy and largely a matter of subjective consideration; the changes within them—the intense Kierkegaardian subjectivity—is what really matters. It remains for the clinician to appraise the changes brought about within the intrapsychic state by the turmoils of the external world [20].

Historical Change

It is only retrospectively that one obtains a true appreciation of the nature of change. The past becomes punctuated by an endless series of events, so that history appears like a succession of stories fabricated in different ways by different historians. This is also true of biography pathography, where once again the story-telling propensity takes over and adds logic and segmentation to the flux. In truth, history does no more than try to explain how and why one situation changes into another. All that history can do is to instruct us how to foster beneficial changes and how to avoid the repetition of malignant ones.

In the not too distant past, not only did history move on leaden boots, but the impact of historical change was imperceptible to the larger part of the people. Without the help of the electronic media, revolutionary changes were often confined for long periods to small local areas, and dissemination, if it occurred at all, took decades to cross national boundaries. Change was thus experienced at the upper levels of society and filtered only very gradually down through the feudal system. This is one way of looking at historical change as it seeps through different levels of the social economy or passed through to different cultures. When seen against the immense background of known history, change develops a dynamic of its own, imperceptible within day to day transactions. History is made up not only of change but also of resistance to change, so that there are times when time seems set in the doldrums. During eras of stagnation, it would seem (at least from a particular reading of history) that inner changes of a morbid nonproductive character are more striking so that the documents of the time become replete with visions and witchcraft. On the other hand, when the flow of change of human affairs becomes rapid, a more extroversive development tends to occur, and transformations of a practical, scientific, and productive nature are more likely to take place. At such times the filtration of change through the population is swifter, so that nations as a whole become conscious of transformation. One might speculate that models of change, whether Heraclitean or Parmenedean, are equally products of variations in the flow of change.

The major challenge today is whether our conservative habits can keep pace with the changes in the environment and its resources. What is taking place in the history of man's management of his environment is an extraordinary acceleration in the harnessing of power: a harnessing of wind power for driving ships began 5000 years ago, of waterpower for driving mills 2000 years ago, of electric power for driving trains 120 years ago, of oil power for heating our homes and energizing our cars 70 years ago, and of atomic power that seems destined to revolutionize our whole manner of material existence hardly 30 years ago.

The historian Toynbee [17] sees the forces of changes metaphorically located in the head and the heart, always pulling in two different directions and moving at different rates. The head's pace has always been faster than that of the heart, and consequently, a widening gap has arisen between these two change agents that threatens to disintegrate the human psyche unless special adaptations can be made to it. The head is constantly taking the heart by surprise through confronting it with revolutionary new technological situations for which the heart is ill prepared, but there is a saving grace built into the situation: the head cannot translate its knowledge into action unless it can more or less persuade the heart to cooperate with it. All head and no heart makes Jack into a technocrat, but all heart and no head does away with our plumbing which represents one of the acmes of present-day existence. This hazardous interplay between heart and head has led to dangerous situations in developing countries all over the world.

Concomitant with the speeding up of change in human life, there has been an equally remarkable alteration in the attitudes and behavior manifested toward women and children. Psychohistorical studies have disclosed what it is still hard for us to believe, that in past centuries and even in certain cultures today, the notion of childhood as we understand it simply does not exist. There is no awareness of the particular nature of children distinguishing them from adults. It is only through the work of Freud, Piaget, Erikson, and other developmental psychologists that childhood has earned its special segment in the life cycle during which it occupies the world conceived to its own image and likeness. If children are responsive to the nuclear age or to the natural disasters that abound around them, it is mainly because of what they learn from parents and teachers and from that great surrogate parent and teacher, the television set. Their political inclinations, like their sexual proclivities, undergo the characteristic development from fantasy to fact—from exuberant political fantasy to the somewhat deadened politics of everyday life. It is clear that the technological age is catching up with the child, invading his internal world, contaminating his fantasy, and providing him with ready-made images to structure his daydreams. It may be that change will end up paradoxically making everyone alike.

Cultural Change

Societies are as prone to change as individuals, and the rate and extent of change can be considerable. Individuals who enter the society also undergo changes in the psychosocial spheres, and once again the tempo of change will largely determine the effects produced. There are thus two types of change related to the social environment: the individual may change along with a changing society or an individual may change as a result of entering a new society. Furthermore, societies, like individuals, accept change, adapt to change, or resist change. The effects of acculturation can be best studied by means of a follow-up. Two examples illuminate the differences:

1. Mead studied the Manus first in 1928 and returned twenty-five years later [10]. At the time of the first visit, the people lived in pile dwellings in a lagoon. The women wore aprons of sago leaves, while the men had bark cloth g-strings. Their religion involved a cult of the recently deceased family head, and diviners and mediums were consulted to learn the disposition of the spirit. In less than three decades, Manus lived on land, wore Western-style clothing imported from Australia in cellophane packages, and attended Christian churches.

2. For centuries, traditional Hindu society limited the individual's opportunities for making significant decisions. A person could only do what he was allowed to do as a member of a particular caste and his behavior was described by Sovani [19] as "devoid of personal initiative, purposefulness and involvement." In 1948 [15] such conformity continued to flourish, and a decade later, Carstairs [6] remarked on the complete subordination of the individual to his family and religion. It was in most instances the women who were the preservers of tradition. Upward mobility rendered things even more complicated. The educated Indian male appeared to live in a bifurcated world: while outside at work, he could be in complete command of his staff, but the minute he entered his home, he was once again the child whose father decided how the grandchildren should be educated and how the family income should be spent.

A Psychology of Change

In constructing the large-scale edifice of psychoanalysis, Freud worked at times clinically and at times psychologically. He examined the gross manifestations of hysteria, but at the same time he began to examine normal phenomena such as dreams, parapraxes, transference and group behavior. Psychoanalysts, like Hartmann, have yearned to establish a psychoanalytic psychology as an underpinning to the clinical work. It would be logical, therefore, to start with psychology and end with psychopathology, although it is difficult for clinicians to keep these areas separate because of overlapping mechanisms. Van den Berg [18] has put forward an argument for the establishment of what he terms "metabletics," that is, a general psychology of change. It would seem that any theory of change requires that certain essential features be taken into account:

1. That both change and constancy are related and reciprocal aspects of development.
2. That the individual, during the course of his development, can undergo massive change and yet remain quintessentially the same.
3. That there is a persistent and mysterious sense of selfness that continues unaltered throughout life.
4. That changes within the individual may be correlated with changes in his immediate and remote environment.
5. That changes may involve every aspect of personal and social living and that the tempo of change may be a function of both the individual and his environment.
6. That it is the summation of changes in the individual and in his environment that generates the phenomenological experience of change. Similarly, the summation of resistance by the individual and his environment to change creates a total experience of constancy and stability.
7. That change is a variable entity, being rapid at one time and slow at another; massive at one time and minimal at another, so that human development may pass through phases of changeability and relative changelessness. Since change often seems to inspire a spirit of optimism, it is well to remember that it can be retrogressive as well as progressive, detrimental as well as positive.

A systematic metatheory of change must, therefore, include a variety of subconstructs: rates of change (acute, critical, sudden, unexpected, rapid or slow, gradual, chronic; static or stagnant; accelerating or decelerating), direction of change (backward, forward, or spiral), amount of change (ranging from slight to massive), type of change such as social (upward or downward mobility), geographical (residential mobility or immobility), and environmental (urbanization, militarization, artificial land and water transformations), and mechanisms of change (plasticity, rigidity, resilience, vulnerability, adaptation, coping, awareness, addiction to, sensitivity to, defense against, mastery of, denial of, and reversal of).

All these features can be incorporated into a general dynamics of change with its own self-perpetuating processes within which change acts at times as a stimulus, at times as a stress, and at times as a disaster. The correlations between individual and environmental changes are hard to determine at any moment on the continuum, with occasionally one or the other predominating.

Measures of change, either psychological or psychopathological, have still to demonstrate their efficacy in generating data and subsequent theory. Any theory of change must take into account the relationship between change in the individual and change in the environment, and in order to study this relationship, measures of both types are required. Psychosocial measures of individual variation are not uncommon, but we still need to develop adequate measures of environmental variation. What impedes work in this area is that we are not at all sure as yet what change aspects of the environment are relevant to change aspects within the individual. Furthermore, objective and external judgments seem at times to bear no relation whatsoever to internal and subjective experiences. Thus in the evaluation of any change phenomena one must have at least some assessment of the changing environment, some evaluation of the changing individual, and some measure of the particular attribute or characteristic under consideration.

Those who have worked in this field will appreciate the fact that the phenomena we are trying to quantify are amorphous and intangible so that only the very crudest characteristics of individual and environment at the present time when the instruments available are generally far from adequate are assessable.

The Changing Environment

Environment has been defined as the set of conditions surrounding and impinging on the individual that shapes and reinforces the tendencies within him. The trouble with the environment is that it has no clear boundaries. One can postulate that it starts from the surface of the individual but thereafter drifts into infinity, and, hypothetically, almost every factor operating from China to Peru may exert an influence on the individual. In general terms, we may all occupy the same space under the sun, but it can be claimed with some truth that no two individuals have experienced the same combination of environmental, interactional, and experiential forces.

No more than the individual does the environment stay the same from moment to moment. The term "developmental environment" [1] refers to the significant forces acting on the individual at any point in his development. Any such description of the environment must include not only the supplies available to the individual but also the extent to which he can make use of them.

Under ordinary circumstances of everyday life, environments appear for the most part benign and unthreatening, but crises and catastrophes can rapidly turn the most placid milieu into something disturbing, destructive, and elemental.

The Psychopathology of Change

Investigation into the psychopathology of change has opened up for us today a new form of risk research in which prospective studies can be carried out, predictions made, and hypotheses of causality confirmed or disconfirmed. Studies of change, like studies of risk, are opening up a new field in the understanding of normal and abnormal human behavior. The extent to which the human individual succumbs to a change experience would seem to depend on an inherent sensitivity to change, the history of which goes back to his beginnings in life. Caplan [5] has also put forward the suggestion that the tolerance for change is largely a function of a three-generation family support system and that where this is fragmented or insufficient the impingement of change can be devastating. The support system provided by an extended family caters to the continually developing biological, psychosocial, and economic needs of the individual members of the family and buffers the individual from exorbitant external demands. The family gradually educates the individual so that new knowledge does not burst on it catastrophically; the family provides the individual with a preliminary resonance board to test out his affects before trying them out on the world at large; the family, through its constant reality testing, helps the individual master both culture and future shock. The family can absorb change and transmit it more gently to its members; where massive changes occur by death and unemployment, a family can help its members to accomplish "worry-work" and bereavement-work both during and after the crisis. It can help also to counteract despair and helplessness by maintaining hope in eventual mastery. However, the family can only operate effectively as a support system, according to Caplan, if it remains in open and valid communication with the world around it.

Within the setting of the family, the individual members can experiment with change, since they are assured of a sufficient degree of stability and constancy.

If sociocultural changes are too rapid, they will limit the capacity of families to act optimally as support systems and thus render them more liable to change pathology. In a world that is changing radically and rapidly, the individual becomes caught up in the accelerated change and finds it difficult to cope with it. Harmful world changes include population movements (often involving separation of family members and the loss of familiar neighborhoods), urban conglomerations (with overcrowding and high population density leading to increased vulnerability to both psychiatric and physical illness), to the sad phenomenon of displaced individuals living in strange worlds that are largely unpredictable.

Even more disturbing than the psychopathology of acculturation is the pathology induced by future shock [16] resulting from excessively rapid and radical changes that take their toll on a significant number of change-sensitive individuals. We do not know as yet what specific patterns of personality disorders occur in children of different ages who are exposed to such situations of rapid change, but one's clinical expectation would be to find symptoms similar to cultural shock—disorientation, insecurity, apathy, depression, poor impulse control, and autistic withdrawal.

A Tentative Nosology of Change

Even at this early stage in our understanding of a change psychopathology, one might attempt, for heuristic purposes, to construct a tentative nosology of change that will not please everyone but might very well stimulate someone to further work and elaboration in this new area.

1. Change generating psychopathology: such as Durkheim's anomie, cultural shock, "future shock," fear of change or change phobia.
2. Psychopathology creating change: deterioration in school performance, psychosocial downward mobility, changes in interactional behavior, drug addiction, delinquency.
3. Developmental changes creating specific developmental crises over periods of transition: psychosexual, educational, biological, emergence of identity confusions and diffusions.
4. Changes in the nature of the presenting psychopathology (or "Whatever happened to Dora?"): a shift away from the classical, somewhat gross earlier conversions and clinical transmogrifications to somewhat pallid dependency, narcissistic, characterological disorders.
5. Changes brought about by resistance to change: oppositional syndromes, authoritarian personalities, obsessive-compulsive behavior, the "just so" rituals of autism, negativism and catatonia.

There is no doubt that close observations of infants reveal very early on in life a disposition to react excessively to even minimal changes in the environmental circumstances. There is an oversensitivity to changes in routine, to changes in caretakers, to transient separations, to the appearance of strangers. As if colluding with the infant's "constitutional" tendency, parents attempt to provide the child with a relatively changeless environment: everything is kept "just so"; rituals are preserved at bedtime and throughout the day; transitional objects and treasures are always around and in the right place; nothing is altered without prior consultation; and every departure from routine and ritual is prepared for apprehensively by the parents. Such children grow up fearful of change, fearful of satisfying their natural curiosities, fearful of attempting something novel, fearful of exploration, fearful of taking chances, and living their self-protected lives within wide margins of safety. One can pick these infants up quite early, as they balk at the edge of the "visual cliff."

Changes in the Support System

Any change in family structure and function, whether through separation, desertion, illness, hospitalization, or death, creates prolonged reverberations in the vulnerable change-sensitive child, and it takes him time to recover not only from the beginning of change but also with the termination of change. Any form of separation from the family milieu or the family members brings about acute nostalgia, anxiety or even severe panic.

Winnik [20] has called attention to the ways in which external changes have led to modifications in internal structure, particularly the superego and its ensuing pathology. According to Winnik, this particular structure does not end its development at the end of the first 5 years of childhood; it simply enters a different phase, where it changes its objects and substitutes the parental influence for those of educators, teachers, and other possible models. He notes that the superego, by virtue of its genesis, must have a contradictory character, since it owes its emergence on the one hand to the severing of the infantile ties and yet through the process of internalization it maintains the parental influence internally. It is, therefore, far from being an integrated and consistently functioning mental structure. Apart from Freud, who spoke of changes in the collective superego, Sachs [13] also dealt with the psychological resistances to technological developments. World changes within the present century associated with increasing urbanization—the emancipation of women, the creation of new job possibilities, automation, and the so-called "acceleration phenomenon" characterized by early puberty, shortening latency, and lengthening adolescence—all have had far-reaching influences on the formation of the superego, such as a diminution of personal factors in favor of institutional ones in its composition.

He feels that the greater impact of the collective superego has helped to enhance feelings of guilt, isolation, and varying forms of anxiety, and this has certainly been exaggerated by the diminution in the size of the family. Another major change has been the fading of the father figure in the process of identification toward building the superego, as described by Mitscherlich [11].

Attempts have been made to alter the course of change psychopathology through religion, art, and philosophy by restoring some sense of inner stability, but they have had limited success. Freud himself [8] felt that religion as a collective solution could no longer affect the combined impact of historical events, cultural changes, and inner psychic new constellations. Individuals, accustomed to gradual autoplastic mastery of change, have found it increasingly difficult without the help of prolonged treatment to deal with massive alloplastic changes.

Therapeutic Change

Change is the essential element of therapy, and the degree of change brought about by therapy depends not only on the nature of the disorder, the confidence and competence of the therapist, the time given to treatment, but also to certain dispositional factors, not least being that of dispositional plasticity. Kubie [9] drew attention to this from the point of view of the psychotherapist, pointing out, at the same time, that frequently striking changes may be obtained in the symptomatic picture of the patient leaving the underlying process of illness relatively unchanged. He said that the secondary consequences of neurotic symptoms and traits were often so great that even the slightest change in them could make enormous differences to the life of the patient so that they may appear less sick from the outside. This led him to make a basic distinction between a sick life and a sick person with respect to the potential for change. Kubie sees it as one of life's deep tragedies that man tends to lose his psychological plasticity on his path through life, and he regards neurotic and psychotic illness as functions of this impairment and limitation in the ability to change. For him, therefore, the change factor is central to human psychopathology from infancy onward. To keep well, the individual has to keep changing or rather keep being able to change. Changes in the degree of freedom to change is the indicator of basic change, and this is what a psychotherapist must look for at the termination of his treatment.

Wallerstein [19], along with others, has also been concerned with the assessment of change through the process of psychotherapy and ascribes changes not only to the variables of treatment but also to events in the patient's life situation. The interplay between situational and therapeutic variables determines the overall course and outcome of treatment. He uses situational measures, therefore, not merely as criteria of therapeutic outcome but also as factors that impinge on the patient and make for change and that may in turn be changed themselves by the changes occurring in the patient. Judgments are made as to the extent and direction of change in any particular criterion variable over time, but global assessments with regard to change in the direction of greater mental health are also made. Changes with regard to the expression of anxiety, the tolerance of separation, the reactions of guilt, and the increase in insight may not necessarily vary in the same direction and may not correlate highly with the overall assessment of mental adjustment. Unfortunately, change is so pervasive and so much a part of living and developing that it is extremely difficult to ascribe particular changes to particular intervention procedures.

Dispositional plasticity has had a long and distinguished history. The gestalt psychologists, exploring the motility and sensitivity of newborn infants, were struck with the variability in responsiveness, although individual infants could be differentiated in terms of rigidity and flexibility. They felt that plasticity was not something that could be learned and retained in the memory but were creative recombinations by virtue of which man became "superior to all other living creatures." It not only increased his adaptability to novel situations but also helped in the resolution of conflicts.

Research on Change

Studies of change, like studies of genetic risk, are opening up a new field in the understanding of human behavior. Change, whether acute or gradual, represents a significant risk for the individual at any age but especially at the two extremes of life. Currently, the dearth of environmental measures constitutes a serious problem in change research. Investigators have frequently limited themselves to simple rating scales of observation so that the final appraisal is distinctly lacking in subtlety of the elements involved. Yet instruments are hard to come by, and naturalistic observations are inclined to focus on persons. It is not easy to interview the environment!

In one such study of the environment [12], dealing with identical twins separated early in infancy, an attempt was made to delineate the environment in which each of the separated twins lived. The measurements, however, were so gross that the findings were altogether suspect. All that could be inferred from this study was that the dimension of an environment that related highly to one human characteristic was comparatively unrelated to another. Before-and-after studies, such as this one, are inclined to overlook all the intervening environments in which the child has lived.

Another group of studies have helped to illuminate the change mechanisms involved in environmental shifts and are of two kinds:

1. Change from the comparatively normal environment to a very powerful and extreme one, identified as very abundant or very deprived can produce deleterious effects, especially on little children who are unable to escape physically or psychologically from the overpowering experience.
2. The reverse shift, crowded and busy environment to one of comparative changelessness, may also conduce to maladjustment characterized by boredom, restlessness, and acting out.

A third set of studies has had to deal with the question of vulnerability to the risks of change. Susceptible individuals are especially liable to undergo disequilibrium in the process of leaving one environment for another. This "freshman" experience becomes critical when it takes place before the individual has time to discover subenvironments to which he can retreat [3] or before he can develop a set of defenses against the initial stranger discomforts. The less susceptible individuals are those who almost immediately set about molding the new environment to their needs, detaching themselves from its pressures and demands, or establishing subenvironments compatible with their style of life. A further group of individuals become rapidly alienated both from themselves and their environment and respond to the change by developing severe identity problems. The clinician who sees them at this point may be likely to diagnose them as schizoid, internally rigid, and quite unable to make the necessary shifts required for change. Specific psychopathologies are now being recognized as sequelae to residential and social mobility, urbanization, migration, immigration, and the havoc wrought by natural disasters.

Some tentative conclusions can be drawn between change and the genesis of psychopathology:

1. That the impact of change is a function of the rate, magnitude, quality, and kind of change.
2. That changes relating to temporal or spacial distancing between individuals decrease in potency and malignancy with increasing age.
3. That an adequate support system comprising family, neighborhood, school, and community may help to offset even massive and catastrophic changes.
4. That although dispositional rigidity may amplify the effects of change to pathological proportions, it is not always easy to predict outcome from such innate givens.
5. That habituation is an important counteractive effect to change and even mitigates recurrent episodes of dislocation.
6. That the core experience of a "facilitating" environment over the first 5 years of life can be very effective in inoculating the child against the ravages of time and change. In this context, one would say that a "facilitating" environment is not merely one that provides for the attainment of satisfactory emotional and social adjustment, an understanding and enjoyment of one's environment, a harmonious family life, and a set of parents who instinctively know how to be parents and enjoy their parenthood. A facilitating environment is also one that prepares the child from infancy onward for the experience and prospect of change, not as a stress but as a stimulus, not as a threat but as a constructive impetus. In the hands of competent parents, change is graduated to occur at a rate not too rapid to be disruptive and not too rapid to discount the sense of stability. The well-developing child must be given a taste from very early on of the experience of change as well as the experience of stability so that he comes to regard both as essential attributes of the healthy and desirable environment.

The same is true of developmental change that is normally punctuated by manageable crises not catastrophies. At each change of
developmental status, a new way of life must almost imperceptibly
become the possession of the growing child. Even when running
smoothly, developmental changes can prove mystifying so that the
changes occurring within the child are frequently confused with
the changes occurring in the world outside. This is beautifully illustrated by the Spanish writer, Barea [2] who tells the story of a boy
beginning to feel at variance with his environment and approaches
his teacher, Father Joaquin, for an explanation:

"It's very funny. Everything seems changed. Even the stones of the cloisters,
which I know by heart, . . . Everybody seems changed to me, the boys, you, the
school. Even the street. When I walked through it this morning I found it
changed. To me, the men, the women, the kids, the houses, everything—absolutely everything—seems changed. I don't know how, and I can't explain it."

Father Joaquin looks at him for a while and then remarks:

"Of course you see everything changed. But everything is just the same as before,
only you have changed. Let's see what you've got in your pockets."

The boy is bewildered by the request but eventually pulls out a silk
handkerchief, a smart new leather wallet, a silver watch, a folded
handkerchief, two pesetas, a fancy magazine pencil and small note-
book. Father Joaquin asks him:

"Haven't you anything else?"
"No, sir."
"Well, well! And what have you done with your marbles and your spinning top?
Don't you carry brass chips, or matchboxes, or printed pictures, or string for play-
ing cops and robbers?"

He then put both his hands on my shoulders and looked me straight
in the face.

"Do you understand now what has happened to you?"
"Yes, sir."
"If you go now to see Father Vesga, he'll tell you that you have lost the condition
of purity. I tell you simply that you are no longer a child."

When parents and teachers are loving and understanding, when
the environment is facilitating and sustaining, when society is evolving gently and evenly, and when traditions and novel experiences

are both treated without excessive respect or fear, then change, whether acute or chronic, massive or insignificant, will bring about progressive psychological rather than psychopathological developments.

References

1. Anthony, E. J. The influence of a manic-depressive environment on the developing child. In *Depression and Human Existence,* E. J. Anthony and T. Benedek, Eds. Little, Brown, Boston, 1975.
2. Barea, A. *The Forging of a Rebel.* Reynal and Hitchcock, New York, 1946.
3. Bloom, J. *Stability and Change.* Wiley, New York, 1964.
4. Butler, Samuel. *Characters and Passages from Notebooks.* Somerset, New York, 1908.
5. Caplan, G., Killilea, M., et al. *Support Systems and Mutual Help.* Grune and Stratton, New York, 1976.
6. Carstairs, G. M. *The Twice-Born. A Study of a Community of High-Caste Hindus.* Indiana University Press, Bloomington, 1962.
7. Erikson, K. *Everything in its Path.* Simon and Schuster, New York, 1976.
8. Freud, S. *The Future of an Illusion,* 1927, Standard Edition, Volume 21. Hogarth Press, London, 1961.
9. Kubie, L. S. The Concept of Change in Psychology. Summary of Scientific Meeting of the Boston Psychoanalytic Society, Jan. 27, 1965. *Bull. Phil. Psych. Assoc.* 15:43–47, 1965.
10. Mead, M. *New Lives for Old—Cultural Transformations—Manus, 1928–1953.* William Morrow, New York, 1956.
11. Mitscherlich, A. *Society Without the Father.* Schocken, New York, 1970.
12. Newman, H. H., Freeman, F. N., and Holzinger, K. J. *Twins: A Study of Heredity and Environment.* University of Chicago Press, Chicago, 1937.
13. Sachs, G. Die Verspaetung des Maschinenzeitaltus. *Images,* 20 (1934), 78.
14. Sovani, N. V. Non-economic aspects of India's economic development. In *Administration and Economic Development in India.* Duke University Commonwealth Study Center, Durham, 1962.
15. Taylor, W. S. Basic personality in orthodox Hindu culture patterns. *J. Abnorm. Soc. Psychol.,* 43 (1948) , 3–12.
16. Toffler, A. *Future Shock.* Random House, New York, 1970.
17. Toynbee, A. *Change and Habit: The Challenge of Our Time.* Oxford University Press, London, 1966.
18. Van den Berg *The Changing Nature of Man.* Norton, New York, 1961.
19. Wallerstein, R. The problem of the assessment of change in psychotherapy. *Int. J. Psychoanal.,* 44 (1963), 31–41.
20. Winnik, H. Social changes and changing psychopathology. In *Mental Health in a Rapidly Changing Society.* Jerusalem Academic Press, Jerusalem, 1971.

Change and the Sense of Time

Albert J. Solnit, M.D. (U.S.A.)

The following perspective by Loren Eiseley [4] sets the mood for my presentation.

> . . . that cut was a perfect cross section through 10 million years of time. I hoped to find at least a bone, but I was not quite prepared for the sight I finally came upon. Staring straight out at me, as I slid farther and deeper into the green twilight, was a skull embedded in the solid sandstone.
>
> It was not, of course, human. I was deep, deep below the time of man in a remote age near the beginning of the reign of mammals.
>
> "Whirl is king," said Aristophanes, and never since life began was Whirl more truly kind than 80 million years ago in the dawn of the Age of the Mammals.
>
> Perhaps the Slit, with its exposed bones and its far off vanishing sky, has come to stand symbolically in my mind for a dimension denied to man, the dimension of time. Like the wisteria on the garden wall he is rooted in his particular century. Out of it—forward or backward—he cannot run. As he stands on his circumscribed pinpoint of time, his sight for the past is growing longer, and even the shadowing outlines of the galactic future are growing clearer, though his own fate he cannot see. Along the dimension of time, man, like the rooted vine in space, may never pass in person.
>
> Through how many dimensions and how many media will life have to pass? Down how many roads among the stars must man propel himself in search of the final secret? The journey is difficult, immense, at times impossible, yet that will not deter some of us from attempting it. "We cannot know all that has happened in the past, or the reason for all of these events any more than we can with surety discern what lies ahead. We have joined the caravan, you might say, at a certain point; we will travel as far as we can, but we cannot in one lifetime see all that we would like to see or learn all that we hunger to know."

To understand change takes time, but what is understood about change is already dated by the changes that have already taken place since we took the time to understand change.

Change is an essential characteristic of life and human development. When there is no change in the individual, the family, the group, or the society, we speak of death or an absence of life. Change may be in the direction of unfolding structures and capacities, the direction in which there is growth, development, and increasing capabilities of independence, of self-starting capacities, of increasing tolerances, and of enduring. Change may be in the direction of slowing down, losing capabilities, regression, less activity, and of folding in or cutting back on tolerances, endurance, and continuity. Change without continuity puts integrity and personal resources at risk.

Change has a qualitative and quantitative aspect. So many functions and structures change over a given period of time. On the whole, a child's inner changes, maturation, and development are relatively resistant to accelerating forces, though enzymes can be evoked earlier than expected by particular stimuli and demands, and a child's capability of achieving a new physical intellectual or emotional capability can be speeded up somewhat in an analogous fashion. On the other hand, through deprivation, inner and outer changes can be slowed down, distorted, and stunted.

Rousseau advised us not to force or speed up development, lest the "fruit" become over-ripe and pulpy.[1] Piaget has referred to a tendency by Bruner and other psychologists to speed up cognitive elements of development as the "American Disease." He challenged in an effective way the assumption that faster is better. On the other hand, there is less controversy over the concept that slower development may be a sign of difficulty, especially in regard to phase specific functions, such as language and speech or in the ripening of major perceptual capacities.

The concept of phase specificity is to some extent based on the embryological model in which certain structures and functions will never unfold to their optimum capacity if they are not activated and elaborated within a given time, a critical period for the emergence of those structures and functions according to the genetic templates which we inherit and which characterize us as a human

[1] *Emile.*

organism. For example, in studies of children that are deprived by long-term institutionalization without adequate maternal care, stimulation, and approving expectations, there is convincing evidence that for most young children there is likely to be a permanent loss of intellectual and emotional capacities that could be expected if they were raised in the well-functioning family.

Historical Perspectives

In medieval times, when the child was openly viewed as chattel, the family consisted of parents and children under the ages of 7 or 8 (Aries, 1962). As soon as the child could control his sphincters, feed himself, dress and undress himself, and be responsible for avoiding obvious dangers, he became a working member of the household. As a worker he was placed in the fields or in the shops where he worked along with others and where his teacher was the field boss or the master artisan to whom he was apprenticed. The adult who instructed the child and demanded work from him was now in the parental role vis-a-vis authority and responsibility to govern the child's behavior, opportunities, and work.

In those days there were many children born of a mating, a large percentage of whom died from infection and pestilence. Those who survived left the immediate family at a young age to work. As Rousseau wrote in *Emile,* "The less one has lived the less one may expect to live. Of all the children, not more than one-half will reach youth." The concept of adolescence in the family and normative conflicts between the generations did not then exist in their present form.

As the Industrial Revolution took place and as the concept of parenthood changed, children stayed with their families beyond the ages of 6 to 8 years. Increasingly, parents were in a position to become advocates for their children. An intuitive effort was made to accommodate to these continuities in family living with institutions and traditions that reflected the impact of these changes on the community. Parents relegated to other adults their authority to instruct, guide, nurture, stimulate, and protect their children.

In contrast to underdeveloped and developing nations, another change also had a complex and enduring influence on the family. As we in the Western world were able to improve our nutrition and cure or overcome infectious and certain surgical diseases, infant mortality sharply decreased. (The expectation of longevity for each human being has more than doubled over the past several hundred years.) More and more the fate of the child was not being decided by mysterious invisible forces of illness, deprivation, and destruction but by parents who could order the nutrition, immunization, sanitation, and medical care needed to assure a longer life for their children. Dependency was extended and intensified. This, in turn, tended to determine many other parental attitudes, both positive and negative. The meaning of parenthood as a developmental phase was extended and increased in complexity.

As each child's survival and development to adulthood within the family became more common, as the Industrial Revolution introduced an epoch of technology, and as democratic values became societal goals in this country, there was an increased need and urge for more education for all our children. As parents attached themselves emotionally to their children as intimate members of their household for 16 or 18 years, rather than 7 or 8 years, not only the meaning of parenthood but the sense of family changed.

Now, each parent could invest more in each child as a carrier of his aspirations for the future. Our increased psychological understanding has revealed that in the family, as we know it, children have come to represent both our replacements and our hopes for immortality. These representations are powerful, and ambivalent, having a potential that ranges from the most intense love for children to the most fearful resentment of them.

Adults have deeply ingrained, irrational reservations about the primacy of children's needs, because they expect to be replaced by them. At the same time, adults have a deep love and concern for children, because parents hope their children's lives will fulfill their own values and aspirations. Unwittingly, in this way parents express their wishes for immortality and reduce their fear of death. Thus parents universally experience children as representatives of their mortality as well as their immortality. In each subculture certain ethnic, political, and social patterns of a given historical period will reflect the balance of these ambivalent parental attitudes through the priorities assigned to the societal resources provided for children.

Developmental Perspectives

Children are born helpless, and the personal relationships that are optimal for their physical and social development are rooted in their biological immaturity at birth. If a newborn child is not fed, kept warm and dry, protected from noxious environmental agents, and stimulated and soothed emotionally (i.e., taken care of totally), he will die. As the child's biological stability is established and as he makes progress in development, the adults who care for him become a presence known in increasingly specific ways: first, by association with predictable events and later in terms of the unique human appearances and behavior (i.e., personality) that shapes and is the anchor of a personal relationship with the child. The helplessness of the newborn and our patterns of socializing and living together are crucial, unchanging forces associated with children's needs for parents who will assure them of survival and of the unfolding of their potential as persons in their own right. Thus even if we all decided that the family unit had outlived its usefulness and that we could create a better setting for children and adults based on our best knowledge of human development, it is predictable that we would rediscover the dynamic human arrangement we call the family. The family is a nourishing, protective, guiding group that also provides a meaningful bridge from the past to the future. Human beings have a deep yearning and need for a sense of continuity as well as for the sense of themselves that is derived from feeling loved and wanted in their own childhoods.

This changing meaning of childhood and adolescence in developed countries reflects not only changes in the structure and functions of the family but also alterations in the timetable and quality of the adolescent experience. As mentioned previously, childhood is physically more secure, and more education is demanded to prepare for fulfillment and success as an adult. These tendencies intensify many of the conflictual aspects of adolescence.

Changes in adolescence have created pressures to change the age of emancipation for various adult privileges. The relationship between the changing social environment and adolescent development has raised confusing questions about how to assert and protect the rights of children and adolescents without destroying these rights through burdening them with decisions and consequences for which they are not prepared.

It may be helpful to outline some of the criteria for healthy mental development in childhood in order to see how changes of the child are responsive to inner, innate capacities interacting with the expectations, affection, guidance, and protection of the adults who provide the care without which the child would die.

The changes in the structure and functions of family are largely a function of the internal, developmental changes evolving as a long-term result of the socializing of the human infant born helpless. These evolutionary aspects of the unfolding human personality are facilitated, distorted, and impaired by the social, medical, and industrial (economic and technological) changes of the social environment. Marriage and reproducing the family are also a function of the effort to reproduce at the adult level the closeness, intimacy, and satisfactions (or frustrations) of the infant.

Children are born helpless, and their survival depends on being protected, nourished, stimulated, guided, and loved by adults. What starts for them as biological helplessness and dependency becomes psychological dependency and attachment to those adults who continually care for them—adults whom we call parents. What starts as a biological demand becomes as well a psychological demand for continuity of care generally expected of and provided by parents for their children [9]. What starts as the parents' adaptation to the helpless infant gradually becomes a state of mutual adaptation. This mutuality [5] becomes the means through which the young child's social development is guided and moulded by the parental persons who in their nurturing—first in feeding, bathing, clothing, playing, and curbing and later with each developmental phase through adolescence, in education, religious training, and discipline—transmit their expectations and demands. The child with his unique makeup and temperament influences, in turn, the unfolding personality and sense of fulfillment of his parents. The mental health of a child is thus a product of his biological and psychological heritage and of his experiences. Therefore, when we assess the mental health of any child we must examine and understand the pattern and quality of interaction between child and parent at each stage of his growth and development [20].

Mental health assessments are designed to identify developmental gains and deficits [8]. Based on clinical observations that are organized according to theoretical constructs, such evaluations provide an inventory of a particular·child's strengths and weaknesses that are measured against rather wide standards of what is normally characteristic of children of the same developmental period. An evaluation may guide the concerned parents in their efforts to maximize their child's potential for healthy growth and development into adulthood.

The ultimate measure of mental health is the extent to which the child is maturing, changing over a period of time, becoming a person who in adulthood is likely to be relatively free of internal conflict about the quality and style of life [10, 12]. The healthy adult has a realistic self-regard that enables him to gauge and react with confidence to environmental demands and at other times to criticize and make sustained efforts to change the society in order to improve or protect his preferred values. Mental health, therefore, is a relative concept in which the balance between individual expression and adaptation to the demands of family and community, and changes in social environment varies over time and from culture to culture.

Observed behavior, without more, is not enough for assessing a child's state of mental health. Evaluations of a child, or for that matter of an adult, that simply equate social compliance and conformity with mental health or that simply equate social deviance and noncompliance with mental illness ignore a fundamental finding of psychoanalysis: What appears to be similar behavior, whether as a symptom of illness or a sign of health, may for different children be a reflection of and response to a wide range of different and even opposite psychic factors. Thus the test of mental health is not to be found in any particular style of life but rather in the sense of self—the sense of autonomy that provides one with a sense of authenticity as an individual who is unique and worthy and who adapts, criticizes, protests, and at all times has access to the self one is becoming. How does this look at times of social crises, at times of technological change, and under other circumstances of rapid change?

The current state of knowledge of child development is sufficient —and there is a reliable and growing body of evidence—to justify the establishment of planned *opportunities,* as opposed to coercive interventions, for child-health-care facilities and educational services that are likely to comport with healthy growth and development. The viability of such opportunities ultimately must rest on their usefulness and attractiveness to parents in furtherance of their own life styles and value preferences. But the state of knowledge is not sufficiently advanced to justify the utilization of diagnostic or prognostic criteria of mental illness or mental health as a basis for coercive state intervention into family privacy. Recognition of how limited is our knowledge should caution against using the power of the state to intrude on parental autonomy by requiring that certain "preferred" child-rearing practices be followed or by imposing a monolithic educational curriculum.

Some Mental Health Concepts and Assumptions About Developing Capacities for Mediating and Responding to Internal and External Forces

Maturation is an unfolding of innate capacities that are evoked, shaped, and learned by the stimulation of, and responses to, the human environment [17]. It is a pushing and pulling experience which gives meaning to each child's humanness. The push comes from within the child, created by inner, instinctual, appetitive longings for development [18]. Parents, primarily, but also other family members as well as teachers, mediate the social environment and assume the task of pulling the child forward in his or her development. From an individual child's point of view, such external pulls may also be perceived as pushes. Rhythm and tempo of pulls and pushes —do they clash or are they synchronized?

Healthy development in the mental and emotional spheres is not conceptualized as a straight-line affair. It is marked by advances, plateaus and temporary regressions. For example, rapid advances are often associated with the advent of a new phase of development (latency, adolescence) which is usually preceded by a period of stability and consolidation (latency before adolescence) or by transient regressions (adolescence before adulthood). It is as though a developmental push requires a child to step back and rest in order to mobilize his energies and consolidate newly won capacities in preparation for the next move forward [8].

The biological and psychological timetables are assumed to complement each other in providing each child with an opportunity for forming a personality of his own. Under the impact of early environmental influences the child develops a capability for differentiating and mediating internal and external demands. The mental agency of mediation that enables him to gradually integrate and adapt to his life experiences is in psychoanalytic theory called the *ego*. In infancy the child's immaturity, expressed in terms of discomforts, tensions, appetitive needs, and helplessness (dependency), evokes the regulating, organizing, soothing, gratifying care of the parents. Metaphorically, this is spoken by psychoanalysts as the parents serving as an auxiliary ego for the infant. In effect, the adults lend their ego capacity to supplement the infant's primitive ego capacities. Gradually the child's ego takes over by exercising the mental functions of perceiving, registering, storing, and reacting to the patterns of his experiences and needs in a manner that normatively enables him to use his memory and to differentiate his external from his internal environment.

The capacity for differentiating his inner psychic life from his social experience enables the child to develop other capabilities that are essential for mental health. These later developments include the capacities for thinking logically, remembering selectively, solving problems, and responding to most instinctual needs by delaying their direct gratification or by finding alternate pathways to achieve gratification. These ego capacities begin to become discernable from infancy or as a child begins to harness his instinctual energies for learning, for expressing his ideas, and for developing his repertoire of affects—including affection, anger, humor, sadness, and concern (empathy). The ego enables the child to form defenses and to use anxiety to mobilize them as a means of protecting himself from external as well as internal threats to his well being. The healthy development of these ego capacities and functions in otherwise normal children is placed in jeopardy if the external environment is chaotic, overstimulating, disorganized, or lacking in continuity of affectionate care [13]. For the more vulnerable child, who at birth is constitutionally disadvantaged, such deprivations may be even more detrimental [2]. In any event, all children, whatever their biological or constitutional equipment, require being wanted by at least one and preferably two adults who will continuously and affectionately provide them with care throughout their childhood. "Physical, emotional, intellectual, social, and moral growth does not happen without causing the child inevitable internal difficulties. The instability of all mental processes during the period of development needs to be offset by stability and uninterrupted support from external sources. Smooth growth is arrested or disrupted when upheavals and changes in the external world are added to the internal ones" ([9], p. 32).

Major Developmental Epochs

The unique way in which each child mediates internal and social forces and develops his adaptive capacities can be viewed in terms of tasks he confronts during the following major developmental epochs [17]:

1. The newborn and young infant (birth to 6 months).
2. The older infant (6–18 months).
3. The toddler and preschool age (under 5 years).
4. School age and preadolescence (5–12 years).
5. Adolescence.

In the newborn period the rhythm and characteristics of an infant's sleeping, eating, and fussing, as well as his reactions to love, to soothing, to frustrations, to discomfort, are key observations in determining normative or healthy functioning. The newborn who cannot be aroused easily or who cannot be soothed may be indicating significant developmental difficulties that may lead to the discovery of either environmental or biological deficits [13]. However, biological and environmental influences often complement each other. In fact, constitutional and external factors that fit well usually promote healthy development. The mother responding with ease and satisfaction to a vigorous, demanding newborn, for example, usually creates a positive setting for healthy mutual adaptation; whereas the mother whose responses are conflicted and confused places obstacles in the path of an unfolding of adaptive capabilities.

An infant attains his first social accomplishment with the development of a responsive smile sometime between the ages of 4 and 8 weeks. This preparatory step toward socialization is accompanied by other physical-psychological phenomena, such as an increasing capacity to utilize sight and hearing in a coordinated and discriminating manner. At the same time other neuromuscular functions gradually unfold, and the child increases specific capacities, for example, to grasp objects, and his general overall capacity to control his body [21].

During the second half of the first year of life, the parent, particularly the primary nurturing one, changes for the child from just a global need-satisfying presence to a more constant identifiable particular person [11]. By this state of development the child has attained sufficient mental resources to maintain a positive mental representation of the nurturing parent, usually the mother, as a living object that both provides love and becomes the object of the child's love and expectations. The child becomes dependent on the protective, stimulating, pleasurable, affectionate attention of this one care-taking person, the mother or the mother surrogate. The father, who becomes important in his own unique way, may in our society initially be, though he is usually not, the most important maternal figure in an infant's life. A grandparent, mother's helper, or older sibling may also become an important source of healthy maternal care.

The mutual adaptation between mother and child becomes the psychological basis for his gradual social development. As the child moves from infancy into the preschool period, he becomes active on his own behalf—transforming what has been passively experienced as being fed or clothed, for example, into such self-initiated activity as feeding and dressing himself. These changes and exchanges are usually acknowledged as achievements and are accompanied by further investments of energy and hope by parents who find fulfillment in their child's development.

In the second, third, and fourth years of life the child's increasing neuromuscular and mental resources enable him to explore his social world physically and verbally. In this period of development the child elaborates his capacities for deferment of immediate satisfaction of impulsive urges and wishes and also elaborates his repertoire of substitutive activities and gratifications leading to increasing autonomy via play and learning. These detour activities secure the child's capacity to tame the demands of his impulses and to achieve partial gratifications that are socially acceptable and that, in fact, promote social development. This sublimation process can be observed when a child waits patiently, despite his hunger, to eat with his family or when he doodles and draws as a way of warding off a not necessarily conscious urge to mess. As he modifies his urges, he simultaneously achieves partial gratification of his impulsive wish and the approval of his parents through such sublimated activity.

Through his developing capability for deferring the demands of the instinctual drives, for transforming them, and for accepting partial and substitutive gratifications, the older child can gradually extend his environment beyond the family with assurance and trust in his capacity to meet societal demands. By being able to master physical and mental challenges and by being able to form firm empathetic personal relationships, the child acquires the ability to persist—even in the face of adversity—in efforts to change or control his ever-enlarging environment.

Education that gradually begins with well-managed pre-kindergarten opportunities can assist the child in mastering separation experiences. Children usually spend no more than a half a day in such nursery schools. The mother's and father's feelings and reactions to the child's experience are critical factors in his overcoming the fears of separation, the temporary breaks in continuity of care [14, 15, 16]. In a healthy situation the child who is 2 or 3 years of age will feel anxious and require a gradual separation in order to be able to keep his parents in mind and form an attachment to his teacher. Later, as he finds satisfaction in his play at school, he will form attachments to his classmates. He will initially play side by side with the other children, finding a variety of activities inviting and satisfying. As he becomes more comfortable with separation from his parents, as he strengthens his attachments to his teachers and becomes free to invest his energies in play activities, the 4- and 5-year-old child begins to play with, not just next to, classmates. In these developments one can observe the beginning of empathy, of an awareness and of some understanding of how a classmate feels or thinks about a particular situation.

When young children (under the age of 2½ years) are enrolled in day-care programs, 6 to 12 hours per day, it becomes even more important that the child is gradually prepared for such long—by a child's sense of time—separations from his parents. The younger the child, the more vulnerable he is to unprepared-for sudden and long separations. For this reason, day-care facilities for children under 2½ years should be located where mothers and fathers can spend their free time with their children and where staff encourage parents to visit and make them feel welcome. The risks in full-day-care programs for young children must be recognized in order to assure adequate family support resources to mitigate, if not avoid, detrimental consequences.

Kindergartens offer the day care and nursery school graduate an opportunity further to test and consolidate his capacity for physically separating from his parents [3, 6]. Better equipped to draw on his internal image of his parents, the kindergarten child identifies with them while he functions as a member of a group and comes to accept and trust the teacher as a guiding, protecting adult. He can repeatedly draw on past experiences with his parents and siblings in forming new relationships outside of the family with teachers and schoolmates in a selective and discriminating manner.

The school-age child gradually begins to develop ideals and values on his own [17]. He views the teacher, school, and class as uniquely related to himself, and he invests himself—his energies—in learning about a larger social scene through the use of symbolic communications which his development enables him to master. In this period social meaning and values are implicit in the cognitive as well as in the play and social activities of the school. Thought may become a substitute for direct action or at least precede it. Such mental activity appears in many forms, including fantasy, memory, and planning (anticipatory thinking), that enlarge and enrich the child's contact with his social as well as with his physical world.

In preparation for becoming an adult, the preadolescent figuratively takes a lingering look at the past. Before the "die is cast"—biologically, psychologically, and socially—the child in pubertal crisis often demonstrates his nostalgia by regressing. He retreats to an earlier position of dependency and appetitive expression as he prepares to mobilize himself into the powerfully dynamic phases of full adolescence. Social development seems at a halt or even in reverse as his standards of behavior are temporarily relaxed. He may experiment with lying, stealing, messy behavior, overeating, and passivity as he prepares to enter his teens and to rebel and to explore life and the world in a bold and experimental manner [17].

Adolescence can be a time in which the individual child is given an opportunity to make up for past deficits, or it can be a time in which vigorous forward development is hindered and past deficits become hardened [7]. According to Goldstein, Freud, and Solnit [9]:

> With adolescents, the superficial observations of their behavior may convey the idea that what they desire is discontinuation of parental relationships rather than their preservation and stability. Nevertheless, this impression is misleading in this simple form. It is true that their revolt against any parental authority is normal developmentally since it is the adolescent's way toward establishing his own independent adult identity. But for a successful outcome it is important that the breaks and disruptions of attachment should come exclusively from his side and not be imposed on him by any form of abandonment or rejection on the psychological parents' part (p. 32).

The instability and outcome of adolescent development can be understood in terms of synchrony and dysynchrony. As the first pubertal changes are sensed, various parts of the personality begin to mature at different rates. The growth spurt may be accompanied by volcanic-like eruptions and increases in appetite for food, sexual gratification, and aggressive outlets. Meanwhile, the intellectual and judgmental aspects of the personality seem to be changing slowly and steadily and thus become out of phase with or fail to keep up with the heightened instinctual pressures. As adolescence proceeds these pressures seem to subside and become relatively quiescent, while the central and social aspects of personality development appear to move ahead rapidly. At such times the adolescent gives the impression of being intellectually vigorous and independent but relatively inhibited with regard to sexuality and social encounters. The adolescent period is marked, then, by unevenness and by the transient discrepancies between the mature and immature or regressed parts of the personality. Adolescence is thus a time of rapid change that does not unfold in a balanced and synchronous way.

On reaching *adulthood* balance and stability are restored, and a developmental plateau is reached. In the healthy adult personality the intellect, the emotions, and the capacity for personal relations and social awareness come into a synchrony. It is accompanied by a realistic self-esteem and a sense of proportion between the need to adapt to the community and the need to change that community because of dissatisfaction with it, not with one's self. Such a level of functioning, inferred on empirical grounds, is usually given a chronological marker, for example 18 or 21, for the legal presumption that a person has both the capacity and authority to fully exercise his rights free of parental control and responsibility. No longer entitled by law to depend on his parents for care and support or to make decisions on his behalf, he now is presumed to have the capacity, for example, to make binding contracts, to acquire and dispose of property, to marry, to vote, to hold public office, to consent to or reject medical care, to commit crime, to make wills—that is, to engage in any activity and to be held responsible for it. The child has become adult in law, and his mental health is presumed unless he is otherwise disqualified or seeks professional help on his own accord because of his belief that he is mentally ill [19].

Concluding Concerns About Children and Mental Health

No consideration of children and developmental changes should conclude without noting the danger to children that has come with society's uncritical application of knowledge about child development. In dealing with children in "trouble" and in trying to be guided by the best interests of the child, often parents, educators, physicians, social workers, and judges have been either too ready to intervene or, when intervention is appropriate, too quick to focus exclusively on what is "wrong" with the child. Instead of asking about the child and his environment, mental health professionals have tended to ask either about the one or the other. Instead of asking whether the child's behavior and development are appropriate for coping with the conflicts and trauma created by his environment, there has been a tendency of those concerned with children to overlook in what ways school, court, or other community institutions and adults, as well as the family itself, may be interfering with the healthy unfolding of a child's capacities. It would be better, once the functions of intervention have been clarified, to begin by asking who or what is standing in the way of allowing a particular child to develop and grow. It would be better to consider what can be done to reduce the impersonal nature and the assembly-line atmosphere and attitude in educational and social service programs. We must be alert to the misuse and abuse of knowledge that comes with attaching unwarranted significance to achievement of standard and standardized goals as evidence of mental health and the failure to achieve those goals as evidence of illness.

Just as we should be sensitive to how the social environment can impede or distort healthy development, we should be sensitive to how little external observations of children say about their internal well being, about their mental health. Respect for individuality and complexity is essential for humane, sophisticated understanding of children and their mental health.

References

1. Aries, P. *Centuries of Childhood*. Knopf, New York, 1962.
2. Chandler, C., Lourie, R., Peters, A. In *Early Child Care—The New Perspective*, Laura Kittmann, Ed. Atherton, New York, 1968.
3. Cohen, D. J. (in collaboration with A. S. Brandegee). *Day Care. 3 Serving Preschool Children*. DHEW Publication No. (OHD) 74-1057. Washington, D.C.: Office of Human Development and Office of Child Development. U.S. Department of Health, Education, and Welfare, 1974.
4. Eiseley, Loren. The Slit, *The Immense Journey*. New York: Random House, 1946, 1956.
5. Erikson, E. H. *Childhood and Society*. Norton, New York, 1950.
6. Fein, G. G. and Clarke-Stewart, A. *Day Care in Context*. Wiley, New York, 1973.
7. Freud, A. Adolescence. *Psychoanal. Study Child*, 13 (1958), 255–278.
8. Freud, A. *Normality and Pathology in Childhood*. International Universities Press, New York, 1965.
9. Goldstein, J., Freud, A., Solnit, A. J. *Beyond the Best Interests of the Child*. The Free Press, New York, 1973, p. 32.
10. Hartmann, H. "Psychoanalysis and the Concept of Health. *Int. J. Psychoanal.*, 20 (1939), 308–321; *Essays on Ego Psychology*, International Universities Press, New York, 1964, pp. 1–18.
11. Hartmann, H. The mutual influences in the development of ego and id, *Psychoanal. Study Child*, 7 (1952), 9–30; *Essays on Ego Psychology*, International Universities Press, New York, 1964, pp. 155–181.
12. Hartmann, H. Toward a concept of mental health. *Brit. J. Med. Psychol.*, 33 (1960), 293–298.
13. Provence, S. and Lipton, R., *Infants in Institutions*. International Universities Press, New York, 1965.

14. Robertson, J. Some responses of young children to loss of maternal care. *Nursing Times,* 49 (1953), 382–386.
15. Robertson, J. *Young Children in Hospital.* Tavistock Publications, London; Basic Books, New York, 1959.
16. Robertson, J. and Robertson, J., Young children in brief separation. *Psychoanal. Study Child,* (1971) , 264–315. Vol. 26.
17. Senn, M. J. E. and Solnit, A. J. *Problems in Child Behavior and Development.* Lea and Febiger, Philadelphia, 1968.
18. Solnit, A. J. Early childhood: Pushing and pulling. In *What We Can Learn from Infants.* National Association for the Education of Young Children, Washington, D.C., 1970, pp. 49–68.
19. Solnit, A. J. Changing psychological perspectives about children and their families. *Children Today,* 5 (3) May-June, (1976), 5–9, 44.
20. Solnit, A. J. and Schowalter, J. Criteria for healthy psychological development in childhood. Unpublished manuscript.
21. Spitz, R. A. (in collaboration with W. Godfrey Cobliner). *The First Year of Life.* International Universities Press, New York, 1965.

Family Support Systems in a Changing World

Gerald Caplan, M.D. (Israel)

The Support Systems Model

In three recent publications [1, 2, 3] we have proposed a new conceptual model we have called *support systems*. Its purpose is to supplement existing models in providing a systematic guide for planning programs of community mental health.

Support systems are defined as attachments among individuals, or between individuals and groups or institutions, that serve to improve adaptive competence in dealing with short-term crises and life transitions, as well as long-term challenges, stresses, and privations, through (a) offering cognitive guidance regarding the field of relevant forces involved in expectable problems and methods of dealing with them, (b) providing information to help understand the feedback cues of other people as well as providing feedback about the individual's behavior that validates his conception of his own identity and fosters improved performance based on adequate self-evaluation, and (c) promoting emotional mastery.

Support systems operate naturally and spontaneously in most societies and include families, friends and neighbors, informal caregivers, mutual-help organizations, and religious denominations. Our model guides community mental health practitioners in recognizing the power of these natural, nonprofessional, person-to-person, strengthening forces in the population; in developing ways of working together with them instead of ignoring them or competing with them; and in stimulating the creation of similar nonprofessional networks, such as mutual-help groups of people who share a particular challenge or privation (e.g., widowhood or having a retarded child) in localities where no natural supportive organizations have developed spontaneously. Since many persons with mental disorders are peripheral to society and become more alienated as a consequence of their disturbed behavior and the stigma associated by society to their condition, our model challenges community mental health workers to build communication bridges between them and the natural supportive networks of their communities. It also encourages sufferers to overcome their own resistance to developing relationships with others "in the same boat," so that they can help each other overcome the weakening effects of stigma and isolation and pool their knowledge and other resources in mastering their difficulties.

The special merit of this model from a population-oriented point of view is that for the first time numbers do not work against us, as they do in all programs based on the approach of intervention by professionals. Since support systems, particularly mutual-help groups, are mainly composed of persons who themselves suffer from the disorder, deprivation, or other form of stress, the more there are of them in a locality the bigger the pool from which can be drawn those who may help their fellows, and in so doing help themselves, by switching from the role of passive victim to that of active helper. Our role as specialists is restricted to both catalyzing this process and doing so with care, so that we do not play too big a part and obtrude our professional values and traditions in a process that derives its main power from the nonprofessional approach of mutual person-to-person identification and strength through unity. This contrasts with even the most efficient model of traditional community mental health practice, consultation, where there is the necessity for a significantly large group of specialists to offer consultation to caregiving professionals, who in turn intervene in the lives of their clients. Population-wide coverage by this approach is limited by the fact that it is very expensive to train and deploy the consultants, so that there will always be too few of them to help enough care-giving professionals to intervene with more than a small proportion of the huge number of persons in need of help in grappling with their acute and chronic life problems.

The Family as a Support System

We have no intention in our model of reducing the meaning of families entirely to their operation as support systems. Families are complicated social units that fulfill many overlapping functions, both for their members and for society, that vary during the lifetime of the members. They cater to the continually developing biological, psychosocial, and economic needs of individual members, and they mediate between society and the individual members as agents of socialization and control. The support system characteristics of families are only one of their main sets of functions, and we conceptually isolate them only in order to sharpen our analysis and understanding.

With this proviso in mind, let me summarize briefly some of the main support systems characteristics of families that we have dealt with more extensively in a previous publication [2]:

1. The family acts as a collector and disseminator of information about the world. In a multigenerational family, information about the past, present, and future world is fed into the family data pool by the different age groups. In traditional, stable families the process is mostly unidirectional from parent to child, but in rapidly changing times it becomes more reciprocal.
2. The family acts as a feedback guidance system. In new settings or when there is a speedup of historical change, the family buffers the shocks of acculturation and cultural acceleration and provides a sounding board or training ground for undefensive testing out and understanding the chains of action and reaction.
3. The family acts as a source of ideology, providing beliefs, values, and codes of behavior that determine the individual's conception of his environment and his own place in it. This internalized map of the universe helps to direct his goals in life. Under conditions of change it functions like a compass and helps him to find his way.
4. The family acts as guide and mediator in problem solving, making the individual's problem the family's problem, adding its collective strength and experience to the situation. Within

the multigenerational setting the family roles are constantly changing and thus accustom the individual to rapid role changes under changing world conditions. In this way the family prepares the individual for change, teaching him to develop the necessary flexibility and skills needed for adjustment. The interplay of generations is important in this respect: children are more sensitive but less experienced with regard to change; parents are more resistant to change and more interested in stability. Within the extended family all the elements are present for helping the group as a whole to face the necessity for change and to learn how to change and assist one another to accomplish this as safely and as smoothly as possible.

5. The family acts as a source of practical service and concrete aid, since tradition, law, and religion in most cultures require parents and children to serve and provide for each other. Such mutual obligations constitute, in effect, a primitive type of insurance system.

6. The family acts as a haven for rest and recuperation where the individual members can relax and unwind from the tensions generated by the changing demands of the outside world. The members monitor each other's state of fatigue and afford moratoria by temporarily assessing the other's role.

7. The family acts as a reference and control group by continually monitoring and judging the individual's conduct and rewarding and punishing him in accordance with the family code, buttressing the internal censor. When individual and family values are consonant, the individual can rely on the family's ability to take account of both his reality and his capacity.

8. The family acts as a source and validator of identity by helping first to form and then to consolidate and clarify the self-image during crises of confusion brought about by change and transition. During such periods of uncertainty, it can remind him of his past achievements and furnish him with the confidence to stand firm.

9. The family can contribute to the individual's emotional mastery by helping with "worry-work" and "grief-work" during periods of crisis and privation when anxiety, depression, anger, shame, and guilt threaten to overwhelm him. It counteracts despair and helplessness through sustained expressions of love, solidarity, comfort, and hopefulness. Such support is of particular value during the debilitating reduction of personal worth that follows on object loss or loss of bodily integrity.

Factors Limiting the Functioning of the Family as a Support System

1. Disturbed relationships among the family members may not only be directly harmful in themselves but may be indirectly pathogenic by interfering with the smooth functioning of the family as a support system. For the system to work the members must be sensitive to one another's needs and perceive each other realistically and not paratactically because of unresolved personal and family problems.

2. Disturbed communication involving contradictory, conflicting, or double-bind messages will also not allow the family to function adequately as a support system. This holds not only for horizontal communication between peers but also for vertical communication across generations.

3. The breaking up of the intergenerational pattern, with its opportunities for healthy relationships with members at many different stages of the life cycle, can also be an impediment to the functioning of the support system. This does not imply that members must live together in the same dwelling but that frequent close interaction is possible.

4. The support system has operated inadequately when the bond of mutual obligations, shared values and traditions, and membership in the same religious denomination no longer exists because the society of which they form a part ceases to be cohesive.

5. The support system becomes limited when power and property are withdrawn from the control of parents and entrusted to other agents of society.

6. A superordinate limiting factor is the extent to which family members fundamentally accept their interdependence and the surveillance and control by the family of important aspects of their lives, that the boundary of their privacy is not their skin but the walls of their home, and that what is good for the family is good for them. Thus the members must be prepared to pay a significant price if they wish to retain family support.

The Effects of World Change

Rapid sociocultural change will have a major effect on most of these factors that enhance or limit the capacity of the family to act optimally as a support system. In a world that is changing rapidly and radically, the individual is exposed to a variety of stresses the family support system may help them to master but which may also reduce the capacity of the family as a support system.

World change can have either a pathogenic or orthogenic influence on the child and his family, and the support systems model provides an effective guide to understanding the various effects and to developing social policy and programs that will foster optimal adaptation.

Pathogenic Effects of World Change

POPULATION MOVEMENT

Economic development often changes the location of major industries and services in a country. This leads to the movement of people from rural to urban areas and from established metropolitan areas to distant parts of the country where new forms of natural resources are being exploited. People have less possibility of sinking roots in a particular residential area, of becoming accustomed to its physical and social milieu. They also are exposed to periods of disorganization in transit from place to place. Such job mobility involves the risk of geographical separation from loved ones. The noxious effect not only relates to loss or separation but also to the loss of a familiar place and ecological setting.

This burden does not affect infants and small children directly from a mental health point of view, except if it involves parent-child separation. Nevertheless, young children are indirectly affected because of the psychosocial upheavals and insecurity of the family group. Older children will also be affected by the significant interruption of attachments to friends and to educators, as well as burdened by being forced to adjust to a new school. The age group that will be most affected will be the adolescents, especially those who have just left school. They may find no jobs available when their family moves to a new place that has perhaps been geared to providing occupation to their elders.

URBAN AND METROPOLITAN CONGLOMERATION

Developments in our modern world are likely to lead to the crowding of people in metropolitan areas or in smaller towns with a high population density. There is evidence that this is likely to have harmful mental health consequences, especially for people who are not used to it. Cassel [4] has shown that the noxious effects are not due to crowding per se but to the increased likelihood in such situations that the individual will every day come in contact with many strangers whose feelings toward him he cannot assess because he does not understand their behavioral cues. In such a situation, where there is no well-ingrained culture, there is usually also a general normlessness and lowered control over hostility. The net result is that the individual must maintain a high level of hormonal and autonomic arousal, be continually on his guard to fend off or escape hostile acts on the part of potentially dangerous strangers. This continuing organismic arousal leads to depletion and to increased vulnerability to both psychiatric and physical illness as well as to a pervasive hostile tension and lack of well-being.

Among children and adolescents this situation is likely to lead to feelings of personal insecurity that may be defended against either by excessive timidity or by aggressiveness.

CULTURE SHOCK

In a new place, and even more so in a familiar place that has changed rapidly, the individual lives in an unpredictable world. He is continually insecure because his old maps of reality do not work, and he cannot depend on knowing what is about to take place not only in the distant future but even from one minute to the next. This is profoundly unsettling; the disorientation and confusion, although fundamentally cognitive, has a major emotional impact. In a world of rapid change, if the change is radical and rapid enough, there is a recurrent danger of such culture shock, which Toffler has renamed "future shock" [5]. Most people after a while learn how to cope, mainly by reducing their investment and involvement in the outside world, as well as by learning to understand it; but a significant number are likely to suffer ill effects. There are, as yet, no studies of the specific patterns of personality disorders that occur in children of different ages who are exposed to such situations of rapid change, but the assumption that the pattern of personality in children will show deviations similar to those of adults suffering from culture shock—disorientation, insecurity, apathy, depression, poor impulse control, and autistic withdrawal—would appear to have face validity.

BUREAUCRATIC COMPLEXITY AND DEHUMANIZATION

The rapid building up of new population centers inhabited by newcomers or transients is usually associated with complex bureaucratic patterns of organization because these represent one relatively simple way of quickly producing order and achieving control over people, supplies, and services. This usually leads to a relatively dull, dehumanized social and physical environment in which the individual feels that he can exercise little, if any, control over essential elements of his life setting. This in turn may lead him to become passive or alienated—to "turn off" and "drop out" as our young people so aptly term it. Such a reaction is all the more likely during the adolescent years when the individual, who has been entitled throughout childhood to be and feel passive and dependent, tries to move actively toward becoming the independent master of his own fate and yet is not able to envision the shape of the future nor to see how he can affect it by his individual efforts. From this point of view withdrawal from a world of reality, which offers no handholds or effective leverage points toward goals that can be envisioned and valued, into the never-never land of drugs, hippiedom, or antisocial rebellion and adventure becomes an understandable choice for many young people.

RAPID OBSOLESCENCE OF ROLE AND SKILL

Rapid technological change, even apart from residential movement, is likely to lead to rapid obsolescence of many previous occupational skills. The main pathogenic impact of this factor is felt in middle age—the parent group—who have achieved status and earning capacity through study and hard work. When their industry suddenly changes its pattern and this role becomes redundant, they are called upon to change or be extruded from the work force. Not only is it difficult for them to change to a radically different role, but from a psychosocial point of view it involves mastering the burden of suddenly having to go back to becoming an insecure and unskilled trainee after having achieved the stability of being a competent specialist. When this happens to a parent it has two types of bad effects on the children: (1) parenting is likely to be upset as a consequence of the blow to the adult's self-respect, social status, and earning capacity and (2) a powerful message is conveyed to the children that we live in a world so unstable and insecure that hard work, thrift, achievement, and careful planning do not guarantee continued future reward, thus reducing the motivation to master the demands of immediate impulse gratification in the service of an occupational and social career.

In addition to these indirect effects that are likely to be felt throughout childhood, adolescents are more directly affected by this situation. In a rapidly changing world the usual complications of initial career choice become much more burdensome, and since technological advances probably increase the need for a high level of skill and sophistication in most branches of the economy, they make specialization more necessary. Thus to succeed in the job market, the adolescent faces a kind of double-bind: he must work intensively in a specialized area to get an appropriate and meaningful job, and if he does so he will become more vulnerable to redundancy when technological development leads to a radically different industrial pattern. On the other hand, if he tries to achieve flexibility and readiness for rapid change of role by not committing himself as a specialist, he probably will not be able to get one of the attractive jobs that are available immediately or in the near future. This is a difficult situation for many adolescents to master. What may well happen is that some will drop out while others will specialize but live insecurely in the hope that they can remain sufficiently flexible to switch and retrain rapidly when the inevitable change occurs, which in turn will probably lower their occupational commitment and involvement. Many may well opt for human service jobs, because though there may be rapid changes also in this field, they may well be less radical, since people are likely to alter less drastically than machines.

INCREASING LEISURE

Despite the possibility of historical discontinuities, it seems as though the manpower to produce the material goods needed in the world of the future will be inexorably reduced as people are replaced by machines. The result will be that people will start working later, retire earlier, and work a shorter week. This process is already well underway in post-industrial western societies. The implication is that in the world of the future people will have to find ways of achieving meaning in life in addition to those derived from occupational productivity. If we enlarge our view of leisure to include this, it follows that people must learn how to utilize their leisure hours and their leisure years in ways that give them the feeling they are making a sufficiently significant contribution to maintain their self-respect and not feel redundant.

Orthogenic Effects

Although the focus of this presentation so far has been on the increased possibilities of pathology in children and adolescents because of the rapidly changing nature of our world, it is very necessary to add that all the factors already discussed may also stimulate a positive, ego-strengthening response in many young people. The mastery of difficulties is likely to lead to stronger and more resilient personalities in individuals who will glory in the excitement of facing the unpredictable, who will learn how to avoid premature closure in situations of confusion and frustration, and who will commit themselves, despite the likelihood of future loss, because they are confident in their flexibility and competence to adjust to new conditions. According to our support systems model, one of the major sources of such strength will be the family and the support provided by it during the earlier years.

Counteracting Harmful Effects on Families of a Changing World

It must be stressed that this is an explicitly speculative presentation, a stimulus to research and program development and not a review of existing knowledge. Therefore, a number of suggestions regarding social policy and program planning based on the support systems model are offered without the research data to validate all of them. Such an approach is called for because of the current state of our field. Sociopolitical and socioeconomic developments are proceeding rapidly and will not be held back until systematic studies have been carried out.

I now briefly summarize the probable weakening effect on the family support system that is likely to be exerted by certain aspects of our rapidly changing world and then suggest how this problem might be met.

FAMILY FRAGMENTATION CAUSED
BY DEMOGRAPHIC CHANGE

The maintenance of three-generation proximity is an important source of the strength of a family as a support system. Until recently we used to believe that the three-generational, extended family was fast disappearing in such urbanized countries as the United States. As soon as we take into account that the crucial issue is not living under the same roof but frequency of interaction, we discover that in most cases grandparents, parents, and children live sufficiently close together to interact frequently and continue to form integrated multigenerational units.

Recent findings would indicate that the bonds between family members have proved so strong that most families have so far managed to overcome the disintegrating forces of the rural-urban shift and the smallness of urban dwellings. Since, however, increased residential mobility is likely to be a prominent feature of our changing world and since the rapidity of change is accelerating, we may predict that at the very least the proportion of fragmented families will increase and that during the crucial early adaptation phases of moving to a new residential area, when the intactness of the three-generational family structure is particularly necessary in providing needed support, it may well be missing.

Suggested Remedies   Planners of new towns or new neighborhoods should make certain that homes should provide space for three generations of family members or that suitable dwellings for grandparents and possibly greatgrandparents should be available near the homes of parents and children.

Amenities and occupational opportunities should be planned as a package for all the age groups of a population, instead of just providing living accommodation for those adult workers who are directly needed for a new industry.

Wherever possible, population recruitment for new or relocated industries should attempt to move networks of families and not individual families, and certainly not just individuals.

Since constraints of the real world may not allow planners to accomplish these tasks in one phase, the highest priority should be given to guaranteeing communication among spatially separated members of families.

THE GENERATION GAP

A rapidly changing world exacerbates normal difficulties of communication among generations in a family, even one that lives in the same home or in adjoining dwellings. The difficulties are likely to be most pronounced between adults and adolescents and between grandparents and their children. Factors include: (1) radical differences in life experience because of major changes that involve the generations differentially, (2) differences in values and vocabulary derived from membership in extrafamilial cultural groups with differing life situations, (3) because of socioeconomic discontinuities, the inability of older generations to act as occupational role models for the younger family members or guide them on the basis of personal experience, which fosters loss of mutual respect, (4) the development of vicious circles that cause the different generations, leading separate lives in the outside world, to stop communicating with each other inside the family, so that the family data pool becomes increasingly impoverished and irrelevant, which further lowers the motivation of members to utilize it and to communicate meaningfully with each other.

Suggested Remedies   Educational programs in schools and through radio, television, and the press should systematically inform each generation about the realities of the others. Children should learn authentic details about the world of their parents and grandparents—its values, preoccupations, and excitements—at least as much as about the lives of historical figures; likewise, young people should be involved in programs of adult education that interpret to the older generations the preoccupations and realities of their current lives, including the inner meaning of their language and art forms.

Whenever possible, planning and management groups and committees should be multigenerational, as should discussion panels on radio and television; the challenge for each generation to learn the other's language and to understand the other's values should continually be confronted.

Whenever possible, social events should involve entire multigenerational family units. From this point of view, I see family diagnosis and family therapy in child psychiatry not merely as a valuable development in technique because it maximizes our understanding of relevant harmful and helpful forces impinging on child patients, but also as one further opportunity of convening an entire family group so that we may help them improve their communication with one another as they work together to achieve a common goal. Similarly, schools should move from parent-teacher sessions to family-teacher sessions, in which the teachers of all the children of a family would sit with the total family group to review relevant educational issues of their classrooms and their home.

PROFESSIONAL AND BUREAUCRATIC
ENCROACHMENT ON FAMILY DOMAINS

The family as an operational unit is likely to be weakened if our social policies establish professional and bureaucratic units that take over important functions in nurturing, guiding, and helping individuals, particularly if these programs exclude the rest of the family from the process.

Suggested Remedies   Medical, mental health, and social agencies should make more use of the family group as an intermediary in offering help to individuals. This would be of particular importance in dealing with adolescent children and grandparents, who in today's world are most likely to be extruded or to wish to be helped in isolation from their family. Agencies should strengthen the positive aspects of the ambivalent relationship of the adolescent to his family or of the family to the grandparent by accepting integration of the family unit as a major immediate goal of their intervention.

The increased demand for women in the labor force and the changing interests of women, which make more of them than in the past seek employment outside the home during the childbearing years, will result in the increasing provision of day-care centers for young children. This substitute mothering should be shared as much as possible by the family—in particular by the older siblings and the grandparents. Both are likely to be ambivalent, and rightly so, and we must beware of unduly burdening them.

Lastly, there is the possibility of supplementing professional social work by stimulating the development of nonprofessional family-to-family support groups. In a rapidly developing new residential and occupational area some families are more successful in helping their children and grandparents find a satisfying place for themselves in

the local economy and society than others. Instead of agencies intervening directly themselves, they might, in certain cases, convene
meetings of successfully adapting families with the families having
adjustment problems and catalyze the establishment of a family-to-
family support group.

THE HARMFUL EFFECT OF SECULARIZATION ON
THE SUPPORTIVE MATRIX OF FAMILIES

The importance of religious denominations as a source of the values and traditions that define and legitimize the family's role as a
support system and promote the mutual obligations of effective family life should not be overlooked. The prophet Malachi puts this well
when he says of God, "He will turn the hearts of parents to their children and the hearts of children to their parents" (Malachi, IV, 6).
Apparently, the need for the prophet to say this was derived from the
breakdown of family bonds and mutual responsibility in his day,
which was in turn linked to a general turning away from religion.

Suggested Remedies Religious leaders usually do not wait for
community mental health workers to stimulate them to action, nor
do they expect the latter to validate their mission, but irrespective of
individual religious beliefs, the professionals should make common
cause with them, since many of the goals are shared. As authorities in
the secular world, mental health workers should continually emphasize the importance in community mental health religion and religious organizations in fostering the humane values and mores that
strengthen family life and provide meaning to individual existence.
Whenever possible mental health workers should collaborate with
religious leaders both in dealing with populations and with individual families.

Furthermore, they could be particularly helpful in persuading
planners to establish places of worship in new settlements as a matter
of mental health significance.

Educators, journalists, broadcasters, and community leaders should
be encouraged to foster the development of decent codes of interpersonal behavior, sensitivity to the needs of others, and commitment to
helping them. As a central part of all such organizational and educational activity, information should be spread to and about families as

support systems, emphasizing the benefits that may be derived by individuals and family groups from working out acceptable codes of mutual obligation to help one another in times of need.

References

1. Caplan, G. *Support Systems and Community Mental Health*. Behavioral Publications, New York, 1974.
2. Caplan, G. and Killilea, M., et al. *Support Systems and Mutual Help*. Grune and Stratton, New York, 1976.
3. Caplan, R. B., et al. *Helping the Helpers to Help*. The Seabury Press, New York, 1972.
4. Cassel, J. C. Psychiatric Epidemiology. In *American Handbook of Psychiatry, Vol. II*. G. Caplan, Ed. Basic Books, New York, 1973.
5. Toffler, A. *Future Shock*. Random House, New York, 1970.

Children and Their Families in the U.S.A.: Three Profiles of Change with a Commentary on Stress, Coping, and Relative Vulnerabilities

S. P. Hersh, M.D. (U.S.A.)

We observe our surroundings, those around us, and ourselves becoming different. We label this "becoming different" as change.

We observe the different rates of change for living and nonliving things. We wonder about "becoming different" and through our wondering react to change. Change thus is an interactive phenomenon with the potentials for modifying as well as generating further change.

Classifying change as good or bad, as challenging and illuminating or distorting and hindering, is an attribution of worth—a statement of one's perspective and values. A different approach involves thinking of change in terms of the stress on both the individual human being and the system within which that person exists. Such an approach allows one to characterize the struggle that individuals, families, and social and cultural systems are engaged in as they try to maintain states of relative equilibrium, of homeostasis. We call the successful struggle—not necessarily directed toward resisting change—to maintain such homeostasis *coping*.

There are times in history when change is so dramatic in magnitude and rapidity that states of relative equilibrium are difficult to maintain. Such times are important to identify and study, for through such study we can improve both our potential and our skills in coping.

What follows are three profiles of changes in the United States over two decades, 1956 through 1976. The changes presented relate to each other on the basis of their effects on children and families. The details are unique to the United States.

Profile A: The Population, Distribution, Economics, and Age Profile

In January 1976 the total population of the United States reached 214.5 million people. This represents slightly more than a doubling of the population over a quarter of a century [1].

However, since 1970 the rate of population growth has declined with a steadily decreasing fertility rate (27 percent decline between 1970 and 1975) [2]. If the present fertility rate continues or declines further, the population's age profile will alter dramatically. The current fertility rate is well below that required for natural replacement of the population [3].

In the United States the population distribution is presented as those living in metropolitan and those living in nonmetropolitan areas. Metropolitan areas, described in terms of standard metropolitan statistical areas (SMSA), represent counties (governing units) with populations greater than 50,000 people and thus include both central cities and their suburbs.

There were 168 SMSAs in 1950. They represented approximately 7 percent of the total United States land area and held 56 percent of the total population. By 1975 there were 243 SMSAs. They represented approximately 14 percent of the total land area and 73 percent of the population [4].

Recall that SMSAs are divided into central city and suburban components. During the 1970s the total central city population declined to a level representing 43 percent of the total SMSA population while the suburban population increased to represent 57 percent of the total [5]. The increased white population in the SMSAs has occurred exclusively in the suburbs, while the number of blacks in the suburbs increased by 16 percent. Despite the increase in blacks in the suburban part of the SMSAs, at a national level blacks still only represent 5 percent of the total suburban population. This represents absolutely no change over a period of 10 years [6].

During this recent period of out-migration from the central cities, one notes several economic facts. First, the average income of the out-migrants was higher than the in-migrants, representing a mean difference to the central city of over a $1000 loss per family between 1970 and 1974 [7]. Blacks represented a high proportion (57 percent) of the low-income central-city residents. Moreover, 56 percent of the total black city population in 1973 lived in city poverty areas and represented approximately three-fourths of all United States blacks living below the poverty level [8]. Black males represent 18 percent of the United States civilian labor force, but 32 percent of the city unemployed were black in 1974.

Concerning the out-migration to the suburbs, there now is considerable evidence to suggest that the number of jobs is increasing at a faster rate in the suburban areas of SMSAs than in the central cities [9]. Women seem to be occupying an increasing percentage of the suburban work force (42 to 46 percent from 1970 to 1974).

Between 1960 and 1975 there has been a doubling in the number of one-person households [10]. This increase has altered the proportion they represent of the total United States households: one-person households now represent 20 percent of all the households in the United States. Only two-thirds of the United States households now include a head and a spouse; this is a drop from three-quarters of the United States households 15 years ago [11].

Family size is decreasing. It is most obvious for families with five or more persons. The trends toward smaller families seem associated with other trends: "High rates of marital disruption by divorce or separation have been resulting in a rapid growth of female-headed families; and changes in the age structure of family heads have been resulting in increasing members of young families who have not completed their childbearing experiences and older families where children have grown and left home" [12]. There is no significant difference between cities and suburbs in terms of the average size of the family in 1974 [13].

The increase in divorces is worth noting, both alone and in association with other trends. In 1960 there were 35 divorces per 1000 marriages; 15 years later there were 69 divorces for every 1000 marriages [14]. In 1975 approximately one person divorced for every two individuals who married. This situation has heavily, but not exclusively (there has been an increase in the female heads of families *never* married), contributed to the increasing number of female-headed families. Just for the years 1970 through 1975 this growth was from 11 to 13 percent of all families, a figure in absolute numbers of 1.2 million families [15]. All racial and economic groups experienced an increase in single-parent families. However, the increase was most dramatic among the blacks. The incidence of families headed by females in central cities was nearly two times that found in the suburbs. In 1974 metropolitan areas held 74 percent of all such families.

Although the central city population declined between 1970 and 1973, the total number of adults (over 18 years of age) did not change. The number of young adults 25 to 34 years old increased. The number of older adults 35 to 64 decreased, as did the number of children under 14 years of age. Similarly, the suburban areas have lost population in the under-14 age group [16]. In March 1975, 66,087,000 people in the United States were under 18 years of age; 99.4 percent of these lived in families; 80 percent with both parents; 15.5 percent lived in families with a mother only as the head; 1.5 percent with a father only as the head. For white children, 85.4 percent lived with both parents; for nonwhite children (all races) 53.5 percent lived with both parents [17].

SUMMARY OF PROFILE A

What we see is a United States with a decreasing rate of population growth. This change in rate is producing a different age profile for the population: although there will be, over the next 10 years, an absolute increase in the number of children and youth, their percentage of the total population will decrease. In some way this decrease will alter both their roles and status in our society.

We also note that there has been a considerable growth in metropolitan living in the United States. This in part has been a function of the increase in the sizes of the communities. Associated with this increase in metropolitan living is an out-migration from the central cities, with people, jobs, and money pouring into the suburbs. Remaining in the central cities is a concentration of poor and minorities. The central cities are also losing their children as well as their older adults.

Women have become an increasingly important part of the work force of the United States. This change applies to minority and non-minority women. However, it is most apparent in the suburbs, with their majority caucasion population.

The family and household structure has changed dramatically. The size has decreased. Marriages are being put off. The divorce rates are very high. One fallout of this is the increased number of children who are living in single-parent families. This increase in the number of children living with single parents is most dramatic in the minority population, where the greatest increase in the number of female-headed households also occurred.

Profile B: Mental Disorders in Children and Youth

The standard diagnostic profile used for epidemiologic studies of mental disorders in the United States includes mental retardation, organic brain syndromes, schizophrenia, depressive disorders, other psychoses, alcohol disorders, drug disorders, all other disorders, and undiagnosed conditions. Applying this diagnostic profile to the under-18-year-old population of the United States (approximately 32 percent of the population) yields a conservative estimate of 7 million young people in need of intervention by the mental health professionals [18]. The National Institute of Mental Health's case utilization projection studies indicate that only 9.5 percent of these young people are receiving treatment.

When one considers the diagnoses for admission to all inpatient and outpatient facilities, 80 percent of them are made in the "all other disorder" category. This category includes personality disorders, transient situational disturbances, behavior disorders, and social maladjustment without manifest psychiatric disorder. Even among hospitalized children, 56 percent of them carry such diagnoses [19]. These children do not represent the same children over and over coming into contact with the mental health system. Indeed, more than 50 percent of the inpatient admissions have not had previous inpatient care, and more than 75 percent of the outpatients have not had such care before [20].

The site of treatment for all mental disorder patients changed dramatically in the United States between 1955 and 1973. This shift is attributed in part to the introduction of the phenothiazines and in part to the establishment throughout the country, beginning in 1963, of a previously nonexistent source of treatment, the community mental health center. State and county mental hospitals handled 49 percent of the patient care episodes in 1955. During the same year, outpatient psychiatric services handled 23 percent of the patient care episodes. By 1973 the situation had changed dramatically, with state and county mental hospitals handling 12 percent of the patient care episodes, the previously nonexistent community mental health centers handling 23 percent, and outpatient psychiatric services handling 49 percent [21]. For those under 18 years of age, the community mental health center outpatient facilities were handling the largest number of patient care episodes [22].

Between the years 1955 and 1973 there was a rapid increase in the number of resident patients in the 15-to-24-year-old age range. This increase now seems to be leveling off. However, during the same period the number of resident patients under 15 years of age has more than doubled. This pace seems to be continuing [23]. In 1973, of the total (25,830) mental disorder admissions to the United States state and county hospitals, one-third were 10 to 14 years old [24]. There also was an increase of 38 percent in the resident rate of training schools for juvenile delinquents [25]. Nonwhites have a four times greater probability of being "cared for" in the juvenile justice/training schools system than whites [26].

Drug abuse is a well-publicized problem among youth. Less carefully examined is alcohol abuse. A recent review of this problem in the United States [27] reveals that of the 13-to-18-year-old population, 23 percent drink regularly (more than once per week), and 8 percent are problem drinkers or alcoholics.

Runaway children and youth have been identified as a national problem only since 1974 [28]. No accurate figures exist. It is estimated that 1 to 2 million children are runaways, over half of them female; 15,000 per week are identified as seeking help and shelter in the runaway houses and through the hotline networks.

Suicides have been increasing in the 15-to-24-year-old group. In 1955 they were 4 per 100,000; in 1969, 8 per 100,000; in 1973, 10.6 per 100,000. The year 1974 yielded 4258 deaths and an estimated 15,000 to 20,000 suicide attempts [29]. These figures are exclusive of accidents, which represent 53 percent of the mortality of the youth group [30].

Given the observed change in fertility rate (Series D projection of the U.S. Census Bureau), by 1985 we expect to have approximately 242 million people in the United States. The segment of the population showing the greatest increase is represented by those between the ages of 25 and 34 years. However, there will be an increase, though less dramatic, in those under 18 years of age. Thus large increases will be seen in the age groups (under 18, 25–34, and over 65) which from past experience are "characterized by high admission rates to the psychiatric facilities, correctional institutions, training schools for juvenile delinquents, homes for the aged and dependent, homes and schools for the mentally handicapped" [31]. A specific example is that one can expect an increase in the number of schizophrenics, because "the highest incidence rates for schizophrenia occur in those age groups where the expected relative increase in population is also the highest: 15–24 years; 25–34 years; and 35–44 years" [32]. The greatest increase in population will be among the nonwhites (18 percent versus 27 percent) [33].

Finally, it is interesting to note family structure and its relationship to contacts with the mental health system. For children under 14 years of age, those residing with only one or with no parent are more apt to have psychiatric admissions to outpatient facilities. With only one parent, the outpatient admission rate is two and a half times greater than with two parents. Living with neither parent is related to a three times greater admission rate than living with both parents [34].

SUMMARY OF PROFILE B

Children and youth represent approximately one-third of the population of the United States. One notes that despite the shift of the entire population, including children, from inpatient to outpatient care over the past 15 years, in absolute numbers there is apparently an increase in inpatient care for children and youth, especially for those under 15 years of age. The fact that the number of contacts with the mental health care community are for the most part new contacts indicates a fairly high rate of turnover and may be a statement of the large number of children in need of care as well as perhaps a statement of the benefits that those who receive care find they obtain.

Most contacts (80 percent) on the basis of an analysis of the labels they are given seem to indicate problems derivative of social and family dysfunction. This hypothesis may be further supported by the continued active abuse with both drugs and alcohol, the increasing problem with runaway children and youth, the increasing percentage of accidents especially automobile accidents, and the increasing numbers of suicides and suicide attempts (a reflection of hopelessness?). Family structure does seem to have something to do with probability of contact with mental health care facilities. The absence of one or more parents significantly increases one's possibility of being directed toward such intervention. Finally, it must be noted for the United States that, dependent on ones race, there is a rather dramatic difference as to where one receives attention for social and psychological dysfunction, the minority person being much more likely to receive attention for similar behaviors from the legal system.

Profile C: Medical Technology and Chronic Yet Fatal Illness

Besides the near-eradication of many infectious diseases and the control of others, this century has seen the medical profession gain the ability to prolong significantly the lives of people who without intervention would quickly die. Cure may dangle beyond current reach, but hope for it is purchased at the price of an existence tied to a medical center, pain-producing tests and treatments, physical alterations, and changes in energy levels.

Acute lymphocytic (leukocytic) leukemia in childhood represents one of the most dramatic examples of change in the course of a chronic yet fatal disease.

In the 1950's no more than 30 percent of children with ALL lived one year from their diagnosis. By 1972, 90 percent survived the first year. 25 to 35 percent now survive at five years post diagnosis. . . . Modern treatment . . . demands complete disruption of the patient's and the family's life. Partial disruption never ceases while the child lives. . . . Procedures include multiple finger-sticks, lumbar punctures, infusions of antimetabolites into the cerebrospinal fluid and blood, x-rays, (irradiation of the central nervous system), intravenous infusions, and bone marrow punctures. Medications can produce burning sensations during the infusions. Blood veins eventually sclerose. Side effects from treatment include: nausea, vomiting, gastric burning, loss of appetite, bronchospasm, itching, hematuria, cardiac toxicity, peripheral neuropathies . . . mouth ulcers, rectal fissures, fluid retention, rashes, hair loss, and rarely blindness [35].

Initial treatment usually lasts a very busy 6 months. After this, if the child is in remission, maintenance treatment usually lasts 2½ to 3 years. When there is a relapse, the entire process begins again, sometimes with new drugs and new side effects.

This illness and its modern treatment creates a series of demands as well as new and expanded roles for the patient and his family. Among these demands are intellectual familiarity with the diagnoses, treatment protocols, and side effects; adjustment to the diagnosis and to the aggressive treatment with its concomitant assaults on body, integrity, and privacy; physical changes, deformity, and stigma; adjustment to the chronic remission/relapse course; the challenges of life planning for the family and patient, with necessary involvement of the school systems, relatives, employers, peers, and neighbors.

Demands on the health care professionals who treat the leukemias expand their responsibilities and roles. They must develop ways of sharing the diagnosis, treatment protocols, and information concerning side effects. A capacity to repeat the same information many times and in many different ways needs to be sharpened. An increasing understanding and ability to deal with such issues as informed consent, the quality of life, stigma, prejudice, and ostracism is called for. Clinical and human skills must be developed to help patients and families deal with panic states, denial, rage, mourning, depression, hopelessness, self-destructive wishes and behavior, magical thinking, and rituals. Members of the medical staff get angry, depressed, hopeless, occasionally self-destructive; some find themselves during periods of high stress in a hypomanic state (on buying sprees and with increased sexual activity). Thus an ability to recognize and share the influence of such work on one's self becomes a major coping tool [36].

David Kaplan of Stanford University has evaluated some of the psychosocial changes found in the families of children treated on an oncology service. Of 173 families studied, he found that among the children with leukemia 53 percent had problems with their parents, 43 percent with school, and 23 percent in the community. The problems either were new or although existing prior to the diagnosis of leukemia had been aggravated. Since that diagnosis, 88 percent of the parents had either grief reactions that impaired their social/work functioning or alcoholism (40 percent) or clinical psychiatric problems (35 percent). Of the fathers 60 percent had work difficulties, and 43 percent of the mothers had problems maintaining the home; 40 percent of the marriages were in trouble, an aggravation of preexisting difficulties; 18 percent separated and 5 percent divorced. Of the siblings 40 percent had school problems [37].

SUMMARY OF PROFILE C

This profile shows that medical technology over the past two decades has resulted for some illnesses, in this case the acute leukemias of childhood, in dramatic change. One finds a situation in which prolonged life and the hope for an almost normal life span are exchanged by patients and their families for significant psychosocial and physical stress over time, uncertainty, as well as continuous struggles to maintain the equilibrium of self and family. For those involved in delivering medical care, the changes are also dramatic, since they too face demands to become involved with issues and ways of relating to patients for which they are not particularly trained. Examples of this are the new dimensions of responsibility concerning informed consent as well as the dramatic nature of the illness and its treatment, which call upon the health professionals to engage in a cooperative sharing of selected responsibilities with the families and with the patients that does not exist in most areas of medicine. Many similar examples could be drawn for other diseases— chronic renal disease, familial dysautonomia, sickle cell disease, cystic fibrosis, hemophilia, to give just a short list.

Commentary: On Change, Coping, Vulnerabilities and Strengths

The three profiles of change (population, mental disorders, medical technology and chronic illness) reveal some dramatic examples of becoming different in the United States. Of particular note are the low-fertility rate that will produce a major shift in the population profile, the migrations and economic shifts from central cities to suburbs, and the increase in one-person households and single-parent families. Examination of mental disorders reveals a shift in locus of treatment and the fact that most such disorders in children are in some significant way probably derivative of family and social dysfunction. Examination of medical technology and many chronic illnesses shows an institutionalization of the "trading off" of quality of life and autonomy for hope and prolonged physical existence. Changes produce other changes. And where such events begin and end is often difficult to dissect out.

By definition, change disrupts any state of equilibrium. Such disruption is a force that can grow until the entire system, which was in some state of active balance, is destroyed. Such disruption is also a force that, when joined by other forces, flows toward the reestablishment of a state of equilibrium in the particular system similar to or different from that which existed before.

Such shifts create stresses. Thus changes, especially when rapid, elicit from some individuals cries of crisis. However, accepting change as an essence of our physical universe, of our biological and social world, promotes coping and psychosocial strength. Cultures as well as individuals have their self-esteem. How well one copes with change becomes an integral part of that self-esteem.

The above process differentially affects people, groups, cultures. This differential influence is a function of the vulnerability of these people, groups, and cultures. In turn, such relative vulnerabilities are a function of the developmental stage of the individual or group or culture within the context of their particular environments [38]. Such relationship of vulnerabilities to the developmental stages accounts, I hypothesize, in part, for some of the clustering of vulnerabilities traced by the changes presented in the preceding profiles:

1. Adolescents—runaways; accidents; suicide.
2. Family structure—divorce; mental health contacts.
3. Chronic illness—anger and relative psychosocial dysfunction.

Much literature exists in the biomedical and behavioral sciences on stress and the stresses change produces within individuals. Less is known about the stress produced by external social change on individuals. Documented is the fact that at least in technological societies significant external change produces in individuals affective and autonomic arousal which in turn relates to an increased secretion of catecholamines [39]. Indeed, a "consistently higher prevalence of hypertension has been found in populations undergoing rapid cultural change, urbanization, migration and socioeconomic mobility . . ." [40]. The arena of stress studies now includes the disciplines of economics and social history. For example, stress in relationship to the economy is a subject that interests a number of individuals. One such is M. Harvey Brenner, Ph.D., who goes so far as to state ". . . it was found that national economic trends were the single most important factor in trends of admissions to mental hospitals in New York State annually from 1841 to 1967" [41]. And studies of religious movements during the middle ages have produced similar observations: "The areas in which the age-old prophecies about the Last Days took on a new, revolutionary meaning and a new, explosive force were the areas which were becoming seriously overpopulated and were involved in a process of rapid economic and social change" [42].

There is some general agreement about social shifts that produce high stress. Dr. Gerald Caplan of Harvard lists what he feels to be pathogenic features of world change to children and their families: (1) population movement, (2) urban conglomeration, (3) culture shock, (4) bureaucratic complexity and dehumanization, (5) rapid obsolescence of role and skill (technological advance), and (6) increased leisure (nonproductions of goods and services) of rapidly developing societies. I find it important to note that in discussing these "pathogenic features of world change," Caplan reminds us that such change can also result in a very healthy outcome for individuals and groups when both the process and effects of change are mastered. Such mastery results in greater individual self-esteem and social strength.

What we have discussed is a new awareness of rapid social change in many areas at once. Unlike other periods of Western history, this situation is not related to a plague, nor is it solely related to a war. But, like plagues and wars, the current changes strike at the future through their challenges to the most vulnerable, particularly children, and to our basic social unit, the family.

It is important for not only leaders and planners but Mr. and Mrs. Everyman to approach change through recognition of its existence and a basic acceptance of the consequent stress as a given in all the processes of life. We can train children to this reality. Such acceptance and recognition releases one to focus energies on delineating coping strategies at the individual and social level. The intellectual effort of delineating coping strategies, whether performed singly or when done in concert with others (as in the family), helps reduce vulnerability. It improves coping through the enhancement of predictability, the reduction of uncertainty.

I am convinced that an objective examination of change and human responses to it throughout history reveals an extraordinary human ability to cope with the resultant stresses. Two elements, however, are necessary, if not sufficient, for such "strength." One element is the recognition of the future resource our children represent. Only through such recognition do we attend to training our children to the realities of both change and stress, as well as to the utilization of the tools they have for dealing with significant shifts. The other necessary element is our recognition, acceptance, and working within our need for social structures, structures represented by the family. Such training of oneself and one's children to the realities of existence within the social context of the family or family-like structures has produced throughout human history high tensile strength—a truly remarkable ability to deal with high stress and even cataclysmic change.

References

1. *Current Population Reports, Population Characteristics. Population Profile of the United States: 1975.* U.S. Department of Commerce, Bureau of the Census, Series P-20, No. 292, March 1976, p. 1.
2. Ibid., pp. 1 and 3.
3. Ibid., p. 3.
4. *Current Population Reports, Social and Economic Characteristics of the Metropolitan and Non-Metropolitan Population: 1974 and 1970.* U.S. Department of Comerce, Bureau of the Census, Special Studies Series P-23, No. 25, September 1975, p. 1.
5. Ibid., p. 4.
6. Ibid., Table F, p. 6.
7. Ibid., Table I, p. 8.
8. Ibid., p. 17.
9. Ibid., p. 12.
10. *Current Population Reports, Population Characteristics, Household and*

Family Characteristics: March 1975. U.S. Department of Commerce, Bureau of the Census, Series P-20, No. 291, February 1976, p. 2.

11. Ibid., p. 1.
12. Ibid., p. 3.
13. Ibid., p. 10.
14. *Current Population Reports, Population Characteristics. Population Profile of the United States: 1975.* U.S. Department of Commerce, Bureau of the Census, Series P-20, No. 292, March 1976, p. 9.
15. Ibid., p. 10.
16. *Current Population Reports. Social and Economic Characteristics of the Metropolitan and Non-Metropolitan Population: 1974 and 1970.* U.S. Department of Commerce, Bureau of the Census, Special Studies Series P-23, No. 25, September 1975, p. 4.
17. *Current Population Reports. Population Characteristics, Marital Status and Living Arrangements: March 1975.* U.S. Department of Commerce, Bureau of the Census, Series P-20, No. 287, December 1975, Table 4, p. 9.
18. NIMH Statistical Note 90, July 1973.
19. Kramer, Morton, "Psychiatric services and the changing institutional scene," Presentation to the President's Biomedical and Behavioral Science Research Panel, NIH, Bethesda, Md., November 25, 1975, p. 3.
20. Ibid.
21. Ibid., p. 32.
22. Ibid., Figure 9, p. 40.
23. NIMH Statistical Note 90, July 1973.
24. NIMH Statistical Note 90, July 1973.
25. Kramer, M. loc. cit., p. 14.
26. NAMHC Report 1974.
27. *A National Study of Adolescent Drinking Behavior Attitudes and Co-relates.* Research Triangle Institute, Contract No. HSM-42-78-80(NIA), Chapter 6, pp. 140–156.
28. Runaway Youth Act, Public Law 93-415 Title III, 93rd Congress, S. 821, September 7, 1974.
29. (a) Vital and Health Statistics Suicides in the United States, Series 20 Number 5, August 1967; (b) National Center for Health Statistics Annual Report for 1969; (c) National Center for Health Statistics (unpublished).
30. Annual Vital Statistics of the United States, Volume A.
31. Kramer, M. loc. cit., p. 18.
32. Ibid., p. 21.
33. Ibid., p. 21.
34. Statistical Note No. 100, February 1974.
35. Hersh, Stephen P. Psychosocial aspects of chronic yet fatal illness in children. In *Mental Health in Children,* Vol. 2, PJD Publications, Ltd., Westbury, N.Y., 1976, pp. 430–431.
36. Artiss, K. L. and Levine, A. S. Doctor-patient relation in severe illness: A seminar for oncology fellows, *New Eng. J. Med.* 288 (1973), 1210–1214.
37. Kaplan, David M. (Dept. of Pediatrics, Stanford University School of Medicine). Presentation to Pediatric Oncology Branch, National Cancer Institute, Bethesda, Maryland, 1974.
38. Coelho, George V. and Stein, Janet J., "Coping with stress of an urban planet: impacts of uprooting and overcrowding," Presentation made at a

panel on Behavioral Responses to Urbanization held at the Annual Meetings of the American Association for the Advancement of Science, Boston, Mass., February 1976.

39. Groen, J. J. *The Psychosomatic Specificity Hypothesis For the Etiology of Peptic Ulcer in Psychotherapy and Psychosomatics,* Vol. 19, 295–1971.

40. Freedman, Alfred M., *Comprehensive Textbook of Psychiatry,* Vol. 2, Second Edition, 1975, pp. 1664. Williams & Wilkins, Baltimore.

41. Brenner, Meyer H., Abstract of Mental Illness and the Economy, Harvard University Press 1973. Cited in *Congressional Record-Senate* S. 78, January 19, 1976.

42. Cohn, Norman. *Pursuit of the Millennium* (rev. ed.). Oxford University Press, London, 1970, p. 68.

Discussion

A. Potamianou, Ph.D. (Greece)

May I start by telling Dr. Hersch how much I enjoyed the precise-ness of his presentation and the richness of his data. His exceedingly well-documented paper indeed gave a dramatic picture of changes in process. I must, however, add that he made me feel that we are all in for a pretty difficult time!!

I will not attempt to go back on all the points I would like to have the time to discuss, especially those pertaining to stress created by the shift of energies and also other problems such as that of the one-parent family, the disquieting aspect of the steps taken toward easy divorce, or the impact of population mobility. I will merely take up a few of the questions he is raising in order to stimulate the discussion.

1. Concerning the problem of the change in population profile, I am in total agreement with Dr. Hersch's conclusion that it intro-duces new dimensions in the social plegma, the young people being expected to engage in more and more demanding positions and be-ing asked to take over heavier social roles in terms of responsibilities much earlier than they do now. Undoubtedly, the power struggle be-tween the young and the "not so old" elders (expected to give up their authority positions earlier than now) will be harsh. But the question remains open as to what inner differences such external changes will introduce for the youngsters. Will the changes act as a channel toward more self-assertiveness, or will they enhance anxiety and flight defenses? What is the meaning of something that has been affirmed here in our meetings, that there is a flow of young people

toward the "Kibbutz" structure of life? Is it in order to avoid the struggle for autonomous life? Is it because of the security provided by an already familiar frame?

A research project implemented by the Center for Mental Health in Greece pertaining to a population of first-year university students came out with trends showing that these youngsters have rather conservative attitudes toward expectations from their children with regard to educational and professional achievement, marriage, and relationship between spouses. They define a successful relationship between spouses more according to obligations toward family than as a love or self-fulfilling experience. All of them consider marriage and family life as an indispensable social institution. The "living together" arrangement is rejected.

It is striking to note that in spite of the many social changes that are taking place in Greece, Greek students seem still relatively untouched by the current ideologies concerning men-women relations, although they are quite influenced by the current political ideologies. The majority of males and females define the role of the man, in a couple, as the decision maker and protector, whereas the woman's role is mainly seen in its "maternal" aspect.

Are these conservative attitudes the sign that young Greeks are resistant to allowing themselves to be permeated by the world-over changing perception of a couple's life? Are their attitudes a reflection of fear, or is change rejected because it has not, as yet, produced satisfactory new models?

2. The second point I want to raise is related to the remark that the size of families is decreasing. Here we are dealing with a problem the confirmation of which, consciously or unconsciously, could raise unexpressed fears not only because of the affective stability and security the family group is supposed to provide for human beings but also because it cannot but be equated to the problem of population decrease.

If we try to think objectively about this last issue, we realize that the earth is fast reaching its limits in terms of feeding its population. Approximately 200,000 babies are born every day, and that exceeds by far the capacity to provide means of support for them. Yet, the idea of population reduction, when viewed in terms of our immediate territory, seems difficult to assume. We are facing here a situation which raises in us profound castration and death anxiety. Can mental health practitioners ever hope to succeed in helping people control these deeply rooted fears? Or will we have to accept the fact that such a reality will always be an extremely traumatic one whenever it has to do with our immediate country boundaries? How does inner ambivalence toward the question of birth control affect the applications of birth-control policy? In countries such as Israel or Greece, both being countries constantly threatened as regards their boundaries, we speak in one and the same breath of the necessity for birth control and of the wish to increase our professionally and socially active population. For example, in Greece the question of bringing back emigrants makes headlines in newspapers, journals, parliament, and the like.

And again: what is the role of mental health practitioners in countries such as India, in which one state is trying to pass a law making sterility compulsory after any family has had three children?

3. I am now coming to the disquieting fact that more young people are being taken in for treatment. I feel, at this point, that one should take into consideration the fact that in the last decades we have been trying hard to refine our diagnostic techniques and that we have not been totally unsuccessful in so doing. We have been trained to "hear" what was not heard, or understood, before.

Therefore, we are taking young people in for treatment who, in former days, would have been considered only as somewhat peculiar and dismissed as such. Moreover, we are multiplying the variety of mental health devices to be put to the service of individuals, families, communities.

This could account for the fact that young individuals unconsciously look out for channels through which to displace responsibilities and regain satisfaction for their passive dependent needs.

I think that the dependency needs of youngsters manifest themselves more forcefully to the exact analogous proportions we are trying to develop their autonomy and have them function efficiently in schools or in professions which daily augment their demands for efficacy.

After all, we are perhaps getting what we are looking for! It could well be that the crises of youth are no worse today, although expressed in more spectacular ways, than those of the past.

4. I am now coming to my last point: Dr. Hersch proposes the idea that intellectual effort toward delineating strategies to cope with the anxieties raised by stressful situations reduces anxiety. To a certain extent I agree with him but only to a limited extent. I think that the slightest provocation will always raise in us deeply rooted, unsurpassable fears.

No doubt that to perceive, and to live through, change is the fate of mankind. But to retain homeostasis is stitched in our skin, too, as Freud has showed us. Pulled between these two conflicting trends and forced by his destiny to face the fact that, as Heraclitus said, "everything flows," man will always be tempted to use numbers, figures, and systems to maintain the illusion that something may be done to give him control over his destiny of flow and inevitable change.

Changes in a Sample of Parisian Children Studied Longitudinally

Colette Chiland, M.D., Ph.D. (France)

Preamble

The title of this paper was inspired by a longitudinal study[1] of a group of 66 children begun when they were 6 years old; we were able to follow 44 of them until the age of 21 and so to learn, in privileged conditions, something about their adolescence in a changing world. The reflections which follow exceed the contributions of this longitudinal study and are elicited by our daily practice as a child and adult psychiatrist and psychoanalyst and by our activity as a university professor.

The longitudinal study cited and our daily psychiatric practice are located in Paris' 13th "arrondissement." An arrondissement in Paris (they number 20) corresponds to an administrative demarcation (official registry of personal data, postal address, etc.), but does not have the reality of a true community. Most of the changes which have taken place in the environment of today's adolescents since their birth, that is, in the last 20 years, do not specifically concern the 13th arrondissement, but rather Paris and, still more, life in a large me-

[1] Research carried out with a grant from the I.N.S.E.R.M. (Institut National de la Santé et de la Recherche Médicale, National Institute for Health and Medical Research). Team research around René Diathine: Colette Chiland, Lia Coppel, Marceline Gabel.

tropolis of Europe. Certain changes are more specific to our arrondissement.

I have been working in this arrondissement for exactly 20 years, and the most spectacular change is that of the buildings. In 1957 the 13th arrondissement counted a few middle-class buildings, numerous decayed and even unhealthy houses, and factories. The factories have been closed in Paris and decentralized; that is, they have been moved to the outskirts of Paris and to the provinces. The old houses have been demolished, and in their place new residences have been built: rental units for moderate-income families (*Habitations à Loyer Modéré*) or apartments to buy. A certain number of these new buildings are thirty or so stories tall and are called towers. Without being exactly skyscrapers—like the Maine-Montparnasse Tower, the highest in Europe at 209.13 meters and with 58 levels—these towers have transformed the appearance of the district, have "Americanized" it. Together with the *Front-de-Seine* in the 15th arrondissement and *La Défense* in the west of Paris, the 13th arrondissement is one of the areas where these towers are concentrated. The current President of the Republic, Valéry Giscard d'Estaing, has put a halt to the construction of towers in Paris.

For anyone who knew the streets, the alleys, the old stables, the wine market (the Halle-aux-Vins) on the edges of the 13th arrondissement, in short, this bit of the old Paris that Balzac described, it is an important architectural and ecological change.

It brings with it a change in the population which inhabits the quarter. The data furnished by three censuses taken in 1962, 1968, and 1975 allow us to objectify this change (Table 1), which is marked essentially by the increase in the upper and middle classes and the diminution of the working class in the distribution of professional categories. The group of children seen at the Alfred Binet Center constituted a noticeably representative sample of the population in 1962 and 1968; its composition remains the same in 1975 and therefore ceases to be representative, since the upper and middle classes consult us less often than do the lower classes. We notice in the group of patients an improvement of the living conditions; the percentage of well-housed families increases, although there remain some who live in distressing conditions; we also see a change in the distribution of the diagnoses. The latter change is due to very different causes: a

Table 1. Percentages of the Principal Professional Categories
in the 13th Arrondissement

Survey	1962	1968	1975
Upper-level management, liberal professions, industrialists and large merchants	10.5	11	17
Middle management	13.4	15	19
Office workers	14.3	25	25
Artisans and small merchants	6.4	6	4
Foremen, skilled workers	25.5	16	12
Semiskilled workers, laborers, domestic workers	26.2	25	19
Artists, clergy, army	3.5	2	3
Other	0.2	—	1

change in the views of the team of psychiatrists who must fill out an epidemiological card for each patient (thus the diagnosis "reaction disorders" is used less and less) and a change in the children who are referred to us (the school takes more and more charge of learning difficulties, dyslexia, and scholastic failures) so that we have to treat more psychiatric and fewer pedagogical problems.

Do these changes we have just described in the appearance of the district and in its population bring about any changes in the way of life that might have repercussions on the psychological organization of children and adolescents?

A certain number of fundamental parameters of daily life have not changed. I am thinking particularly of the working-class families, whose children are more exposed to the risk of scholastic failure and the difficulties of sociological integration and to the troubles this failure engenders. The nature of the work, the working hours, the time it takes to get around have not changed. If comfort in the home has improved, traffic is more difficult and the atmosphere is more polluted.

Some women do not withstand life in the big new residential compounds which deprive them of easy neighborly relations; sometimes their malaise is so great as to constitute a real phobia. As for the children, they find in the commercial centers and in the vast supermarkets favorite places for pilfering and for loitering after school or when they are playing hooky.

The development of television and its introduction into most homes (if some families do not have one, they are most often from the upper social classes) is, on the other hand, an important parameter. The first tests of television in France date from before World War II. But the creation of television networks took place only after the war: in 1949 there were 178 television sets; in 1950 there were 297 television sets; in 1974 there were 12,924,519 television sets. A second color network went into service in October 1967.

This is an important phenomenon, with both negative and positive aspects. Family life has been changed. The family meal may cease to be a moment for coming together (in some families, where children were forbidden to speak at the table, it never was such a moment): they watch television instead of talking to each other. I leave aside the quarrels regarding the choice of program and the deprivation of television as a new mode of punishing children. Television brings an opening onto the world and shows children what they would not know without it. It could contribute to correcting cultural inequalities. It does this very little if at all, for the use that is made of television depends very much on the attitude and the cultural level of the parents: either the child remains planted for all his leisure hours before the television set, or the programs are chosen for him; either the child is a passive spectator, or the program is an occasion for questions, conversation, exchanges with the parents.

Television has had considerable repercussions on school life. Sometimes the school uses it; there are educational programs. There is also discussion about what the children have seen at home. On the negative side, there are the children who arrive at school in the morning half-asleep, tired because they did not go to bed in order to watch programs to the end, between 11 o'clock and midnight. More profoundly, this easy, seductive, passive means of satisfying one's curiosity devalues the narrower path of "instruction" and culture proposed by the school. The school is not "competitive" in the attraction it can have for children.

The educational crisis, and especially that of secondary schools, is a major one. Each minister of education makes reforms. And we have witnessed a series of changes, which we now describe.

In 1962, when our longitudinal research began, the nursery schools were—and had been since the beginning—coed; secondary schools often were, too, especially those which had been built since World War II; primary schools never were, and boys and girls were separated. It was after 1968 that all the public primary schools in the 13th arrondissement became, rapidly or progressively, coed. The adolescents about whom we speak did not, therefore, experience continuity in coeducation.

The school is an institution that resists change, and any changes take time. Thus minds in France are often hostile to a school week like that in the United States, in which the children would go to school from Monday to Friday and be free on the weekend—it would be bad for the health of the children (the poor English, the poor Americans, etc.). When our lay school originated, when the separation of church and state was instituted, a day was reserved so that the families who wished to could send their children to catechism. That day was Thursday. After 1968 this day off was brought back to Wednesday, and there were no longer any classes on Saturday afternoon. As of the school year beginning in September 1977, the schools were able to choose, with the families, between maintaining the pause in the middle of the week (on Wednesday) and having the complete weekend off.

The configuration of the school year and vacations has been continually modified. And the students are caught between the exigencies of the program which remain great and the diminishing number of class days.

There have been attempts to transform certain teaching, for example, the teaching of mathematics. So-called "modern" mathematics was introduced by a 1968 decree for the first 2 years of secondary studies, by a 1971 decree for the following 2 years, and by a 1970 decree for primary schools. There, too, change and resistance to change have occurred. The teachers must be trained, "recycled"; they accept this and succeed in it more or less well. Parents who have gone through school become incapable of following their children in their schoolwork. Finally, in the course of the last decade mathematics became selective. Only the parents able to buy books and to study "mathematics for Mom" and (at a higher level!) "mathematics for Dad" can help their children in primary school. In the second cycle of secondary school, the classes of the mathematical section called "C" constitute the elite channel through which one must pass in order to be admitted to a number of universities and upper-level schools (écoles supérieures) or in order to pursue a program of study with some chance of success, notably medicine. This program marks the end of the "humanities" which formed the preceding generation and many others before it. It is the end of Latin and Greek, the earlier means of selection, which were just as debatable, moreover. The "letters" are today "feminine" studies, just at Latin and Greek were reserved for the male sex until the end of the 19th century.

Like any change, this one creates a reorganization, even a disarray, especially since access to secondary studies has been considerably broadened. School attendance until the age of 12 has been compulsory since 1932, until the age of 14 since 1936, and until age 16 since 1959 (which involves those children born in 1953 and later). Secondary instruction addressed 10 percent of the population before World War II; it addresses three-fourths of the population now. This means that to avoid the crisis which has rocked education, especially since 1968, it would have been necessary to change the subject matter, the programs, the pedagogical methods. In spite of all the attempts at change in the shape of official reforms and initiatives on the part of the teachers, there has been no real alteration. And too often adolescents do not become involved in their studies; *they are bored.* That might justify certain of the conclusions of Ivan Illich [4] which do not apply at the primary school level.

It cannot be said that those who denounced the problems were not heard. Attempts were made to improve the situation. We have seen the primary school with which we have been working since 1957 change buildings and move from the 19th century (there were stoves which were lit every morning) into the 20th century—into new premises, too noisy, but offering new resources. In 1970 were created the G.A.P.P., the psychopedagogical aid groups, composed of a psychologist and teachers specialized in various types of rehabilitation; the G.A.P.P. give individual help to children in difficulty, in little groups or in adjustment classes with small enrolment, and they focus especially on the early stages of primary education. Wherever a G.A.P.P. is implanted, there is a decrease in the proportion of students who repeat a year.

There was an attempt to transform the structure of secondary schools. Before the war, after primary studies at the district school (école communale) or at the "little high school" ("petit lycée"), children entered high school (Lycée) to pursue secondary studies for 7 years, culminating in the baccalaureate. Some students pursued "upper-level primary studies" until they received the school-leaving certificate. This double track was eliminated in favor of a "single school" and, in order to receive students in large numbers, the secondary school was cut in two by putting the first cycle (4 years, from the age of 11 to 15 years) in colleges of secondary instruction ("collèges d'enseignement secondaire" or C.E.S.), the second cycle (3 years, from 15 to 18 years of age) remaining in the high schools (lycées). I am simplifying the description and the analysis: the attempt to combine in a "comprehensive-school" teachers from the primary, the old upper-level primary, and the old secondary schools has until now been a failure. And the structure of the C.E.S. which was to permit the students to pass easily from a short secondary cycle to a long secondary cycle, from low-level classes to high-level ones, has most often functioned merely as a segregating tool, maintaining each child in his initial track. We are still confronted today with the fact that the school gives insufficient help to the child who comes from a culturally disadvantaged environment and that it contributes to maintaining social segregation.

Again, the adolescents are bored. They smoke, they drink, they take tranquilizers and, after medication, illegal drugs, which the preceding generation did not experience.

The extension of compulsory school attendance prolongs the economic dependence on the parents, even if high-school and university students have begun to take on seasonal or part-time work, very much later than in North America. In contrast with this economic dependence vis-à-vis their families, adolescents enjoy an independence previously unknown. At a very young age they go away on trips with their friends, without their parents, they have a sex life, they leave their parents' homes. The civil and political majority has been lowered from 21 to 18 by the law of July 7, 1974.

The sexuality of young people is probably the most important change. There again there are negative and positive sides. Parents cannot refer to their own history and oscillate between total laxity, which the adolescent experiences as abandonment, and a rigid refusal of change. Young people have more-or-less pleasant sexual relations and often seem not to be any happier for them. But the sexual initiation of the young man is no longer accomplished by a prostitute in a brothel while the young girl is a "white goose" whose innocence one wishes to maintain. Hypocrisy is receding. The young girl, with freedom to live and love, is free to study and to work.

Whether admitted by their families, the sexuality of the young has been becoming more and more precocious. Movies have been becoming more and more daring, more frankly pornographic. In a hypocrisy of a civilization "inciting to crime" ("pousse au crime"), the people demanded the lifting of total or partial restrictions on films (admission forbidden to those under 13 and under 18) in the name of freedom of expression; at the same time they refused minors free access to contraceptive methods. It is true that contraception became legal in France with the Neuwirth law of December 29, 1967, with many restrictions, among them the necessity of parental authorization for minors, until 1974 when the law was liberalized. In fact, many doctors with full awareness broke the law before 1974 and wrote prescriptions for girls who came to ask for them without their parents. The voluntary interruption of pregnancy has become legal with restrictive clauses only since the Simone Weil law of January 17, 1975; parental authorization remains necessary for minors.

French adolescents of today, born after World War II, seem to live a golden life in the eyes of yesterday's adolescents, caught as they were in the upheavals of the war, of the occupation, of restrictions. Today's adolescents have transistors, television, motorbikes, clothes and food, the possibility of travel, peace (since 1962, date of the recognition of Algerian independence). . . . They are bored; they live without hope, without a horizon. What is happening in our "consuming society" ("société de consommation"—the French expression combines the English "consume" and "consummate" and plays on their multiple connotations—tr.)? What is happening in this world that produced concentration camps, the atomic bomb, the Gulag. . . ?

We have sketched a picture of the most visible external changes, we have set out in very general terms some of the impacts of these changes on adolescents. However, the noisy, spectacular demonstrations are the deed of only a minority of adolescents. Inside the "silent majority" the changes are less evident. What are they?

We studied at age six 66 randomly chosen children from the public schools of the 13th arrondissement, 34 boys and 32 girls, and their families. This sample was at that age representative of the population of the district as to the profession of the parents; in its behavior at school it was representative of the educational cursus of French, and more particularly Parisian, pupils; the distribution of the levels of intelligence (IQ measured by the Binet-Simon standardized in 1949) ranged from 74 to 135, with a slight asymmetry in favor of the good levels.

We followed these children and their families from year to year. And in the period from 16 to 21 years of age we were able to see 44 of them again (i.e., two-thirds), which is a good proportion for a longitudinal study. Added to this number are a few cases in which we had indirect news or saw the family but not the adolescent again, which makes available certain data for 59 cases in all.

The interview or interviews we had with the adolescents we saw again differ from our usual practice as psychiatrists. These adolescents did not come to ask for anything, even though two of them subsequently asked for psychotherapy. They knew that they were the object of a study, and they agreed to cooperate, with the exception of one boy. We had not seen him again since the end of primary school, his mother being opposed to it; at age 20, he made his father sufficiently worried that the father persuaded him to come see us. We found ourselves faced with a paranoiac character, and we respected his refusal to engage in an interview, even though he had come to the meeting; at the age of 6, he had seemed to us to be prepsychotic. The other adolescents were remarkably cooperative and on the whole not very curious about this study, which had nonetheless been going forward for many years. Of the beginnings of the study, they had either little recollection or memories reconstructed phantasmatically, such as the boy who spoke to us of troubling feelings he experienced on being received into a room where there was a bed and where we drew the curtains, whereas there was no couch in the schoolroom where we used to meet him; moreover, he blended into a single female image the three women of the team who had examined him.

We let each adolescent speak as he wished; there was no systematic questionnaire. We tried to give renewed impetus to the interview in order to explore the whole of the adolescent's life: high school or work, cultural or political interests, sentimental life, or family. But we could not push the interview in a way that might have been judged indiscreet by an adolescent who was not asking for a consultation.

The first observation was that these adolescents did not seem to have been touched by the phenomenon of drugs. At least, with the exception of only one, about whom we speak later, none of them presented himself as a user of drugs. Neither did any family evoke this problem for their child. That does not mean that drugs had not been occasionally tried; they did not occupy the front of the stage.

The only boy who was an habitual user of hashish told us about it when he was hospitalized for an acute psychotic episode. Born in Algeria, abandoned, taken in by a foster family at 18 months of age (no one knows how he lived until the age of 18 months), he had worried us a lot at age 6, but he seemed to have come out of his prepsychotic state and to have evolved rather favorably. In adolescence he interrupted his business studies and attempted suicide; his preoccupations centered on his identity, because he knows nothing of his origins: to which of the hostile factions of the Algerian population does he belong? After his foster father died, he set out and toured France, lived who knows how, working periodically, leaving his jobs in psychopathic outbursts, staying with "buddies." He smoked tobacco and hash, drank enormous amounts of coffee, became agitated, and was hospitalized in a state of confusion and delirium from which he emerged rather rapidly to restructure himself in a paranoiac mode. The psychopathology overrode the drugs; it is not a question of addiction.

In view of the fact that since 1968 people have denounced the use of drugs by the young, it may seem surprising that we did not encounter this problem in our sample. Our adolescents are distributed in different educational establishments and places of work; it is not the hypothesis of a place protected by chance which can account for this. Perhaps this is one confirmation of the opinion expressed by Fréjaville, Davidson, and Choquet [3]. Fréjaville writes (p. 206): "The drug phenomenon is now—in France at least—of little importance in reality"; and Davidson and Choquet (p. 69): "the increasing use of drugs by the young began to seem intolerable to the national authorities in the years 1969 and 1970. The newspapers, radio and television related almost daily deaths and serious accidents caused by drugs and multiplied warnings based essentially on the desire to dissuade through fear. This dramatization, probably excessive, nonetheless had the advantage of provoking the creation of reflection groups at various levels and a new awareness of certain problems of youth, not new in their essence, but different in their manifestations." The exact percentage of young drug addicts is very difficult to know. One must distinguish the occasional users from those who are intoxicated. The phenomenon is clandestine, and we only know those who come to get help; not all of them come, in spite of the anonymity that is guaranteed them.

Young addicts, under 25 years of age, who have been cared for in specialized establishments and could be studied, often come from broken homes. We can compare the frequency of this break-up of the family in different samples. Table 2 brings together the data from [3] and [2].

Table 2. **Percentage of Broken Homes in Diverse Samples**

Our sample at age 6	14
Our sample at age 21	21
Patients of the A. Binet Center 6 years of age 1961–1963	29
All patients of the A. Binet Center 1962–1963	27
Drug addicts under age 25	44.7
Young delinquents	38.2
Suicidal youth (ages 14–20)	32.5
High school students (ages 14–20)	12.2

Despite the addition of five families broken up by divorces which occurred between the ages of 6 and 21 in our subjects, the figure for broken homes remains low in this group; only the high-school students, a privileged milieu of those who show themselves capable of pursuing long secondary studies, have a lower figure.

The proportion of our adolescents who were able to pursue secondary studies to the completion of the baccalaureate is probably good in relation to the national average; we do not possess any statistics that allow us to calculate how they relate to children born in the same year. One-third received their baccalaureate, 11 out of 34 boys and 12 out of 32 girls; the slightly higher proportion of girls, 52 percent of those graduated in our study, corresponds to the national proportion of 56 percent (in 1973). The girls were consistently better students than the boys. As early as the preparatory course (the first year of compulsory primary education), two girls out of three had learned to read very well, as compared with one boy out of three. That is translated over the course of the primary education: 50 percent of the girls finish without having been held back, contrasted with only 30 percent of the boys. The girls' superiority is less clear; it is even less so at the end of secondary school. Various hypotheses can be advanced by way of explanation. The boys might have a different rhythm of psychological development: what is true of the curves of weight and height and of the age of puberty could be true for the age of acquisition of reading skills and for the early stages of schooling. The girls, for a long time kept away from studies, do very well at them; they are favored at the beginning by their greater aptitude for language, their docility (they are less unstable, hyperkinetic, etc. than the boys). At high school they have but a slight advantage, which will be erased at the level of university studies. It seems difficult to imagine that they become more "stupid," that the aptitudes manifested at the end of their growth diminish much faster among the girls than among the boys. The cultural restraint probably plays a preponderant role there. The education that most families still give their daughters includes less valorization of their intellectual future, and multiple barriers, evident or hidden, are thrown up along their path.

Ten years later we find the conclusions of Bianca Zazzo's 1966 work [5] still valid. She finds that girls give greater weight to sentimental success over professional success (p. 205):

Girls differentiate themselves and withdraw from their own group and tend to become closer to boys. But while rejecting verbally what they believe to be the feminine model, they are deeply dependent on it, when they envisage their own realization, their adult accomplishment. A lesser affirmation of self, a greater dependence on others is apparent from their projects: sentimental success is the objective that they strive for above all, the goal they give themselves, and even when other goals are envisioned, the mode of social integration which they advocate expresses the same attitude of dependence: success in life is for them a function of the reactions of others, of their pleasure (agrément) if not of their despotism ("bon plaisir"—"bon plaisir" is an old expression used particularly by kings in their edicts—tr.), it is the result of a skillful adaptation and not of a conquest" (p. 375). The M.L.F. (Mouvement de Libération des Femmes, French women's Lib—tr.) and Women's Lib are much talked about, but they still have a lot to do!

Girls or boys, their educational future was very broadly sketched as of the end of their first year of primary school. Out of 23 recipients of the baccalaureate, 21 knew how to read well, 2 had had mediocre results. All the children who learned to read easily at 6 or younger did not receive the baccalaureate, only 2 out of 3; but among the children who had difficulty learning to read, there are only 6 percent who have the baccalaureate. And these exceptional successes are encountered only in families of a good sociocultural level who supported their children and succeeded in keeping them channeled toward the long-term education from which they were to be excluded. The intellectual level such as one can measure it at age 6 plays a role, of course (see Table 3). The sociocultural level of origin (see Table 4) also plays a role (given our small sample size our figures should be read as indicating only a tendency).

Thus at the same moment when it becomes more extensive, when compulsory school attendance is prolonged, the school meets with failure: poor learning and restlessness in the primary school, boredom in the secondary program, difficulties of integration at the university. . . . Often the child is not happy at school; if he comes from a culturally deprived family, school does not allow him to compensate for his handicap; the adolescent only rarely finds stimulation

Table 3. Intellectual Quotient at Age 6
and Completion of the Baccalaureate

IQ at Age 6	Sample Size	%
110 and above	16/23	69.5
90–109	7/32	22
89 and under	0/11	0

Table 4. Sociocultural Level of Origin and Completion of the Baccalaureate

Sociocultural Level	Sample Size	%
Upper	12/15	80
Middle	10/24	42
Lower	1/27	3.7

and a prospect for the future there. Is this a problem of the school or a problem of society?

Olivier, who had an IQ of 74 at age 6, the lowest IQ in our sample, lived an unhappy childhood and, far from perceiving the rejection of which he was the object, thought "that he was bad and didn't want to do anything." At the end of his obligatory school attendance, he met a teacher who awakened him. He did an apprenticeship in painting and was transformed. Freed from school, he has blossomed and is one of the adolescents who has the greatest number of varied interests—ice skating, handball, trumpet, and so on—and who expresses himself with the most humor.

The condition of the worker in this last quarter of the 20th century is obviously no longer what it was in the 19th century. Even if many problems remain (the nature of the work, living conditions, salaries, etc.), especially at the lowest end of the scale, the laborers and the semiskilled workers (who, precisely, are not at all "skilled"), indisputable progress has been made: social security, limitation of working hours, 24 working days of paid vacation annually, family allowances, free primary and secondary education, and the like. However, this progress has as yet had very little repercussion on the capacity of children to succeed in school. It is true even for this generation, which is now 20 years old, for which the attempts to transform the structures of secondary education were made and which has been saturated by the mass media, notably television. The possible opening onto the world via television which we pointed out previously remains a superficial dusting and does not correspond to a profound cultural shaping.

We were astonished by the little intellectual curiosity of those very ones among our adolescents who were able to pursue their secondary studies and obtain the baccalaureate. Many made very conformist responses as to their reading; few read with true interest a variety of books. The big source of information is television. Some read articles on economics in *Le Monde,* recommended by their professor. Most read no newspaper. And in spite of all that has been said about the "politicization" of the high schools, few of them have a precise political orientation, to say nothing of a militant participation in a party.

In a survey of a representative sample of 30 adolescents aged 16 to 21, whose sex life she proposed to study, Castaréde [1] makes the same observations we have made:

Very rare are the adolescents of our sample who have a precise center of interest, although many more occasions for cultural, artistic, and athletic development are offered to them. . . . For more than half the study . . . leisure activities are only objects passively consumed: cinema, nightclubs, restaurants. . . . There is no true personal curiosity, still less a critical spirit with regard to these activities. They do not at any time enter into the construction of personal originality, but they distract from the daily greyness (p. 153).

Ambitions are often limited, for example, those of the boy, having difficulty at school despite a normal intellectual level, who had been dreaming since the end of the latency period of nothing more than entering the postal service; he succeeded, he is delighted, and his family is too.

We do not have any reference documents from which to judge whether those who were 20 years old 30 years ago differed significantly from these adolescents of today. It is not enough for each individual to refer to his own personal experience . . . but from what we observe we can draw some conclusions: easier access to cultural means and the development of powerful mass media do not develop intellectual curiosity and personal activity as much as one might have hoped.

In sexual life, adolescents have certainly changed. There, too, our group is "good"; just as the problem of drugs does not appear in this random sample open to all comers, there is no patent case of extremely precocious sexuality. It is between 16 and 18 years of age that they begin to have partners whose existence is known to their parents, with a clear turning point around 18 where some of them begin to live as couples outside their parents' homes. The number of those who marry equals that of nonmarried couples.

Our observations coincide with those of Castaréde. Out of the 30 adolescents she interviewed, 28 wish for a life as part of a couple, and two-thirds of them favor the idea of marriage. "Those who reject marriage (9 adolescents) are all culturally and socially favored: challenging marriage appears, in our sample, intellectual and middle-class" ([1], pp. 135–136).

We are also in agreement with Castaréde [1] about the importance of the family ties which this contesting generation conserves. In her nondirective conversations, the instructions which she gave did not refer to the family: "I would like to have you talk to me as freely as possible about the evolution of girl-boy relations, sexuality; I want you to speak from your own experience, telling me what you personally think about it" (p. 69). For two-thirds of the adolescents the theme of the family concurs with the instructions ([1], p. 113). They insist on the importance of the dialogue with their parents, of the trust between parents and children, either to congratulate themselves on their relations with their parents or to complain of a lack.

In our sample the adolescents whose parents put at their disposal a bedroom outside the family apartment very often continue to come and take their meals at home and are more often present in the parents' home than the parents themselves would like. When there is a break with the parents, it is more often the act of the parents than that of the adolescents. And even then the dependence of the adolescents with regard to parental imagos is striking.

Today's adolescent, like yesterday's, must mourn idealized parental images, and this mourning is not easy for him. His depression is clothed in new forms of expression and would pass unnoticed behind demands for freedom and an active sexuality. Parents today are in greater confusion than in the last generation: they cannot refer to their adolescence as a model; they can no longer incarnate a divine right of authority; they must still play a protective role, which the adolescent asks them for without saying it, without knowing it, without accepting that it be felt.

In the course of this evolution from age 6 to age 21 two moments of eruption of difficulties are apparent: at 6 there were numerous symptoms that had disappeared 2 years later; from 18 on structured disorders and decompensations became manifest: one girl suffers from mental anorexia, another is in prison (we do not know why), one boy had a perforated ulcer, another, whom we have already mentioned, had an acute psychotic episode; for others, lines of fragility stand out, which cause us to formulate reservations for the future. It is probable that when these fragile subjects enter primary school and when their education ends and they enter active life the weight of social changes aggravates that insecurity of fragile subjects.

If, in the course of these 15 years, the world has changed around them, our subjects have continued their evolution while remaining very much like themselves. If it is difficult to predict at 6 what the adult will be, it is possible to situate him in a "bracket" between the best and the worst of his possible evolution. We can rejoice that several have held up relatively well in perturbing family environments. We can be sad that some destinies were already very oriented by the first 6 years of life.

In conclusion, we would like to adopt the term *plurality of adolescence* proposed by Zazzo [5]. The adolescent of today may be defined with reference to the noisy adolescents who are talked about: the protesters of May 1968, the restless high-school students, the drug addicts, those who take trips (both road and drugs), those who are very precocious sexually or are sexually promiscuous, and so on. But the majority of today's adolescents are closer to the adolescents of yesterday than the mass media would have us believe. Their language, their hairstyles, their clothes, their superficial behavior have changed. But they must face the same identity crisis as yesterday, the same mixture of exaltation (everything is possible, "take your dreams for realities," as the slogan of 1968 puts it) and of depression, the same difficulty finding a "joie de vivre" outside of utopia, in this world without *Hinterwelten* (Nietzsche).

References

1. Castaréde, M.-F. *Les adolescents d'aujourd'hui. Aspects de la psycho-sexualité adolescente en 1976*. Thèse de Doctorat en Psychologie, Université René Descartes, Paris, 1977.
2. Chiland, C. *L'enfant de six ans et son avenir*. P.U.F., Paris, 1971.
3. Fréjaville, J.-P., Davidson, F., and Choquet, M. *Les jeunes et la drogue*. P.U.F., Paris, 1977.

4. Illich, I. *Deschooling Society*. New York, Harper and Row, 1971; French edition, *Une société sans école*. Editions du Seuil, Paris, 1971.
5. Zazzo, B. *Psychologie différentielle de l'adolescence. Etude de la représentation de soi*. P.U.F., Paris, 1966.

Discussion

Colette Chiland

Interviewing children in a follow-up study can be interesting from the point of view of the formation of so-called "screen memories." I recall one boy whom I saw as a small child and again at the age of 18 years. When asked whether he recalled his earlier interview he said: "May I speak quite frankly? You must take precautions with children that you see from now on and not do with them what you did with me." ("And what was that?") "You should not have seen me in a bedroom with the curtains drawn!" Actually he was seen in a formal classroom furnished like any schoolroom. Thus what the children remember of an interview can be distorted in the manner of any other early experiences in the service of unfulfilled drives.

Several participants in the study group have inquired about the changing sexual behavior of today's teenagers in France and the effects of this increased freedom. Here I would say that adult fantasies outrun the facts. Paris is not the center for unlicensed fornication among the young! In actual practice, many of the adolescents keep one partner for many years, and the two quite frequently get married in the end, so that a kind of psychological monogamy is maintained. In my opinion, this would appear to be a better initiation into sexuality than the older method of visiting brothels. At least it is based on a relationship. This early living together cannot be held responsible for the rise in the divorce rate, since this antedated the "new sexuality" by many years. The parents do not have to "go along" with this new life style and are better advised to live according to their own standards of right and wrong and not adopt for themselves the changing mores of their children.

Perhaps the most striking finding of this normative study was the high rate of serious psychopathology in the nonpatient children (12% were borderline or psychotic). This has also been found in other studies of the general population and warns us that a significant group of disturbed children are still not being referred for psychiatric help.

The success of the follow-up can be attributed to two factors: (1) the image of our clinic as a community and resource center that opened the school doors to us and (2) the strong "research alliance" established by our social worker with the sample. Unfortunately, however, even with these advantages, we were not able to see about a third of the sample between the ages of 16 to 21 years, although we continued to collect information from other sources such as the school and the family. This represents one of the vicissitudes of longitudinal investigations.

Delinquent Self-Image and Social Change*

James B. Welsh, Ph.D. and
Daniel Offer, M.D. (U.S.A.)

During the past decade, American society has witnessed a number of events so prominently visible that questioning their potential effects on that society has become part of the popular introspection. The suspicion is afoot that this has been a period of notable social change, leading perforce to personal change. Since many of these events implicate the young, a focus of this questioning has been the potential effect of this period on adolescents. The particular focus of this chapter is the potential effect of the period on the self-image of delinquent adolescents.

Unfortunately, empirical investigation of these potential effects is hindered by the paucity of ongoing data collection across a significant period of time. A frequently voiced concern is the lack of replication of large-scale empirical studies of adolescents, which would permit historical comparison. The information which is currently available is largely conveyed in cross-sectional studies, each of which employs different measures to study different problems with different populations of adolescents. Although studies such as those of Douvan and

* Supported in part by the Judith Baskin Offer Fund for Research and Education, Institute for Psychosomatic and Psychiatric Research and Training, Michael Reese Hospital and Medical Center and by grant ST 32 MH 14668 from National Institute of Mental Health.

Adelson [8] or Offer [18] may provide future researchers a baseline for historical comparison, present research is limited by available data on specific populations of adolescents. The population employed in this study was selected (at least in part) because of such limitations.

We intended to study temporal trends in adolescent self-image. In spite of the availability of a large data bank involving the same instrument (the Offer Self-Image Questionnaire for Adolescents), we found the diversity of settings in which the measure was administered over the past 15 years prevented us from attending to the temporal dimension in these data. We, therefore, chose to examine self-image data for a relatively stable setting: an inpatient adolescent psychiatric unit for the treatment of delinquents. This constancy of setting allowed us to look at the temporal dimension in the data, to examine the potential effects of this period of social change upon one specific dimension of adolescent personality, self-image.

Adolescence is characteristically described as the point of transition from childhood to adulthood. This transition entails a personal displacement from the world of the family to the larger social world. Tasks that had previously been attended to by the parents come increasingly into the province of personal responsibility. The period is thus marked by a variety of personal changes.

These changes are effected by a manifold dynamic with biological, psychological, and social components. Such components are, of course, highly interrelated, with the degree of coordination or disjunction among them leading to different patterns of growth. Pubertal development involves not only physical changes but also social growth through hormonally induced affective changes, sexual differentiation and role assumption, and similar consequences of biological maturation. Cognitive abilities undergo changes that allow greater incorporation of others in one's plans and improvement of self-reflective capacities necessary for adult performance. The social dynamics affect in varying degrees the dawning realization of identity and the assumption of a personal place in the collectivity.

Among the multiple tasks incumbent on adolescents, one which has aroused considerable scholarly attention is the attainment of personal identity. Indeed, Erikson [9] has designated this attainment as the central task of adolescence, noting its dependence on previous stages of the life cycle and its influence on subsequent development. Blos [4, 5] ascribes a similarly central role to the process of separation and individuation by which the adolescent transition is accomplished. Under these or most other paradigms, the attainment of individuated identity is subject to multiple influences.

Individual patterns of growth, adjustment, or coping in adolescence are likely, therefore, to be affected by both the family setting from which the transition issues and the social setting to which it aspires. Certain choices made at this time will be more circumscribed by the history of family inputs, whereas others will be more open to social-historical contingencies. Some aspects of adolescent personality are likely to remain rather invariant in the face of shifting social contingencies; others are likely to be more variable. Determination of the relative variance or invariance of adolescent personality in the face of social change is difficult *a priori*. As Keniston [13] has cautioned, "Any global judgment of overall developmental level is based on a profile derived from sector-specific evaluations. Thus if we are to speak precisely about the factors that promote an individual's development, we must specify which sectors or lines of development we are talking about."

Sector-specificity is a concept to be kept in mind when considering the possible effects of social change on adolescence. Certainly, aspects of adolescence most closely controlled by biological process are expected to remain fairly invariant in the face of social change. Here, the effect of such change is severely mitigated by evolutionary conservatism, but is clearly not eliminated, as it can influence diet, health care, or other biological inputs. At the other extreme of reactivity, even the most transient social changes are seen to affect some choices, like musical preference, styles of dress, jargon, or advertising-induced beliefs, all of which have some impact on identity. The vast majority of interesting questions about adolescence lies between such extremes of variance and invariance in the face of social change. Our understanding of the influence of social change in these areas depends on empirically derived information and theoretically derived expectations.

We turn, now, to an empirical study of the question, and subsequently (in the discussion) to the consideration of theoretically divergent expectations.

Method

SUBJECTS

Subjects for the study are referrals to the Illinois State Psychiatric Institute's adolescent unit, who were administered a research battery during the screening, as part of ongoing research activities of the program. The unit accepts male and female patients who are not overtly psychotic, mentally retarded, or brain damaged. Referral sources include the juvenile courts, schools, social service agencies, private psychiatrists, and others. Patients are generally 13 to 17 years old, and they have exhibited some delinquent behavior severe enough to warrant hospitalization. Most have had contact with the police, and many have already been held in detention centers or are on probation. Delinquency is defined as overt or covert violation of the law and includes such behaviors as theft, assault, vandalism, sexual promiscuity, running away, truancy, and drug abuse.

Data are available for 115 subjects during the period 1969 to 1976. The distribution of subjects by race, sex, and age is presented in Table 1.

Table 1. Subject Characteristics: Race, Sex, and Age

| | Age (in years) | | | | | | | |
Race/Sex	12	13	14	15	16	17	18	
White/male	—	5	6	18	8	2	—	(39)
White/female	1	2	9	14	7	8	1	(42)
Black/male	—	1	4	10	5	—	—	(20)
Black/female	—	—	3	9	2	—	—	(14)
Total	(1)	(8)	(22)	(51)	(22)	(10)	(1)	

PROCEDURE

At the screenings, the referrals were administered a research battery that included (among other data) demographic information and a measure of self-image (the Offer Self-Image Questionnaire for Adolescents—OSIQ). The demographic variables used as statistical controls in this study were race, sex, age (in months), and parent's occupation (as a rough measure of socioeconomic position).

The OSIQ is a paper-and-pencil, self-descriptive measure of psychosocial adjustment of adolescents. It was originally designed to select a group of normal or modal adolescents from a larger group of high school students [17]. Subsequently, it has been administered to over 20,000 adolescents at over 40 sites in six countries (cf. [17], [19], [20], [27], [21], and [18] *inter alia)*. Its reliability, as measured by intraclass correlations (alphas) and item-total correlations, is high. Its validity has been established both by its discriminatory ability among the different populations studied and by corroborative evidence from other sources, such as psychiatric interviews. It discriminates older and younger adolescents, male and female respondents, subjects from different cultures, delinquent and normal subjects, disturbed and normal adolescents, and so forth. Details of its construction, reliability, and validity may be found in [17] and [19].

The OSIQ comprises 130 items to which subjects respond on a one- to six scale indicating how well the items described themselves (from 1 = "describes me very well" to 6 = "does not describe me at all"). Items were written to cover 11 content areas considered critical to adolescent development. These 11 component scales are (1) impulse control, (2) emotional tone, (3) body and self image, (4) social attitudes, (5) morals, (6) sexual attitudes, (7) family relations, (8) external mastery, (9) vocational and educational goals, (10) psychopathology, and (11) superior adjustment. The different components allow consideration of specific areas of adolescent adjustment that contribute to self-image.

For the analysis of changes in delinquent self-image across the period 1969 to 1976, subjects were indexed by the month in which the OSIQ was administered. Thus a subject tested in June 1969 was given a value of 6 on month of testing; a subject tested in December 1969 was given a 12; a subject tested in May 1970 was given a 17; and so forth.

The central empirical question was whether the scale scores of our subjects would show a temporal pattern over the period 1969 to 1976. This is a period during which it is commonly assumed that notable social changes occurred in urban American life. If such changes were to have effects on delinquent self-image, we would expect to find correlations between the temporal dimension (month of testing) and the scale scores from the OSIQ. Particularly important is the degree of correlation found after the effects of the four demographic variables have been statistically removed. The direction of any temporal trends and their specificity for certain scales were not matters on which we entertained a priori hypotheses.

Results

Multiple regressions were performed on the scale scores to examine the degree of correlation between self-image and the temporal dimension. In a stepwise procedure the effects of the four demographic variables (race, sex, age, and parent's occupation) were first removed, and then the critical variable month-of-testing was entered. Table 2 presents the results for each of the eleven scales.

The first column of Table 2 reports the multiple R, a measure of the correlation between all five variables (four demographics and month of testing) and the scale score. These values are quite low, indicating only a slight correlation between the scale scores and the total set of variables employed in the analysis. The second column of Table 2 reports the simple r for each regression. This is a measure of the correlation between scale score and month of testing before the effects of the other four variables are controlled. Positive values

Table 2. Multiple Regression Results for OSIQ Scales

	OSIQ Scale	R	r	R^2
1.	Impulse Control	.20	+.14	.02
2.	Emotional Tone	.23	+.09	.01
3.	Body & Self Image	.20	−.04	.00
4.	Social Attitudes	.19	+.05	.00
5.	Morals	.29	+.08	.01
6.	Sexual Attitudes	.39	+.01	.00
7.	Family Relations	.19	−.03	.00
8.	External Mastery	.19	+.03	.00
9.	Vocational & Educational Goals	.23	−.02	.00
10.	Psychopathology	.22	+.06	.00
11.	Superior Adjustment	.13	+.04	.00

R refers to the multiple correlation coefficient;
r refers to the simple correlation coefficient;
R^2 refers to the change in the square of the multiple correlation coefficient attributable to the inclusion of month of testing.

would indicate progressive decrement on self-image across the time period, and negative values would indicate progressive improvement of self-image across the period. It will be seen that these simple correlations are very small, showing virtually no association between month of testing and self-image score. Since demographic variation in the scores might obscure the simple correlation, the third column is the most relevant. In the third column of Table 2, the change in the square of the multiple correlation coefficient is reported. This measures the additional (incremental) contribution of the final variable (month of testing) after the effects of the four demographic variables were removed. The statistic expresses this contribution as the additional reduction in the variance of the self-image scores that is produced by entering the month-of-testing variable. Thus a value of .15 would represent an additional reduction of the variation of test scores by 15 percent when the last piece of information (month-of-testing) was added. It will be seen in the table that the contribution of month of testing is negligible. The highest value for this statistic is 0.2, representing a 2 percent reduction in variance attributable to the entry of the temporal variable. For most scales, month of testing contributes less than 1 percent of the variance of test scores not attributable to the demographic variables.

Thus in these data, no change in self-image of delinquent inpatients was observed across the period 1969 to 1976. Given the range of different components of self-image assessed by the OSIQ, it may be somewhat surprising that a temporal trend was not observed for even those scales which one might expect to be more susceptible to historical fluctuation, such as Morals (scale 5) or Sexual Attitudes (scale 6). Despite certain limitations of sample size and the inherent individual variability of delinquent self-image scores, a robust effect of social change would be expected to manifest at least a diminutive effect in these data. We are led, therefore, to a consideration of the expectations regarding social change and delinquent self-image generated by differing theoretical positions.

Discussion

Our finding that the self-image scores of delinquent adolescents did not correlate with time during a period of presumed social change invites interpretation at two distinct levels. One account of these data would question whether the immediate social environment of our subjects actually underwent significant change during the period reflected in our data. One might assert, for example, that the historical process reflects a gradual accommodation to changing social conditions, such that a much longer time span would be necessary to see effects of social change. Alternatively, one might maintain that the social position of the delinquent subjects is similarly marginal, even during the most rapid periods of social change, and this strongly mitigates any effects of change on such a population. Additionally, the immediate family context may be considered an effective screen against the impact of social change. These matters implicate one's view of the relationship between adolescence and social conditions and one's view of the relevant influences on delinquency.

The second level at which one might account for these data concerns the reactivity of self-image to the social setting. In a discussion of generational differences, Thomas [26] distinguished three levels of beliefs, with corresponding reactivity to the historical dimension. At the level of attitudes, he found the least generational differences, and at the level of values, the most differentiation. At an intermediate level of beliefs, for example, those about authority, he found a differentiation of differences between the generations. This is similar to the view termed "selective continuity" by Bengston et al. [3]. Self-image may be resistant to changes in the social setting because of the relative importance of early childhood events in forming basic character structure. The relatively limited array of psychological defense mechanisms, the limited possibilities of affects and feelings, forces psychotherapists of all persuasions to aim for modest changes in their patients and clients. What has once been imprinted on the individual by a complex, interwoven set of variables from bio-psychosocial systems has become a stable operating unit which we call the character. Psychological structure, therefore, can simply be translated as a set of functions that are stable over time. The complexity and duration of psychoanalytic treatment of basic characterological defects is just another example that such a psychic apparatus is not easily altered by simply shifting external conditions. On the contrary, the essential orientations and defensive structures often seem to exhibit a remarkable tenacity. Self-image may reflect such intransigence imparted by the primacy of early intrafamilial events, leading to the expectation of no real reactivity to changing social conditions.

Thus expectations regarding the effect of social change on delinquent self-image are framed by one's orientation to the relationship between social conditions and adolescence, the relevant influences on self-image, and (secondarily) the dynamics of delinquency.

Competing positions on the relationship between social conditions and adolescence have received their most recent airing in the discussions of generational differences. The essential dichotomy is between advocates of a generational-historical view and advocates of a structural-functional view.

As Goertzel [10] has noted, Mannheim's generational approach is heir to the German romantic-historical tradition: "The romantic-historical thinkers argued that each historical period had its own spirit, or zeitgeist. Generations were important, in this view, because individuals in the same age groups grow up in the same historical period and form their views of the world in terms of the zeitgeist of that era." In this view, social change is the constantly occurring background against which communalities among individuals emerge as generations.

The contrasting orientation is derived, as Goertzel also notes, from French positivism and its contemporary heirs: "Perhaps the most general domain assumption of the structural-functional approach is that societies tend toward integration, and that contradictions within the social structure tend to adjust themselves." In this view a stable social structure provides the background against which communalities arise by virtue of position in that integrated differentiation. The fundamental contrast is between a view in which the changing historical process influences the interpretation of ongoing social structure and a view in which the ongoing social structure influences the interpretation of the historical process.

This contrast is an important influence on one's view of adolescents as a group of social actors. From one perspective, adolescents belong to a particular cohort. Each cohort is distinguished from others by its unique, historically framed view. This leads to the expectation that the adolescent transition is complicated by the disjunction between the adolescent cohort and those with which it must increasingly come into contact. From the other perspective, adolescents belong to a particular age status (cf., [14]). Each age status is distinguished from others by a system of attitudes and values appropriate to a particular position in the social structure. This leads to the expectation that the adolescent transition is complicated by the transformation of attitudes and values accompanying the transition to a different age status.

A study of Meddin [15] examined certain implications of the generational-cohort and the age-status views in the domain of sociopolitical attitudes. Using data from national representative surveys in 1964 and 1970, categorized into four age groupings, he found support for a generational view. At present, no similar confrontation between these two paradigms has been undertaken for self-image. Such a study can be readily imagined in principle. It would require the administration of the self-image measure to different age groupings in different historical periods (which need not be excessively long) and a second administration subsequently to determine whether similarities of self-image follow the same age grouping across time (as cohort phenomena) or adhere to similar ages across time (as suggested by the rival position). In practice, such an undertaking is hindered by the lack of longitudinal investment and by the lack of measurement instruments applicable to different age groups. Since the instrument used in the present study is designed expressly for adolescents, it could be employed to study differences within the rather wide age span currently included in discussions of adolescents. Periods of social change would be of interest in such a study to see if their effect is principally that of modifying the size of the cohort or altering the values for particular age statuses.

One's expectations regarding such a historical study of self-image are further colored by one's view of the relevant inputs on self-image. From the panorama of differing foci, four positions can be extracted to illustrate the differing attention accorded psychological and sociological emphases.

One view focuses on the intrapsychic genesis of self-image. For example, psychoanalytic approaches attend to the early childhood influences as determining the particular resolution of the search for identity. This view attends more to familial dynamics and less to prevailing social conditions. It leads to the expectation that individual variation will not readily appear as reaction to social change. The idiosyncratic resolution of self-image will be viewed as a response to fairly universal concerns, and once formed will not readily be modified by the forces of history.

A somewhat different set of expectations is obtained by attention to the reflected appraisals of others as influences on self-image. Although this position would accord importance to the family context as an early source of such reflections, the adolescent transition would involve peer inputs as well. The effects of social change would be expected to appear as mediated by the particular peer groups individuals fill. Attention would, therefore, be directed at the immediate social context within which the adolescent transition is shaped.

A third view would attend to the differences across contexts as a determinant of self-image. This position hinges on a process of social comparison between members of one group and groups of different membership within the social structure. For example, Rosenberg's concern [22] with adolescent self-image highlights the disjunction between one's own position and that of significant other groups as a determinant of negative self-image. Social change periods may alter the relative discrepancies between such groups or alter the availability of groups to serve the comparison process.

Finally, it is possible to conceive self-image as influenced directly by social ecology. Similarities among individuals would be sought in terms of demographic parallels in terms of socioeconomic variation. In some ways, such a view would expect the greatest reactivity to social change, since the immediate ecological context may be the most rapidly altered, with ideological or other variation seen as a delayed consequence.

The study of delinquent self-image is informed by similar theoretical foci on the dynamics of delinquency. Here, too, a bewildering variety of views have been expressed. For the present purposes, it is sufficient to note parallels to the above views of self-image.

For example, the intrapsychic vantage point has been used to study delinquency under psychoanalytic propositions. The work of Aichorn [1] and Alexander and Staub [2], among others, accords a principal role to the early childhood dynamics and minimizes the social dimension.

The view of self-image that accords importance to the role of reflected appraisals, and consequently to the peer group, is consonant with several orientations to delinquency. Cohen's work [7] on gangs proposed that "the crucial condition for the emergence of new cultural forms is the existence, in effective interaction with one another, of a number of actors with similar problems of adjustment." Sutherland's theory [24] of differential association highlights the acquisition of criminal skills and beliefs in the intimate social context of criminal association. In his view, delinquency results from such association when definitions of the social situation favorable to violation of the law are in excess over those against its violation. The acquisition of such definitions of situation and self are addressable in terms of reflected appraisals, and the modification of Sutherland's view by Glazer [11] into a theory of differential identification emphasized this link within a Meadian perspective.

Attention to contextual dissonance, under the third view outlined above, has informed delinquency theorists as well. One could place Haskell's reference-group theory [12] here with its note of the distinction between the rejected norms and values of the family and the adherence to norms and values of the new reference group toward which the delinquent aspires. More germane to this third orientation, however, is Cloward and Ohlin's proposal [6] on delinquent opportunity structure. They emphasized the discrepancy between aspirations of the lower class for material success and the expectations for its attainment through legitimate means. The comparison context influences both the level of aspiration and the available opportunities for adjustment to the discrepancy.

Finally, the social ecology position outlined above is well represented in the work of Shaw and McKay [23] and Thrasher [25], which emphasizes the economic and geographic correlates of delinquency. Periods of social change may well affect such important considerations under this view as mobility and neighborhood decay.

The importance of contrasting positions on issues like the foregoing for research is the limitation imposed on where one looks. Research is always limited by the uninvited source of variation that arouses post-hoc attention. Research on a period of personal change (adolescence) within a period of social change greatly increases the likelihood that something has been overlooked. In the study reported here, it seemed reasonable to expect that changes in the social milieu would have a greater effect on subjects whose adaptation to that milieu had already shown signs of deterioration. A case can be made, however, for the view that these delinquent subjects were more isolated from the impact of social change, either by virtue of their earliest endowment or by their social position as marginal within the social structure. Whether such an absence of temporal trend would be observed in normal adolescents is, of course, an inviting question for research.

The possibilities for adequate research on the influence of social change on adolescence rest on two developments. One is the design of studies that permits the separation of social change from the personal change associated with development. Nessleroade and Baltes [16] have undertaken such a study for certain aspects of adolescent personality during the period 1970 to 1972. They (and others) have proposed the study of cohorts (or age groups) longitudinally to attend to developmental differences and historical differences. Their study implicated historical or cultural factors more strongly than age factors in the aspects of adolescent personality investigated. Whether self-image is such a reactive dimension is an empirically resolvable question, which points to the importance of the second recent development. Findings for one particular aspect of development are little more than suggestions for other lines of developmental research. The specificity of such research extends not only to the content area examined, but also to the population. We are increasingly reminded that adolescence conceals important differences only intuited by the division into early, middle, and late adolescence. Extensions into differences between normal and disturbed adolescence, between the sexes, and between social classes will be necessary considerations in deciding the relative merits of the differing views related above. Attention to limitations of design and of population will help to move the study of adolescence from a period of adolescent enthusiasm to a period of more reality-based maturity.

References

1. Aichorn, A. *Wayward Youth*. Meridian Books, New York, 1955.
2. Alexander, F. and Staub, H. *The Criminal, the Judge, and the Public*. (rev. ed.). Free Press, Glencoe, Ill., 1956.
3. Bengston, V., Furlong, M., Laufer, R. Time, aging, and the continuity of social structure: themes and issues in generational analysis. *J. Soc. Issues,* 30 (2) (1974), 1–30.
4. Blos, P. *On Adolescence*. The Free Press of Glencoe, New York, 1961.
5. Blos, P. The second individuation process of adolescence. *Psychoanal. Study Child,* 22 (1967), 162–186.

6. Cloward, R. and Ohlin, L. *Delinquency and Opportunity: A Theory of Delinquent Gangs.* Free Press, Glencoe, Ill., 1960.
7. Cohen, A. *Delinquent Boys.* Free Press, Glencoe, Ill., 1955.
8. Douvan, E. and Adelson, J. *The Adolescent Experience.* Wiley, New York, 1966.
9. Erikson, E. *Identity: Youth and Crisis.* Norton, New York, 1968.
10. Goertzel, T. Generational conflict and social change. *Youth Soc.* 3 (3) (1972), 327–352.
11. Glazer, D. Criminality theories and behavioral images. *Amer. J. Sociol.* 61 (1956), 433–444.
12. Haskell, M. Toward a reference-group theory of juvenile delinquency. *Soc. Problems,* 8 (Winter 1960–1961), 220–230.
13. Keniston, K. Psychological development and historical change. In *Explorations in Psychohistory,* R. Lifton, Ed. Simon and Schuster, New York, 1974.
14. Linton, R. Age and sex categories. *Amer. Sociol. Rev.* 7 (1942), 589–603.
15. Meddin, J. Generations and aging: a longitudinal study. *Int. J. Aging Human Dev.* 6 (2) (1975), 85–101.
16. Nessleroade, J. and Baltes, P. Adolescent personality development and historical change: 1970–1972. *Monographs of the Society for Research in Child Development,* 39 (1974), 1 (Ser. No. 154).
17. Offer, D. *The Psychological World of the Teenager.* Basic Books, New York, 1969.
18. Offer, D. The Offer Self-Image Questionnaire for Adolescents: Revised Manual, (mimeograph), Chicago, 1977.
19. Offer, D. and Howard, K. An empirical analysis of the Offer Self-Image Questionnaire for Adolescents. *Arch. Gen. Psychiat.* 27 (1972), 529–537.
20. Offer, D. and Offer, J. *From Teenage to Young Manhood: A Psychological Study.* Basic Books, New York, 1975.
21. Offer, D., Ostrov, E., and Howard, K. The self-image of adolescents: A study of four cultures. *J. Youth Adolescence,* 6 (3), (1977), 265–279.
22. Rosenberg, M. *Society and Adolescent Self-image.* Princeton University Press, Princeton, 1965.
23. Shaw, C. and McKay, H. *Juvenile Delinquency in Urban Areas.* University of Chicago Press, Chicago, 1942.
24. Sutherland, E. *Principles of Criminology* (fifth edition, prepared by D. Cressey). Lippincott, Chicago, 1955.
25. Thrasher, F. *The Gang.* University of Chicago Press, Chicago, 1927.
26. Thomas, L. Generational discontinuity in beliefs: an exploration of the generation gap. *J. Soc. Issues,* 30 (3) (1974), 1–22.
27. Offer, D., Marohn, R. C., Ostrov, E. Violence among hospitalized delinquents. *Arch. Gen. Psychiatry* 32 (9) :1180–6, Sep. 75.

America's Babylift of Vietnam Children: What Is To Be Learned for a Psychology of Change

Edward Zigler, Ph.D. (U.S.A.)

How do you work to change a nation's social policy toward children? As a person working at the interface between the fields of child development and social policy, I have long been concerned with this question. I would like to offer some critical factors in constructing enlightened social policy for children and their families, factors that come not from a textbook but from experience.

First of all, I cannot overemphasize how important it is for a nation's leaders to be concerned with children and families. The leadership's involvement immediately gives the enterprise of child development and family life a very high priority in a nation's policies. This particular conference began with the presentation by Mrs. Yitzhak Rabin, wife of the Prime Minister. Not only was her talk of substantive value, but her association with an effort of this type clearly states that children and families are indeed important, and they are important to important people.

Attitudes at the high level of leadership vary among nations. My colleague Urie Bronfenbrenner relates a story told to him by the Prime Minister of Sweden, Olaf Palme. Palme answered the door of his home to find a woman, quite upset, accompanied by two children she was babysitting. "Their mother was supposed to be back at 6:00," she said. "It is now 8:30, and there's no mother. What should I do?" The Prime Minister responded by sending his own 18-year-old son to take the children back home, feed them, and sit with them until the mother finally arrived. It is meaningful that, in a busy, industrialized nation, a Prime Minister took the time to act in this manner. Bronfenbrenner, in writing up this anecdote, asks the rhetorical question, "I wonder what would happen if a babysitter showed up at Henry Kissinger's door and knocked?"

It is necessary to mobilize the very top leadership of a nation if social policy makers are to be effective. In the early days of America's Head Start program, for example, it was highly significant that the wife of the President of the United States, Lady Bird Johnson, assumed the role of Honorary Chairman. At her invitation, women came from all over the country to gather in the East Room of the White House to launch the Head Start program. Later, they held a meeting in the Rose Garden. That kind of national leadership involvement was critical to Head Start's success, and to that of any social policy program.

In addition to securing the involvement of national leaders, we must be sensitive to the importance of symbolic events. We must be ready to utilize such events. Textbooks do not devote much space to the importance of symbolic events, but in our lives we recognize their significance. Unfortunately, we too often miss opportunities to capitalize on such events as catalysts for social change.

Change has meaning only when one thinks of continuity. There are long periods of status quo, and then suddenly things begin to happen. What accounts for the change? Although the climate must be conducive, change often springs from a single symbolic event, such as the freeing of the hostages in Entebbe.

We all know that 100 lives are important. Indeed, one life is very important. Even when one thinks of the thousands of children dying in Biafra, one can still say that 100 lives are important. But in a world of 4 billion people, it is not so much the 100 lives that are important; it is their symbolism, and what their rescue means to a nation. Perhaps in the long run, more important than the 100 lives may be the thousands, if not the millions, of lives that can be influenced by the national sense of optimism and accomplishment that comes from a symbolic event. A nation said, "If this is possible, all things are possible. If we have this courage and this intelligence, then every problem can be solved." To decision makers concerned with social policy, the sense that problems are solvable is crucial.

The importance of America's Head Start program may be more symbolic than substantive. Despite all of the literature about Head Start, it serves only some 200,000 children out of the 3 million who qualify for the program, to say nothing of the many millions of children in the country who do not qualify. But the Head Start program is significant because it focuses attention on children and their needs. Furthermore, Head Start has served as a national laboratory for implementing innovations and evaluating them.

We turn now to discuss Operation Babylift, the airlift of 2000 Vietnamese children that occurred in 1975. I do not have to stretch things to tell you why the babylife effort is pertinent to change, both personal and social. When the babylife occurred, I had high hopes that the effort could serve as a symbolic event around which to mobilize our nation's concern and commitment to all children.

Looking at the babylift from a child's viewpoint, I can imagine no greater change that could occur than to be picked up in one culture in Saigon; placed on a C-5 airplane and brought to San Francisco; shipped across the country to Mobile, Alabama or Boston; and set down in a brand new home in a new culture in a matter of 2 or 3 days. In corresponding with Anna Freud about the babylife, she compared it to the World War II evacuation of children from London. In her letter, she described these children from London:

This was done purely from the safety point of view and with full disregard for the children's bewilderment, separation anxiety, severe regressions in behavior, toilet training, etc. Not surprisingly, many of them were evacuation failures. In the war nurseries there was plenty of opportunity for us to see what it does to children to be torn away from the life where they belong.

Yet, as Anna Freud went on to point out, although the London children experienced severe shock, the Vietnamese children underwent a far more drastic change; at least in England the children moved within the same culture and the same language.

The babylife also tested the ability of America as a nation to change. Were we flexible enough to meet the needs of these children?

I present what is essentially a short case history in social activism, the story of my efforts from my position in a university to change a nation's behavior and shape a nation's policy toward a group of children who need help badly. The case is still open. I wish there was something terribly optimistic to report. There is not. I can just give you the history.

As an academic, my first reaction to the babylift was to write an analytic paper. The paper's conclusion is evident in its title, "The Vietnamese Children's Airlift: Too Little and Too Late." The purpose of this paper was to prepare a solid analysis of the situation so that when I talked to people around Washington in their bureaucratic dens, I would have established my credentials as an advisor on what to do for these 2000 children. The paper essentially concluded, "By any careful analysis we should never have brought the children to America." That point is moot. I then went on to say, "The children are here; now what must we do for them to fulfill our moral obligations to them?"

At the time of the babylift an important symbolic event occurred, one that I tried to use. The President of the United States went to San Francisco to meet one of the many planeloads of children that came in. He went aboard the plane, took one of the Vietnamese babies in his arms, walked down the steps of the plane, and the pictures were taken. It was a moving sight. The President of the United States said, "I guarantee that these children will receive every bit of care that they need to optimize their development."

In my analysis I tried to stress that these children were vulnerable, high-risk children. Many children were likely to be sick on arrival, as indeed many were. It was probable that they would have continuing health problems, and that they would be extremely vulnerable psychologically as well. I presented some background on these babylift children:

In one report, Judith Coburn described an orphanage supervised by South Vietnamese nuns. The 273 children in the orphanage slept in four rooms so crowded that the children near the walls could not get out without crawling over the other children. In such overcrowded facilities, many babies lay in their urine and feces for hours while the overworked caretakers rushed from crib to crib attempting to change them. In such quarters, a single child's illness could quickly generate an epidemic. The senior nun reported to Coburn that the biggest problem in the orphanage was the expiration of young babies in their cribs. This nun felt that many of these dying infants had no visible disease and may have died "from simple lack of love or stimulation."

When one considers the background of the Vietnamese children brought to America, one thinks immediately of Spitz's work on stimulus-deprived infants. In fact, when the children arrived, I had a déjà-vu experience. People described how the children hungered for attention, very much like the socially deprived children that I had been studying in institutions for the past 20 years.

My hypothesis was that these Vietnamese children and their adoptive parents would have many difficulties, a sad hypothesis which, unfortunately, was quickly confirmed. Very early on, people began calling me about the babylift children, one case at a time. An HEW official telephoned to say, "One of these children has become psychotic and nobody can understand the child. He speaks Vietnamese; he's psychotic. What should we do?" And I said, "Do you plan to call me each time one of these children has a problem? You mean to handle each one of them on an ad hoc basis?" Of course, I was attacking the wrong person, who had no other recourse at that time.

Reports started coming in of children with extremely serious physical problems. Not too far from New Haven, one babylift child was reported to be crippled for life. The reports kept coming in. Unfortunately, the headlines were made later: one baby is now dead, the victim of alleged child abuse in the baby's adoptive home. The evidence was quickly documented that these children did indeed need special care.

I decided to work for a two-pronged effort on behalf of these children. First, I was concerned about the children remaining in Vietnam. The airlift of 2000 children was clearly a mere tokenistic effort. The population of Vietnam is now somewhere between 17 and 18 million, and after years of war half of that population consists of children under the age of 15. It is those millions of children that the world (although I can speak only for my own nation) should attend to. In my paper I stated:

Thus the airlift episode was little more than a tokenistic effort. A danger of tokenistic efforts lies in giving the appearance that a great deal is being done which in turn interferes with moving on to more honest and realistic broad scale efforts. We cannot construct a sound social policy to meet the needs of the children of Vietnam if we believe that we have fulfilled our responsibilities to those children by transporting 2000 of them here (meaning the United States).

Thus my Plan A was sort of a Marshall Plan for the children of Vietnam. I even went so far as to suggest Patrick Moynihan to serve as the commissioner of such an effort.

The second prong of my effort, Plan B, was to try to provide some help for the 2000 babylift children we had already brought to America.

To return to my point, mechanisms should be set in place and funded that would permit dealing with the physical health and mental health needs of the babylift children. In regard to physical health, some of these children are handicapped and others will have long term medical problems. I recommend that the federal government supply funds to the American Academy of Pediatrics and charge them with providing medical services to the babylift children where needed. Because of the early deprivation experienced by many of the babylift children and because many adoptive parents could not have anticipated the magnitude of the problems now confronting many of them, mental health services must also be made available to those adoptive families and children requiring assistance of this nature. Funding should be provided by the American Academy of Child Psychiatry for the development and administration of such mental health services. Given the sketchy plan outlined above, I want to make clear that the effort I have in mind should not be limited to the actions of the federal government alone. These 2000 children now live in many communities and localities. What must be done is to program local physical and mental health resources so they can be optimally used by the babylift children and their families. The development of such advocacy and services brokerage functions at all levels of government is consonant with the recommendations of the report of the Joint Commission on the Mental Health of Children, a document that has yet to receive the attention it deserves. The problem is that our nation has yet to develop sound methods of child advocacy and optimal models for providing services to children and their families. Let us not blind ourselves to the fact that the physical and mental health services that I am proposing for the Vietnamese children are also needed by many American children. Perhaps by developing models of advocacy and services delivery for the Vietnamese children, we will learn how such efforts should and could be done. Such models would be readily transferrable and instruct us on how we might better deliver a variety of services to all of America's children. I am suggesting here that by committing ourselves to helping others, we may eventually be helping ourselves.

After presenting these plans to a number of people in Washington, from the White House through HEW to the Hill, I completely abandoned the plan for helping the children in Vietnam. People thought the plan was too radical, too expensive. They advised me that I would only hinder the effort to get funds for the 2000 babylift children if I insisted on tying it to much more expensive programs for children in Vietnam. Being a pragmatist, I concluded that it was better to try for something than wind up with nothing.

I started out mildly optimistic that Plan B for the babylift children would be accepted. First, I thought that it represented the correct and humane thing for a nation to do. Second, the President of the United States was clearly on record as wanting to help these children—an important and politically useful fact. Third, the cost was relatively modest, somewhere between 4 and 8 million dollars.

Nevertheless, Plan B also met with rebuff. Congressmen explained that their constituencies opposed spending money on the Vietnamese. Then, when the 140,000 Vietnamese refugees were brought to America, their problems, of course, overshadowed any concern for the 2000 babylift children.

In an attempt to convince Washington to use some of these funds for the babylift children, I resorted to another Ziglerian principle of social policy activism: I formed a committee. Committees serve to legitimize the efforts of an individual who otherwise may appear to be merely obsessed. That committee included Dr. Al Solnit, Director of the Child Study Center, Norman Lourie of Pennsylvania's State Welfare Department, and Dr. Julius Richmond, Director, Judge Baker Guidance Center, Boston. This committee then wrote its own set of recommendations for the babylift children, and for the refugee children as well.

At this point I have written many letters; I have visited many offices. The plan I outlined is not yet in place. I am still working on it. Recently I have turned my attention away from the Administration people, who started out welcoming me but now find me an embarrassment, and focused on the Congress. Members of the committee concerned with the refugees are giving me a somewhat more positive reception, particularly Senator Edward Kennedy on the Senate side and Representative Joshua Eilberg of the House.

How this will all be resolved, I do not know. There have been many disappointments over the past year. All that can be said is that the effort on behalf of these children will indeed continue.

In retrospect, one might ask, why should a scholar even attempt to work for social change? Social policy will be made with or without us. But I am convinced that if people with even a modest amount of information do not step forward to influence social policy, individuals less knowledgeable will indeed proceed to do so.

Discussion

Phyllis Palgi, Ph.D. (Israel)

Professor Zigler is one of the small group of academicians who is not afraid of confrontation with large-scale tragic human problems which have arisen out of the complex world political situation characteristic of our technologically sophisticated society.

We have from him a many-faceted analysis of America's ambivalent, vacillating role in the past with regard to Vietnam refugee children. He has spelled out carefully the necessity for a feasible comprehensive plan for the future that would be based on "beyond the better interests of the child." To support his argument, he traced the development of and analyzed the motivations behind the highly controversial project, namely the "baby airlift" linked to an adoption program. He saw it, in the main, as a well-meaning, emotional, but simplistic act that was not thought through with regard to its possible consequences. In his words, it represented the best and worst in the ethos of the American nation.

As an Israeli anthropologist whose work for more than 20 years has centered on the motif of uprooting and resettlement, I should like to discuss whether there is anything useful we can learn from different cultural contexts about similar bitter experiences where children and parents have been torn apart under catastrophic circumstances.

There are four points of entry that I believe may lead us to find relevance in the Israeli setting for the problems posed by Professor Zigler:

1. A large proportion of the adult population living in Israel experienced, prior and during World War II, deep deprivation in their childhood. Recent and ongoing research has highlighted the complexity of the effects of such experiences. The unusual positive social adaptation and, on the whole, high-level

functioning of these one-time refugees has been documented. However, it is now emerging that many carry with them permanent psychological scars that are transmitted even to the next generation.

2. Israel has an unconditional commitment toward Jewish victims of persecution, and the saving of children's lives has been a central theme in its ethos.

3. Individual and collective expression of guilt that not enough was done to save lives is expressed from time to time.

4. Some of the many plans for refugee and immigrant rehabilitation in Israel have been well thought-out, whereas others have been based on improvisation due to panic, fear, or ideological commitment.

Israel has for historical and cultural reasons a much deeper, in fact, transcendental involvement with refugees than that of America with Vietnam. But at the same time, one must not underestimate the effect of the Vietnam experience that has probably become internalized in the psychohistory of at least two generations in America. A major theme in the counterculture was, for instance, that American participation in Vietnam was a ghastly mistake. I absolutely support Professor Zigler's implied contention that if there exist feelings of guilt within the society, denial or token projects will only increase tension. Effective action will not only benefit the recipients but will help reduce the "sickness" in the so-called strong and intact society. This has clearly been the experience in Israel. I believe so many people bearing psychic wounds can live together and function because of the basic policy of social commitment towards them.

Professor Zigler recommends that the children of Vietnam should be helped to reconstruct their lives, preferably in Vietnam. In their own country, they have a chance to develop a sense of continuity and belonging. The youth immigration organizations for Jewish refugee children built their entire philosophy on that very principle. In the Jewish reality, orphaned or refugee children had to be transported to Israel so as to ensure them a sense of identity with the past and hope for the future. It was this principle that helped to save the sanity of the numerous bands of children who had wandered through Europe keeping themselves alive without adult care from the age of 6 and 7 years. They had lived by their wits, were deculturated from the point of view of the larger society and yet almost all were subsequently able to accept Israel as their homeland. In Israel, it was possible to make viable for them the symbolic significance of many traditions which had been that of their parents.

Professor Zigler reminded us that in Vietnam the refugee problem involves dispossessed persons of all ages. Separating out only the children for care is, in fact, a counterproductive measure. It took us many years in Israel to realize the fundamental significance of this finding. Fortunately, it is no longer widely believed that a large segment of the parent immigrant generation is a "lost generation" and that it is only worthwhile investing in the children. However, in the meanwhile, Israel paid a price for that misconception. Many of these adults had their confidence, as parents, undermined, leading to negative repercussions on the behavior of the next generation.

I believe social scientists like Professor Zigler should get full support in their efforts to influence social policy makers in their attempts to alleviate large-scale human sufferings. He has shown that there exists a body of knowledge and experience at their disposal that may at least prevent the same mistakes others have made in the past.

A Heritage of Transience: Psychological Effects of Growing Up Overseas

Sidney Werkman, M.D. (U.S.A.)

American children who live overseas for extended periods of time encounter unusual developmental challenges. They face repeated experiences of separation and loss, the hazards of transitions, and confrontations with novel patterns of behavior. Such challenges, generic to the lives of geographically mobile children, can also contribute to the understanding of the ordinary nodal points of child development. Although the effects of geographic mobility on psychological processes are of increasing prevalence and importance in the contemporary world, little has been written about them [1, 2, 3, 4, 5, 6, 7].

The 230,000 American children who attend overseas schools each year comprise an ongoing experiment in an alternate style of growth and differentiation that may be of considerable importance for our understanding of events and stresses that mold typical character development. These American children share many characteristics with a much larger group of people from other native lands. In this historical period of extensive geographic mobility and increasing international travel, the total group constitutes a new category of people of a "third culture" [8]—an international population that has loosened its ties to a home country but does not become totally integrated into the host country. These internationalists, more knowledgeable about each other than either the countries in which they live or their lands or origin, share attitudes, interests, concern, and intrapsychic processes that may well be distinctive and enduring. Some unique aspects of growing up within this population are examined in this chapter.

117

Dimensions of the Population

The children to be considered are the offspring of parents engaged in a wide variety of military, government, and civilian occupations. In 1970 the 1,375,000 military personnel and their families were the largest category of Americans overseas, while 236,000 families worked in private sector activity, and 110,000 overseas families were civilian government employees. The civilian adults were involved in a large range of activities, including religious work, engineering, teaching, scientific disciplines, and technical activities [9]. It should be noted that the overseas population, particularly the parents of those approximately 80,000 children who attend civilian sponsored schools, make up a highly selected group of professionals and college-educated administrators, largely with intact families and high levels of ambition, who probably represent a more than usually stable, educationally and psychologically supportive group of people.

A new element of considerable importance has been added to the "American presence" abroad. Over the last decade a gradual change has been taking place in the type of work done by Americans overseas, with a great increase in the number of people involved in geology, energy exploration, construction, and middle-level management. These careers seem to be replacing some of the more traditional representational and executive ones. Further, the expectation of past generations that a substantial part of a career would be devoted to overseas work may now be superceded by commitments to shorter-term jobs. Children of parents who comprise this new American force abroad undoubtedly will have different developmental needs and, therefore, mold the educational and social systems in which they participate in novel ways.

Since we do not possess adequate incidence and prevalence data on psychiatric disorders among children in the United States, it would be presumptuous to attempt to make conclusive comparisons of the mental health of children reared in the United States with those raised overseas. Because of the great heterogeneity of geographical, cultural, and socioeconomic settings overseas, any generalizing speculations must be tentative ones. Nevertheless, the issues we are considering are important ones that deserve serious though modest attempts at systemization.

Families who choose to live overseas are highly self-selected for many factors that correlate with resistance to overt mental disturbance. Some of these factors would include a high percentage of intact families, relatively low divorce rates, concern for education, high socioeconomic status, and the supports made available by relatively small, highly visible American communities in which most overseas families live. For example, juvenile delinquency, a problem of alarming significance in the United States, is almost nonexistent in overseas communities, unless one includes the relatively mild problems that stem from drug use. The problems that exist tend to be subtle, though at times devastating ones, not easily defined in conventional terms such as schizophrenia or overt depression.

Subjects

The data and observations on which this chapter is based have been derived from the following sources: clinical psychiatric practice with patients whose problems began in relationship to living overseas; adults and adolescents interviewed by the author during consultation trips to international schools overseas; tape-recorded research interviews with university students who have lived overseas; and a research sample of 172 adolescents living overseas compared to a control group in the United States. Though precise data are not available on average length of stay overseas or number of moves, it is a shared clinical impression that by far the largest number of American children live overseas more than 2 years and move several times before they return to the United States for high school or college.

Among the variables involved in overseas experience are age at time of each move, number of moves, sex, country in which a child lives, school situation, father's career, and parents' ways of coping with the stresses of life overseas. All these issues must play important parts in the idiosyncratic life of a child overseas.

Though no final generalizations can be made about such a varied group of children, all share certain distinctive stresses that impinge on their lives.

1. Separations, the individuation of each child, family relationships, educational demands, and personal interactions must be worked out in relatively isolated circumstances, away from usual supports and role models present in the United States. Overseas life forces families to rely on their own resources. Many families develop an unusual degree of closeness and interdependence. Intimately shared encounters with adventure, dazzling sights, isolation, difficul-

ties, and overt danger act as a cohesive force to bind parents and children together. However, the absence of relatives, life-long friends, and trusted mentors forces parents to rely exclusively on their own judgment when making decisions about child-rearing issues. Comparisons cannot easily be made between one's own children and those of a sister or brother. No grandmothers are available to take children to the circus or attend piano recitals. There is no relative to turn to if a child needs to get away from his parents for a weekend with a favorite relative. Thus typical developmental challenges may result in unique solutions. In Thailand, for example, children are carried in the arms of nursemaids until they are approximately 4 years of age. They experience an overprotection in comparison to toddlers raised in the United States. Accepted patterns of sleep, feeding, and aggression differ from country to country. Under such varying conditions developmental milestones will deviate from those typically described in the United States.

2. Fathers are highly selected members of their business or government organizations and many must travel frequently. The visible, representational position of many fathers, together with their unavailability to their children, often places a child in the position of idealizing the absent father yet at the same time feeling rejected by that parent. A greater child-rearing burden is placed on mothers who, themselves, are undergoing a cultural transition. Husbands and wives must work at new relationships between themselves, especially when a wife is left without the support of relatives or close friends in an alien culture in which she has little work to do and little opportunity to pursue a career of her own. The effects of such circumstances on children are often of great significance.

3. Servants, rarely available to families in the United States but quite frequently utilized by Americans overseas, offer a mother welcome relief from household duties, but they all too often introduce concerns about competition in return. The mother in such a household may well find her sense of authority and significance undermined. The child in such a household may gain a built-in playmate, but also the values, habits, and fears of that playmate. Parents who dilute their responsibility for a child by employing a nursemaid introduce complications to a child's development and identifications. Further, when a family must leave a country, the separation problems for both servant and child may be intense.

4. The American child *born* overseas is a special child among spe-

cial children, for he has never known life in the United States. The
country of his birth will forever color his view of what he is. His
reference points and special allegiances will necessarily refer to the
country in which he was born, despite his American nationality. "I
grew up in Peru until I was ten when we moved to Charlotte, North
Carolina," a teenager recalled. "I tried for 2 years to fit into school
and to this country. I still have the ways of a Peruvian and think like
a Peruvian, and even my parents can't understand a part of me because they didn't grow up the way I did."

A young American woman raised overseas described her plight in
this way in an open letter to her parents:

"A particular aspect of my 'heritage' is that unlike most, it's not a shared one. I
don't have anyone to 'swap notes with,' if you know what I mean. Even you and
Daddy experience things in a radically different way—you were adults and already formed, while I was a child malleable, susceptible and unmolded. The
uniqueness, while precious, is also very lonely at times. Being a child, I had a
child's ability to adjust. I learned to assume that things were only temporary,
that upheavals were always around the corner. This enabled me to survive, of
course, but in the process I learned not to trust in "security," not to invest too
much of myself in any one place for fear of losing it—in short, I learned to culti-
vate a sort of inner distance from the world around me. These are things I must
unlearn today for they are handicaps to me as an adult trying to send down roots.
But the habit and conviction of uninvolvement are very hard to break" [10].

5. A childhood lived overseas bypasses much of the homogenized
supermarket, shopping-center, consumer-goods-oriented culture in-
flicted on youngsters in the United States and often substitutes opportunities for creative cultural involvements and character broad-
ening travel. Children overseas typically develop an enviable sense
of tolerance for differences in people and their customs, a respect for
the variety and significance of world cultures. As one teenager put it:
"I don't think that unusualness, ambiguity, even unpleasantness
bother me as much as they do kids in the U.S. And, even though I've
lived well, I think I've learned to tolerate more physical discomfort
than kids in the U.S."

Instead of facing the realities of competition, independence, and
individualism described by Slater [11] in *The Pursuit of Loneliness*
as characteristic of life in the United States, the child abroad is absorbed into a society that is far more group oriented and communally
cohesive. He feels a part of things, responsible to his community as
well as his family, and visible at all times. These are subtle but pow-

erful differences that come into sharp focus on return to the United States.

6. Intimate friendships develop quickly and with great intensity, in part to fill the vacuum left by the loss of the extended network of social, recreational, and athletic activities available to youngsters in the United States. These friendships, almost like shipboard romances, have built-in self-destruct qualities to them. "Never once did I have to break up with a girlfriend," a young veteran of such brief encounters reminisced:

"My love affairs were always beautifully, romantically severed in first flush. Either I was transferred or she was. You could stand at the airport or shipside and wave the relationship away—just like that. When I was in high school I found a girl-friend in February, knowing she was going to leave in June. I took her for what she was on the surface, and she did the same with me, knowing that we didn't have time to change each other or get to know each other very well. There was no sense of history in what we were doing. Even now I still tend to assume in some place deep inside of me that there is no need to confront problems or adjust to them, because I feel they will just sail away when my tour is up."

Another observer described his experience as follows: "There was a separate reality in my mind, a part of me held back. You didn't learn to be tentative or cautious. Instead, you developed an ability to throw yourself totally into a situation, expecting that you were also going to pull yourself out totally at a later date. It was sort of like the total commitment of early childhood, continued forever."

A move overseas with its intoxicating immersion in a foreign language, an exotic culture, and unusual activity, often frees a person to try experiences he would not seek out in his usual home. Impressionable young people may find themselves recurrently drawn to the vividness of new experiences and intense friendships, out of the very intensity of their loneliness and isolation. As one philosophic returnee recalled, "I am forever pursuing experiences as intense, exotic and elemental as the ones I encountered in my youth abroad. I have developed a kind of fearlessness, a kind of survivor's euphoria and optimism."

A Love Affair with a Foreign Way of Life

Some children develop what can best be called a fixation on a stage in their growth and experience, often of a romantic nature, that may result in prolonged grieving or depression when they return to the

United States. A teenager expressed such feelings in a letter to a friend still overseas:

"Vienna, Virginia is about as middle-class as it can be. Our school is gigantic, made up of commuters and freaks, with no sense of spirit and a lot of people just trying to get it over with. It's tough to rise about the general sense of apathy. I sit here with your year book and am so envious of all of you there in Tunisia and think of how lucky you are to be isolated from the mass education we have here in the homeland."

A wise host country teacher summarized the passionate nature of such encounters in this way:

"American teenagers who come to our school develop strong attachments and sometimes intense crushes with Italian youngsters. They become inseparable, for each sees in the other, at a time when both are bursting with vitality, an opportunity to fulfill all of life's wishes. The breaking off of these friendships when the American goes home can be devastating for the visitor and the Italian child alike. Both suffer the effects of separation, as I know from conversation and letters, for such a long time."

Children who develop this syndrome have idealized every aspect of life overseas and repressed the ordinary, boring, or anxiety-provoking components. They dismiss everything in the United States as uninteresting, worthless, or harmful. They are unwilling to integrate themselves into a new school, the pleasure of American sports, or the challenges of making friends when they return to the United States. Instead, there is a desperate clinging to memories that are exquisitely pleasing precisely because they do not need to be tested against the reality of what actually happened. The dynamics of children with such problems bear considerable resemblance to those of cases conceptualized by Fleming [12] as "parent loss" situations, in which a deeply experienced loss results in a kind of freezing of psychological maturation, openness to new experiences, and sense of time.

Return Home to the United States

The most difficult adjustment for many people occurs not in living overseas but when they return to the United States. As one youngster put it, "I had lots of friends and played on the school soccer team overseas. When I got back nobody noticed me and nobody was going to go out of his way to be nice to me in that big school. My marks slipped and I was miserable for 2 years."

On giving up a foreign way of life, returnees must learn to live without cherished friends and accustomed activities at the same time as they struggle to be accepted in American culture. Unfinished tasks, unfulfilled dreams must be dropped or forgotten. The need to abandon intense friendships and cultural supports frequently results in disturbing feelings characteristic of a grieving process.

Though most seem to make a good surface adjustment to this country, that adjustment may, at times, cover over a host of barely contained feelings of uncertainty, alienation, anger, and disappointment. Many returnees describe feelings of discomfort and vague dissatisfaction with their lives, feelings that cannot be attributed to any overt problems. They are able to adjust to the United States, but they are not comfortable with that adjustment. Despite their ability to function effectively in the society and the richness of experience gained from their lives overseas, they typically report feelings of restlessness, loneliness, and rootlessness, even when their external lives are going well. The defining events and attitudes that shape such feelings contribute to the formation of a unique sense of self possibly characteristic of Americans who have lived overseas.

The Sense of Self in Americans Raised Overseas

Identity develops from a combination of the identifications of early childhood and the ability of the adolescent to mold his own distinct, effective, valued qualities into a kind of self-consistency, separate from others, and yet functioning with others in his society. As Erikson [13] pointed out:

The younger person, in order to experience wholeness, must feel a progressive continuity between that which he has come to be during the long years of childhood and that which he promises to become in the anticipated future; between that which he conceives himself to be and that which he perceives others to see in him and to expect of him.

A child growing up in the United States incorporates a considerable part of his identity from the youth culture that surrounds him. This process occurs largely without conscious effort. Only in stressful circumstances does he need to ponder the question of "who am I?" On the other hand, the child from overseas must integrate a heritage of externally prescribed behaviors that may hinder his own personal exploration and differentiation with a uniqueness of experience that makes it necessary for him to seek out his own selfhood in bewildered isolation. For example, he may be told repeatedly that "we are little ambassadors," cautioned against chewing gum in public, and warned never to utter any negative statements about the host country. (A teenager confided to me that "my dying fear will be that a fight I had with a Pakastani boy would affect American relations with the subcontinent.")

A polyglot background may add to the complications involved in developing a coherent sense of self. "My first language was Dutch, my second Greek, and I believe my youngest brother spoke Armenian when he was small," a young returnee confided to me, and added: "I developed certain ways of thinking in Dutch and Greek that remain today more vivid and accessible to me than English." Another said: "I'm two people. The one who uses English is quiet and precise; the Portuguese one gestures and is poetic and free."

The forging of an American identity is made difficult by the lack of authentic role models in adolescence. One youngster remembers his groping concerns in this way:

"We were this whole group of Americans desperate to be Americans, but we were in India. So we would sit around and talk about hamburgers. Really! We would talk about hamburgers and about half of us wouldn't remember what a hamburger tasted like, but we pretended we did. 'Oh Yea! Wow! I really miss a great hamburger.' And I remember we read movie magazines and at one point even decided that our school should have cheerleaders. Our school didn't even have any teams, but we decided we had to have cheerleaders. So there we were having try-outs and learning cheers. In India! Someone who had been a cheerleader in America had just come and she taught us all the cheers. We made these little skirts out of Indian material. It was weird" [14].

In order for a firm sense of identity to develop the adolescent depends on the support of a stable society to confirm the value of his growing sense of inner coherence. The youngster growing up overseas often must move during adolescence—the very time when stability of behavioral expectation and easy availability of role models and ego ideal figures are most needed. As a result, he must make many individual, often lonely decisions that define his being. He cannot fall back on parental experience for guidance, because his parents have grown up in a different societal situation, typically that of the

United States. Because a premium is placed on conforming behavior overseas, the adolescent is both under pressure to adhere to generally rigid American community standards, and at the same time bombarded with the standards and values of the host country. (In some Southeast Asian countries, for example, there may be rigid rules about dating within one's peer group, while at the same time sexual experience with prostitutes is quite acceptable within the community.)

A teenager described another aspect of this complexity this way:

"You end up with a double concept of yourself. There is this sense that you have an extra talent, your knowledge of another language and another culture, that has no value except in planning your later life. I think where people get into trouble is that they tend to come back and know they have this asset, but think that everybody else should know about it and feel 'you should respect me because I've got this extra experience,' but it doesn't apply. What you gain from experience abroad is going to be maintained, but it's better to tuck it away. What you have learned not only doesn't get you anywhere but it tends to threaten or irritate people."

A young adult offered these shrewd observations on the same theme: "When I came back to college I kept observing and adapting my behavior to suit my country, all along feeling something like those transsexuals we hear about who adjust the best way they can to the fact that they seem to have been born into the wrong body. What they have is called gender dysphoria syndrome. What I have might be called culture dysphoria syndrome."

A part of the culture dysphoria syndrome was described as a legacy of "fitting myself into many strange situations and places where I was an outsider but trying somehow to be part of it. It gives you a minority group empathy, being always yourself a foreigner. You are much more sensitive to outsider's needs than most people."

The sense of self developed from such experience can be one of great strength and resilience, but as described by a particularly gifted American who grew up overseas, it must be worked at and won with pain and effort. He wrote: "Once you realize you can never penetrate the hermetically sealed, parochial xenophobia of the natives here in the United States, you breathe a sigh of despair mixed with relief and set out toward a native country you know you must create for yourself, inside."

The paradigm of separation-individuation defined by Mahler [15] is a useful metaphor to place these observations in context. It is as if the overseas-reared youngster retains a symbiotic attachment to his international experiences or returns symbolically to that attachment under the stress of the demands for individuation made by his return to the United States. If the attachment to the overseas life was too intense or too gratifying, the returnee may find it exceedingly difficult to venture into the anxiety-fraught area of new experiences, particularly if the adults involved are, themselves, unable to give up the fantasied gratifications of their overseas past. Conversely, too headlong a rush into new experiences, without having mourned the loss of previous attachments, may leave the returnee with a heritage of concerns with desertion, rejection, and devaluation. A significant portion of life experience may remain isolated and become a hindrance to the development of autonomy and a firm American identity.

Some of the results from a research study conducted with Americans overseas compared to teenagers in the United States [16] corroborate these reports. The data suggest that overseas youngsters are unusually capable of acknowledging potentially disturbing affects. They appear to be less secure and optimistic than adolescents who live exclusively in the United States but, in many ways more psychologically sensitive. The self-concepts of overseas teenagers appear to be less positive, and they seem to show less of a feeling of security and optimism about life in general. These results do not suggest that teenagers who have been raised overseas are less psychologically healthy than those in the United States, but rather that overseas experience does mold their values and attitudes.

Faced with such a bewildering group of what a patient of mine once called "cultural orders," it may be difficult to define a sense of self that is more than a series of changing masks. A youngster who returned from an overseas life to boarding school in the United States, indeed, called the process one of "adopting of expressive masks, hoping to find the core from the various disguises we choose in incestuous emulation of one another."

Yet the overseas child needs to forge an unusually strong and anchoring sense of self in order to sustain some coherence and permanence in the face of perpetual change. This can be accomplished through the development of a character structure that includes wide tolerance for ambiguity and a comfort with the realization that many life shaping events cannot be shared with others.

The splitting highlighted by several of the vignettes in this chapter may be the result of an adaptive need to suppress significant portions of one's developmental experiences. An important part of the self remains foreign, hidden, split-off, except when brought into consciousness through the mediation of someone who has shared similar experience. The American who has grown up overseas typically finds it necessary to create in himself a complex identity, one that includes a freedom to withhold significant ego components without developing feelings of guilt or anxiety, while retaining those components in readiness for expression when the opportunity for a shared relationship becomes available.

References

1. Kantor, M. B. *Mobility and Mental Health.* Charles C. Thomas, Springfield, Ill., 1965.
2. David, H. O. and Elkind, D. Family adaptation overseas, some mental health considerations. *J. Mental Hyg.* 50 (1966), 92.
3. Pedersen, F. A. and Sullivan, E. J. Relationships among geographical mobility, parental attitudes and emotional disturbances in children. *Amer. J. Orthopsychiat.* 34 (1964), 575–580.
4. Werkman, S. L. Hazards of rearing children in foreign countries. *Amer. J. Psychiat.* 128 (1972), 992–997, Werkman, S. L. Over here and back there: American Adolescents overseas. *Foreign Serv. J.* 52 (1975), 13–16.
5. Werkman, S. L. *Bringing up Children Overseas: A Guide for Families.* Basic Books, New York, 1977.
6. Bower, E. M. American children and families in overseas communities. *Amer. J. Orthopsychiat.* 37 (1967), 787–796.
7. Burvill, P. W. Immigration and mental disease. *Aust. N.Z. J. Psychiat.,* 1973, 7:155–162.
8. Useem, J., Useem, R., and Donoghue, J. Men in the middle of the third culture: The roles of American and non-western people in cross cultural administration. *Human Organization,* 22 (3) (Fall 1963) , 169–179.
9. Vuebke, P. T. American elementary and secondary community schools abroad. *Amer. Ass. School Admin.,* 1976.
10. Weiss, S. Letter from Bronxville to New Delhi. *Foreign Serv. J.,* September 1972, 6–8.
11. Slater, P. *The Pursuit of Loneliness.* Beacon Press, Boston, 1970.
12. Fleming, J. Early object deprivation and transference phenomena: The working alliance. *Psychoanal. Quart.* 41 (1972), 23–49.
13. Erikson, E. H. The problem of ego identity. *J. Amer. Psychoanal. Ass.,* 4 (1956), 56–121.
14. Miner, R., personal communication.
15. Mahler, M. S. On human symbiosis and the vicissitudes of individuation. *International Universities Press,* New York, 1968.
16. Werkman, S. and Johnson, R., The effect of geographic mobility on adolescent character structure, unpublished data.

A Television-Fed Child: What Therapists Encounter in a Changed World

D. J. de Levita, Ph.D. (Holland)

All research on television viewing by children seems to agree that television programs alone never have the power to elicit pathological behavior in the child, but only serve to provide the contents for a structure that was already present. Rushton and Owen [1] showed that exposing children to a television model's generous or selfish behavior affects the childrens' subsequent generosity but in a less durable and overall weaker way than a live model. Schramm and others [2] showed 15 years ago that televised instruction is able to stimulate childrens' interest but hardly conveys knowledge in the way a living person can do it.

Compared to the rich literature on television viewing by children, the clinical material that has been presented is scarce. I want to make a few brief notes on television viewing by the children of the inpatient unit of our child psychiatric department of the University of Amsterdam, Holland and present some material on one of the children, who for some time had had television as the only intellectual and cultural nutrition offered to him and whose subsequent development we were able to follow.

In our Amsterdam Child-psychiatric inpatient unit 15 children

are treated, most of them under the diagnosis child psychosis or borderline state. Some of them have suffered from serious parental neg-
lection. Treatment comprises a program carried out by child-care
workers and special teachers, casework with the family, and each
child's having his own individual psychotherapy, which can vary
from two interviews weekly to full psychoanalysis. It has become
common knowledge in the ward that the television set should be
used only for school television, of which we have two kinds: one for
toddlers and one for latency children. The children enjoy these programs and are helped by the child-care workers to digest them. On
all the other programs there is a strict taboo, and we think for good
reasons: when during a weekend at home the children have been allowed to watch television programs they come back full of anxiety
which may continue for many days. Psychotic children obviously
lack an agency that enables them to defend against the emotional
contents of the program or helps them to digest it.

Fred, now 7 years old, was admitted to the unit at the beginning
of this year on request of the day-care center where he had been because of an extreme retardation, especially of his speech and mental
development, although the staff had a strong feeling that his intelligence was normal. The family situation was an unusual one: The father had left the family in 1973 after having seriously mishandled the
mother. She lived in a bare, hardly furnished flat with Fred and his
little sister; her only support was a much older man with whom she
had a very peculiar relationship and who turned out to be a brother
of the lover of her own mother who lived in the flat upstairs. In the
latter family also lived the mother's grandmother who, from her
wheelchair, exerted much influence. During the mother's childhood
the marriage of her parents had also come to grief; the father went
with other women till he had been forced to leave the family.

Fred's mother, a black-haired, frail, highly nervous but not unin-
telligent creature, was quite aware that after her own marriage had
ended she had drifted into a state of mind which could be compared
with that of "Sleeping Beauty" of the well-known fairy tale. She felt
that she had to think about her life, undertook no activities with her
children, hardly spoke to them, never went out with them, didn't offer them any toys, permitted them to watch television until midnight when the program ended. When we saw Fred for the first time

he was a small, pale-looking boy, hardly able to speak, seeming not to notice anything of the world around him, but still quite different from a mentally retarded child. He, his mother, and his sister turned out to have lice which we took up with the mother as a sign of her enormous self-depreciation. It was in handling this problem with the mother in a delicate way that the social worker managed to establish a relationship with her. It was the beginning of a change in the mother's behavior; she had never had any hard feelings against her children and seemed to wake up from a dream.

When I started therapy with Fred, his communications were not understandable, not only because of his broken language but also because of the contents of what he said. For nearly 2 months the puzzle stayed unsolved; he said, for instance, "bears can eat chickens," and when I asked him if he had seen such a thing he neither confirmed nor denied it. We thought that he had hallucinations. Meanwhile he was so pale and tired when he arrived early in the morning from home that we had him examined by our pediatrician on the suspicion of anemia. One day we found out that many fragments in his communications originated from television, that he watched it every night till midnight and got far too little sleep. When I told him that I now understood he was telling me about television programs he had been watching this gave him no relief at all. He just continued to give me his reports of what he had been seeing, a strange mixture of things observed through the window and seen on television. In the unit he kept apart from the other children, was all by himself in a small corner of the garden where he seemed to indulge in fantasies of an uncanny character. What he told the child-care workers in his very rare spontaneous expressions always had to do with death, being eaten, buried, burned, and the like. For another 4 months there was hardly any visible progress in therapy, but the child-care workers reported that he began to enjoy being read to. The main development was in the mother herself, who seemed to have waked up and displayed an incredible lack of knowledge of the commonest things around her. It was like somebody coming out of prison after 20 years. A kind of crisis occurred when both children got scarlatina and the mother undertook, with the help of the social worker, to take care of both of them. For the first time in her life she read to the children and told them simple things about animals. The effect was dramatic.

When Fred came back to the unit after he had recovered from his scarlatina, in his first session he started to tell me everything about milk-giving cows, sheep, and horses. This was a quite sudden improvement for a boy who never had said more than five words. When I complimented him on his knowledge, he said with a very happy smile, blushing, "mother told me." In the next sessions he started to enact burials. He buried small insects and spoke incessantly of killings between animals. When I tried to make use of the situation to explain to him what therapy really was for (i.e., discussing these uncanny fantasies with him) he said, "I don't think these things myself, I have watched them on television." He told me the whole story, how he had been sitting there watching television every night till it was very late, seeing programs that according to him were just endless killings. Meanwhile we have heard from the mother that many fights have happened in the house and that Fred heard many threatening noises without ever reacting to them.

Fred showed an arrest of development while his mother was in a developmental crisis, trying to find ways to restore her life, feeling not consciously hostile toward her children, just putting them outside her existence, seriously understimulating them. Fred was placed in a day center where he was properly taken care of, but this had no effect on his development. Only when, after his admittance to our unit, a social worker started an outreaching casework contact with the mother and was successful in eliciting in her a new interest in her children did Fred start to make new progress in development.

Television seems to have acted (as it has been described by Riley and Riley [3]) as a compensation for the lack of stimulation by the mother; it, so to speak, kept his mental apparatus busy and filled his empty receptors without—as it seems—ever having induced real affective distress. The aggressive feelings that the mother's apathy cannot have failed to have elicited in the children seem to have caused no other effect than Fred's selection of killings in the television material he watched. It is remarkable that in the cognitive area he could initially make no distinction between observations of television material and the real world but that, on the other hand, he was perfectly capable of defending against the emotional contents of the television programs, quite unlike the psychotic and borderline children of the unit who are not able to do this and can have terrible fear afterwards for many weeks. Fred is now developing well and seems to have no fears at all.

References

1. Rushton, J. P. and Owen, Diane, Immediate and delayed effects on TV modelling and preaching on children's generosity. *Brit. J. Soc. Clin. Psychol.,* (1975), 309–310. Vol. 14.
2. Schramm, W., Lyle, J., and Parker, E. B. In *Television in the Lives of Our Children; with a Psychiatrist's Comment on the Effects of Television,* L. Z. Freedman, Ed. Stanford University Press, Stanford, 1961, X, pp. 324.
3. Riley, M. W. and Riley, J. W., A sociological approach to communication research, *Pub. Opin. Quart.,* (1951), 445–460. Vol. 15.

Some Comments on Social Change in Greece

A. Potamianou, Ph.D. (Greece)

In an age of rapid and unbridled progress, such as ours, society calls upon the individual to respond to complicated social necessities and relationships. As a result, the evaluation of given possibilities for social participation and group achievement becomes ever more urgent, as no social, economic, political, or any other type of program can yield the desired results if the persons participating in it are carrying it out unwillingly or if those for whom the program is devised do not understand it or simply resign themselves to it without being duly prepared to cooperate for its success.

In Greece this fact has not yet been fully understood, and indeed, at times, people seem to be completely unaware of it. It often happens that programs are implemented without any previous preparation of those for whom the programs are planned. Moreover, the possibilities for participation of individuals concerned in them have not been properly gauged.

In private discussions, publications, and so on there seems to be general agreement on the existence of certain difficulties concerning the capacity of Greeks for group participation and achievement. For example, it is generally accepted that it is difficult for Greeks to cooperate; that although at first sight they appear endowed with initiative, in fact, within the framework of groups to which they belong, they show a tendency to avoid responsibility. Also, it is evident that they have difficulties in organizing their activities and in following up the subject matter methodically.

These problems have been noted long ago and are interpreted, according to each investigator's point of view, as being due to the well-known historical upheavals through which the country has passed, to defects of the educational system, to lack of preparation of the leaders, and so on. All these reasons do, of course, apply. But the question arises as to why they apply and why they have not been tackled in the past few decades.

Explanations based on Greece's economic difficulties, on wars or political instability, are no longer satisfactory. The fact that through all these years, and despite serious efforts made to deal with these shortcomings, Greece as of today has not been able to overcome them lends color to the argument that the factors generally cited by the investigators are not the only ones and that there are other, deeper causes, which mold the personality of the Greek and determine the level of development of his social awareness as well as his possibilities for group participation and performance.

How does the Greek of today behave in groups? How does he handle his relations with others within the different groups in which he is called on to participate? What follows concerning those questions is based on research material gathered in the framework of the Center for Mental Health as well as on observation and conclusions of discussions systematically promoted within groups of community officials, priests, police officers, presidents of cooperatives, social workers, and the like with which I had the opportunity to work.

One could say that the social behavior of the Greek presents itself under different aspects according to the specific unit that at a given moment takes up his attention, that is, the family, one of the numerous other groups in which he is called on to participate (such as professional groups, associations, and clubs), or the state. Within these different groups the Greek would appear to an observer to adopt a number of particular attitudes, depending on whether he is acting as member of his family, as member of another group, or as citizen.

Within the limits of the family circle, relationships between individuals seem to be determined by a tendency toward mutual protection, by attitudes of dependency, as well as by a strong sense of responsibility. Looking after the family, providing for its moral and material well-being and advancement appear to all Greeks, both men and women, the most important measure of value for many decades.

If such are the attitudes of the average Greek within the framework of the family, what could be said about the behavior of Greeks within other social groups of which he is a member? The point which perhaps mainly determines his attitudes is his belief that the group has been organized by individuals for the benefit of individuals and not that individuals are members of a group that as a unit has its own aims and dynamics to which the individual is called on to contribute and submit.

Generally speaking the participation and the contribution of Greeks as members of professional or other groups are dependent on the existence of personal ties already formed or created immediately after the entry of the person concerned into a specific group. Those personal ties take on an altogether special significance in the case of the leader. Within the framework of different groups the participation and contribution of individual members seem to increase in proportion to their closeness to the person in authority. Some attitudes of Greeks concerning their work are indicative in this line.

The Greek has always looked upon work as a duty that should not interfere with his inner freedom. The individual does not feel that his membership in a professional group compels him to conform to the demands of that group. Whenever he finds himself obliged to do so, he resents it. Greeks wish to apply their own rules and pace in working. The popular dictum "take it easy" is not a sign of laziness. It is the expression of a sense of inner freedom. And in this conception of freedom the impetus appears to be given not by the individual's acceptance of the rules of the professional group to which he belongs as an expression of a certain social reality but rather by his attempt to shape reality according to his own measurements.

It is no exaggeration to say that considerable time is needed for a Greek group to be stirred to action in a way that shows that its activity is the result of the coordinated effort of its members in assuming initiative and responsibilities. The members tend for the most part to relate their performance to the man or woman who leads the group. Their behavior, to a greater or lesser degree—according to the level of those comprising the group—expresses the position "we are doing this for your sake." The members take action not to serve the groups' aims but to please the leader. If private enterprise has been up to now so successful a factor in the economy of the country, it is because the personal touch in business relations fits the Greek character.

Coming now to the consideration of the average Greek's attitude toward the state, it becomes evident that he appears to have difficulties when regarding it as an impersonal power. The law and the state are impersonal, and as such they do not call for loyalty. The average Greek's participation in civic life is expressed mainly by his tendency to criticize or by fluctuations in his political positions. Greek voting is more or less determined by friendship and/or individualistic aims.

Following these observations one could maintain that a very obvious characteristic of the Greeks in their social behavior and their relations within groups is the demand for personal ties and personal contacts whenever the acceptance of responsibilities and obligations (i.e., restrictions set on the individual by his membership to a social group) is entailed.

The emphasis placed on the person of the leader, whether man or woman (i.e., on a father or a mother figure) is certainly not an exclusively Greek phenomenon. It is a stage through which all groups pass. What is peculiar to Greeks is the degree of their dependency and the acuteness of their ambivalent feelings despite their apparently independent attitudes.

What explanation can be given for this type of relationships among Greeks? Interpretations vary. Still, the frame within which their psychological and social development takes place is worthwhile examining. In examining this frame and in trying to define what the conditions of life are actually in Greece, one can easily detect that the development of the country's economic standards are directly linked with the progress of industrialization. But industrialization, though it provides opportunities for technical progress and for the absorption of surplus labor, places the individual within a framework in which conditions of work are, in principle, much more impersonal than the ones involved in agricultural occupations or home crafts. For people who until recently were geared to the increase of agricultural income and the strengthening of the bonds with the soil—in other words, to a system of life proper to small and closed social groups where the human unit has a clearly defined mission—the change is great and appears fraught with danger.

But were one to disregard the industrial and technical framework and examine other economic factors, such as trade or the merchant marine, there again it becomes obvious that the change is impressive. Both international and local conditions of work have so shaped the professional occupations that cooperatives and large companies are more and more depriving the individual of his feeling of personal professional worth.

Changes are also visible in the structure of society. Today this structure is rapidly changing in Greece. Until recently Greek society was definitely patriarchal. In all social groups the dominance of a single figure representing authority was practically unchallenged. The father, the husband, the teacher, the president of the community, the doctor, the oldest brother, and the like were the figures that represented authority and commanded obedience. Nowadays, neither international nor local conditions are conducive to such a social scheme. Facilities in communication between the country and the town are bringing about the gradual abolition of this social structure in both urban and rural areas. Greece is going through the difficult process of abandoning established social values, although, on the other hand, certain groups in the country are still struggling to remain faithful to old types of behavior for many reasons, one being because this gives them the self-deceptive feeling that they are somehow stopping the process of change. Thus on the social level one can observe a current of change combined with strong conflicts linked to its acceptance or efforts tending to its total rejection.

Nowadays every individual in Greece is called on to adapt himself to a constantly changing and as yet not thoroughly studied social, economic, political, and educational frame. But change, even when its results can be predicted as favorable—that is, even when the individual can foresee that he stands to benefit by the change—creates psychological tensions. Also, it imposes on the individual important demands for adaptation. The average Greek protects himself against these tensions either by adhering to the old modes of life or by erecting a wall of indifference within himself expressed in the favorite phrase: "why bother" or by reverting to the rejection of any form of authority and rules or on the opposite side by depending on authority for his performance.

And here we come to the consideration of specific problems pertaining to the relations of Greeks to figures representing authority. The roots of this problem could be sought within the family itself.

The atmosphere of the family in Greece is undoubtedly one of warmth and affection. It is also very demanding. Assumption of responsibilities does not arise from a freedom of choice, and consequently, the acceptance of such responsibilities arouses in the individual exceptionally intense negative feelings for the members of his family, without, of course, excluding the existence of positive ones.

But the free expression of ambivalent and mixed feelings within the family is still incompatible with the moral conscience of the Greek in the climate in which this conscience is developed. Only in such acts as the so-called "crimes of honor" do the feelings of aggressivity and rebellion come into the open, since such crimes cannot be explained by the mere influence of tradition and customs alone.

On a different level of thinking, one could say that castration anxiety might provide the explanation of the Greek's compliance to family imperatives while discharge of aggressivity occurs in relation to groups other than the family.

At this point one should note that recent family studies, conducted in the framework of the research service of our Mental Health Center, showed that there is a relative disruption of the closely knit patriarchally hierarchical family group which comprises the nuclear family and a more extended family constellation due to housing and working conditions. As a result, our research material reflects a splitting in the perception of change by individuals. Change is viewed negatively as far as values having to do with the supportive function of the family are concerned—it is being viewed more positively as far as individual freedom and accomplishment are concerned.

The intensity of ambivalent feelings toward authority figures in spite of the recently changing attitudes in family structure and life still hinders individuals from achieving independence as far as authority is concerned. Thus the Greek needs to have the leader near him; authority must be personalized, and he must be closely linked to it just as the child feels the need for the presence and commands of his guardians for his social achievements.

In stressing the above-mentioned trends of dependency-rebellion and displaced aggression, one must, of course, not overlook the fact that those trends were nurtured in specific historical and national conditions. It should not be forgotten that for many decades governmental power was in the hands of those whom the Greek child, from his earliest age, was accustomed to treat as enemies. To "deceive the state" was equivalent to "deceiving the Turk." Respect for the state was tantamount to national treason. Evasion of orders imposed by the state was not only legitimate but was also necessary.

One should also add that the new Greek state as an expression of authority has not succeeded as yet in creating more mature attitudes in its citizens. It did not present itself as a positive and secure framework that could assist the citizens in the process of political maturation by laying the foundations of true democracy that involves discipline (i.e., assertion of rights but also understanding of obligations). But, of course, state machinery is in the hands of Greeks; consequently, the problem is again to be examined in relation to their personality.

The Transition from Childhood to Adulthood In Old and New Sub-Saharan Africa

E. F. Thebaud, M.D. (Liberia)

Africa is a vast continent, the second largest in the world, in which many climatic conditions—Mediterranean, Desert, the Savanna and the Rain Forest—prevail. It is also a continent of many racial and ethnic groupings. African societies were not static before the European conquest. In the West, through trans-Saharan routes, contact was established with the Arab world and Europe, and the Eastern coast was already trading with the Far East in the Middle Ages. Those contacts resulted in a mixture of races and civilizations.

This chapter deals with sub-Saharan Africa, or black Africa. It is not an homogenous area and comprises many countries and peoples who, nevertheless, share certain similarities at this stage of their history. They all have been submitted to colonization by Western powers, which introduced money economy and imposed new ideologies and institutions on the old traditional system. In the best of cases one can talk of uneasy cohabitation if not of open conflict between the old and the new. Young people who are in a peculiar situation of transition between childhood and adulthood experience this conflict as a loss of communication with their parents' generation.

Considerations of African Demography

There is a lack of reliable data on African population. The reports on census are generally accepted as rough estimations rather than accurate data. In spite of these reservations, one can make the following observations.

1. Looking at the age distribution, it appears that there is a predominantly young population in Africa. For Liberia, where data were obtainable, 51% of the population comprises people under 20.
2. In spite of the trend toward rapid urbanization, the majority of the African population still lives in rural areas. Urban population varies from country to country: from 3.4 percent in Rwanda to 36.3 percent in Zambia.
3. The rate of illiteracy is quite high in most countries: 79 percent in Liberia. In this same country, school attendance is 13.4 percent.

The predominance of young people in the population points to the magnitude of the difficult process of acculturation for the young generation. On the other hand, it would be wrong to conclude from the low urban population that the rural areas have remained untouched by outside influences. There is practically no area that has been spared by the process of acculturation, to the extent that one can only talk of a relatively traditional environment.

The African Family

To get some insight into the potential conflict between children, or more properly between the younger generations and their families, it is important to understand the structure of the traditional extended family, the place assigned to the individual within such structure, and the interaction between the individual and the group.

The natural environment is generally the Dense Forest, where one hardly sees the sky, and the Savanna. It is where one may encounter wild animals and "bad spirits." Very early in life the child learns not to venture too far into this hostile environment without some form of protection: weapon or talisman. Life is very precarious, and daily existence is constantly threatened by natural hazards: draughts, rain, flood, destructive insects. Under these conditions the cohesion of the group is essential for survival. All the upbringing of the individual will prepare him to see himself and to function as an integral part of the group. Tribesmen are also kinsmen and feel that they originated from a common ancestor. The stranger is a factor of disruption. In a village near Monrovia, while a traditional ceremony was taking place, the following sign board was prominently displayed: "Sinner Not Allowed." Understand by sinner, nonmember. This illustrates the uneasiness, if not the suspiciousness, with which strangers are regarded.

The town chief possesses both spiritual and temporal powers. His authority is unchallenged, because he has acquired wisdom and knowledge mainly by the virtue of his age. He is the link between the living and the outer world of the dead, the ancestors and those not yet born. If the group is affected by a calamity, he offers an explanation: ancestors have been neglected and sacrifices should be offered to appease them. The tribal chief also establishes a link between his group and the government. It has happened in some countries that government efforts to force young men into wage-earning labor were implemented by the tribal authorities.

In the tribal organization the goal of education is not to achieve independence of the individual. Instead, sociability and integration into the group are presented as ideals. The individual only exists in relation to others. However, it would be wrong to think that the individual is nonexistent. Everyone has his place, even before birth. A child may be the reincarnation of an ancestor and is entitled to some special privileges from birth.

The ideal tribesman is prepared to fulfill his role by an educational system which deserves some considerations. Some authors have called it an extra uterine symbiosis, the relationship that exists between mother and child. Indeed, through back portage, the child is in constant physical contact with the mother. Children can be seen sleeping on their mother's back while they are cooking, selling in the market, or paddling over the lagoon. Breast feeding lasts from 18 to 24 months. The breast is always available to the child, who can pick it and suck the milk whenever he feels like it. This lack of oral frustration probably leaves deep influences on the organization of the personality of the adult.

The child, besides his mother's, also has access to many females' backs in his immediate environment. Physical contacts are increased as well as other forms of nonverbal communication.

Sphincter control is acquired freely, probably by a process of identification with adults rather than by coercion.

One should be reminded that paternity and maternity are not biological concepts in the African family. Uncles are considered as fathers; aunts and co-wives (where polygamy exists) as mothers.

Adolescence is marked by certain ceremonies, which are meant to reinforce the individual's integration into the group. In some areas beside the age group, we find the "Initiation Schools," also known as "Secret Societies." This is one of the few ways by which nonliterate societies can transmit knowledge orally from generation to generation. This transmission is codified and ensured by the "Secret Societies." The importance of these societies can be illustrated by the fact that Pygmies, who are nomadic and gatherers, leave their children to attend the "Initiation Schools" of their neighboring sendentary tribes.

Secret societies are separate for boys and girls. In Liberia, Sierra Leone, and some areas of Guinea and Ivory Coast, boys attend the Poro society, and girls the Sande society. Those highly structured organizations have a wide variety of functions, ranging from the art of medicine and recreational activities to the rules of sexual conduct. At the end of his initiation the adolescent is prepared to fulfill both his productive and reproductive functions in the society. It is during this period that marriage is arranged for girls. In this case it is not two individuals who unite but two families. The goal of sex is mainly procreation, and the interests of the couple remain subservient to the interests of the group. Husband and wife are accountable for their actions to their families, who will see that the union remains a viable one. The circle is closed, and children born from such unions will be raised to feel as integral parts of the extended family, the clan, and the tribe. There is no sharp delineation between his ego and his kinsmen.

Should we conclude from these observations that the traditional African societies ignored conflicts and anxieties? There was no conflict between generations, because each individual had his life planned beforehand. A system of reference offered an explanation for the more-or-less predictable causes of anxieties and offered the means to cope with them. People did not question the wisdom that inspired a group decision.

Let us now look at the impact of changes on the functioning of the group and its consequences for the young individual.

The African Family in a World of Change

The above-described type of family structure corresponds to a very simple type of society living on subsistence economy and employing very modest technical means to influence the natural environment. The main concerns of the people are fertility of the soil, fecundity for the women, and health for the men. The relatively few tasks to be performed require little specialization and are designed almost once for all.

This cohesiveness remained undisturbed until the Western powers introduced money, wage labor, and capitalistic form of economy on a large scale. Migration started taking place, with large numbers of people moving to cities, plantations, and mines. Attempts have been made by the migrants to congregate according to tribal affinities in the new settlements, but the extended family showed an irreversible trend toward nuclearization. The domination of the traditional economic system by the capitalistic one has its ideological counterpart. The acquisition of book knowledge became a condition of mastering new skills. This new phenomenon, "book learning," affected parent-child relationship adversely, because age used to be the main source of wisdom and knowledge. In schools, conducted mainly by missionaries, the young African started getting acquainted with new values. English and French were now superior to African languages, monogamy to polygamy, competition to reliance on the group and so forth.

The tribal authorities have no choice but to compromise with the new trend. For instance, the duration of initiation classes that used to last for years has been reduced to months if not a couple of weeks, to avoid conflicting with academic programs. The author made the following observation during a "bush breaking ceremony" which means the coming out of an "initiation school." The outfit of most of the pupils was a strange mixture of traditional costume made of a straw and Western necklaces, brooches, or finger rings. Many of them were wearing sunglasses and carrying purses. The facial and body decorations were also a mixture of clay, lipstick, and nailpolish. After all the tribal rites had been observed, the girls were directed to a house where a room was especially prepared for them. One could see a huge fan working at full speed and hear a record player playing pop music. When they were asked about these combinations, the tribal authorities answered that these children had just returned to the world they belong to.

The hesitations and ambivalent feelings of the parents in face of the changes are exemplified by the following story. A man who has been working as a cook in the city for the past 30 years converted to Christianity. All his children were born and have always lived in the city and are also Christian. Against all expectation he decided to send his daughter to an "initiation school" that lasted only 2 weeks, during vacations. He explained his decision in the following manner: "She is not good in school. She cannot get far. If I don't send her to the "bush school," she will belong nowhere."

The Young African In a World of Change

The young individual who has been trained to live and share with others finds himself in the solitary and individualistic life of the city. Every aspect of his social and psychological functioning will be affected by conflicting value systems. In the classroom, if he is caught communicating with a classmate, he will listen with astonishment to the teacher telling him that it is wrong to share his knowledge.

Sometimes the student is the only one among his siblings who has been chosen to attend school. As soon as he can earn some money, younger brothers are sent to him, and the family expects him to send back home some of his earnings. He lives in the fear of failure, and his anxiety increases during the time of examinations, because he is aware that a lot of pride and hope have been invested in him.

Those solitary youngsters anxiously look for one another. A lot of the time that should actually be spent studying is used for frequent visits. Sickness or academic failure give rise to persecutory interpretations. They often think that they have been "witched" by jealous people. A few visits are then made to the village to get some protection, but it often happens that the system of interpretation offered by the families for the misfortunes have lost their convincing power. It is of no surprise, then, that not only persecutory interpretations are more often encountered in the cities, but that new religious sects are proliferating and offering solutions to the new anxieties.

CASE 1

G., a young student nurse, is referred to the psychiatrist because of strange behavior observed at work. Quite often he apologizes to his superiors for faults he has not committed and begs them not to expel him from the school. He always promises to improve his performance. His history reveals that in his tribe it is customary that when a man dies his first son inherits all his wives, with the exception of his own mother because of the incest taboo. Therefore, when his father died, his mother became the wife of his older brother and had children by him. The brother is an alcoholic and cannot live up to his responsibilities. G. lives with the fear of being expelled from the nursing school, because the acquisition of a profession will enable him to support his mother and her children.

Unlike Western cultures, traditional Africa considers sexual initiation as a social affair. During the passage from childhood to adulthood the adolescent undergoes certain ritual performances in groups. Tribal marks are put on his body, and in some tribes, boys undergo circumcision and girls clitoridectomy. The origin and the signification of those practices are still a matter of controversy and speculation. It would be wrong to consider them as a form of punishment. They should be seen symbolically as a form of integration into the world of the adult. Those ceremonies are followed by prearranged marriages for girls. Boys get married at a later stage of their lives, when they can afford to pay the bride price.

Unlike his Western counterpart, the young African is not left alone with the anxieties in his crucial period of his life. Sex is considered as a normal function, approved and codified by the group. However, with exposure to Christian teachings, the adolescent learns that sex is a sinful thing when it is practiced outside of marriage, if not of Christian marriage. He is made to feel that he is born from a sin of his parents and regards them as sinful people. The appraisal of his cultural heritage and of himself is consequently affected. "Native names" are changed to "Christian" or "civilized" names to facilitate a better integration into the norms of the dominant culture.

Sex becomes this mysterious and anxiety-provoking function. Since in traditional Africa the individual feels responsible for the acts he performs in a dream, an erotic or worse an incestuous dream may be the source of anxiety and guilt.

Through readings and mass media, the Westernized young African learns that the choice of a partner can be a very personal affair and finds it now difficult to accept the interference of the family in such matters. In the past parents chose a partner for their daughter not only on the basis of certain criteria such as wealth but also on belonging to a clan, since somebody does not marry a person of an inferior clan. They fail to realize that today, for their Western educated children, the choice of a partner may be based on quite different criteria.

CASE 2

C., a young man, started losing weight. His performance at work started to decline. He always looked lost. He explained his situation by relating the following story: His uncle had chosen a young girl for him to marry before he left the village for further education. The girl also started attending primary school in the village and reached grade nine. In the meantime, the uncle decided to marry her by a mutual arrangement with her family. She escaped from her husband's home because according to her he drinks excessively, is illiterate, and is at least 25 years older than her. She joined C. in town and stated that she would kill herself if forced to return to the husband. When this was learned, the uncle insisted that she return to him, and her family agreed. C. also learnt that the girl's family was powerful and could kill him within a year through "African Science." Although he cares for the girl, he felt for his own well-being that she had to return to the uncle. A family meeting took place in the absence of the girl, and it was decided that she should rejoin her husband, the uncle.

Conclusion

Within the limits of this chapter it has not been possible to deal with all the complexities of the problems facing African parents and their children today. Every day new implications of these rapid social changes are being demonstrated. For instance, kwashiorkor, which is now prevalent in urban areas, used to be considered as a simple protein deficiency. It is now accepted as a form of anorexia nervosa, a reaction of the child to the rejection by the mother when a newborn arrives. We could also mention learning difficulties due to imported teaching methods and academic goals that do not take into consideration the African realities. The high frequency of psychiatric disorders associated with childbirth deserves to be mentioned in this context, since girls may get married and become mothers from the age of 13. In the cities, groups of vagrant marginal adolescents have become associates of delinquents and drug users. Although missionaries are introducing sexual taboos, contraceptive methods are becoming available to larger numbers of young people.

Parents are uncertain about their role and about which attitude to adopt. Some abdicate their responsibilities, while others use coercion, and each attitude is equally harmful. Another group tries to compromise by keeping certain traditional rites, but for many those rites have lost all their meaning. For instance, circumcision that used to punctuate the passage from childhood to adulthood may be now practiced as a medical act.

In spite of the specifity of the African situation, parents and children in Africa are facing the same dilemma as their counterparts, the world over: Which way? There is no magic solution. It is utopic to try to reverse the trend of history and to return to precolonial Africa. Although questioning the value of Western individualism and competition, one has to admit that certain aspects of the traditional culture need a reassessment in a modern society.

However, too often, in their search for material progress African leaders discard traditional values without replacing them with anything meaningful to the people. They must bear in mind that a requirement for the validity of changes affecting their lives is that the people identify with them. Such an approach might help to relieve some of the tensions and dilemmas which face the emerging African nations.

THE JERUSALEM CONFERENCE*
ON THE IMPACT OF CHANGE IN
A RAPIDLY DEVELOPING
SOCIETY

Meeting of the International Study Group on
"Children and Parents in a Changing World"
At Jerusalem, Israel
July 12–16, 1976

Participants

Chairman: Albert Solnit, M.D.,† President, International Association For Child
Psychiatry and Allied Professions

Co-Chairman: E. James Anthony, M.D.†

General Commentator: Reginald Lourie, M.D.

Rapporteur: Peter Neubauer, M.D.

Local Organizer in Israel: Anat Kalir, M.D.

Invited Speakers

Gerald Caplan, M.D. Martin Wolins, Ph.D.
Stephen P. Hersh, M.D. Joseph Noshpitz, M.D.
Edward Zigler, Ph.D.

Official Discussants

Jon Lange, M.D. Reimer Jensen, Ph.D.
Kiyoshi Makita, M.D. Luis E. Prego-Silva, M.D.
Anna Potamianou, Ph.D. Colette Chiland, M.D., Ph.D.
Winston Rickards, M.D. Cyrille Koupernik, M.D.
Lionel Hersov, M.D. Joyce Grant, M.S.W.

* Sponsored by the William T. Grant Foundation.
† Also presented a paper.

Participants from Israel

Mrs. Leah Rabin
Michaela Lifshitz, Ph.D.†
Phyllis Palgi, Ph.D.
Anat Kalir, M.D.
Rafael Moses, M.D.†
Karen Moses, B.S.W.†

Julius Zellermayer, M.D.
Helen Antonovsky, Ph.D.†
Lea Baider, Ph.D.
Tamar Bresnitz, Ph.D.
Jona M. Rosenfeld, Ph.D.
Hillel Klein, M.D.

Kibbutz Adolescents: Changing Aspects of Behavior and Attitudes

Mordecai Kaffman, M.D. (Israel)

> *"If only there were a dogma to believe in.*
> *Everything is contradictory, everything tangential;*
> *there are no certainties anywhere.*
> *Everything can be interpreted one way*
> *and then again interpreted in the opposite sense."*
> (Herman Hesse: Magister Ludi)

The Kibbutz Adolescent: Less to Fight Against

Until a few years ago the consensus of all the investigators who studied the characteristics of kibbutz adolescents was that the attitudes and behavior of most of them indicate a clear identification with the "establishment" positions of the adult world [12, 10, 2, 1]. Among the central characteristics of the kibbutz adolescent, mention was made of the lack of rebelliousness, the absence of conflict in the choice of kibbutz values, the puritanic behavior, and the prevalent sexual codes of "purity" and abstinence. A survey carried out in 1962 [11] on a sample of more than 300 kibbutz adolescents (17 and 18 years old) revealed that the predominant majority of boys and girls was highly satisfied with communal life. More than 90 percent of the sample believed that kibbutz child rearing and education were "the best in the country." They planned to remain in the kibbutz and "to

155

give their children the same kind of upbringing that they have had." Only less than 10 percent of the adolescents were not sure about the kibbutz as their future home. Since this questionnaire was administered anonymously on an individual basis, there is no reason to think that any peer group or adult pressures were operative.

The kibbutz appears to be a confirmation and illustration of the view presented, among others, by Opler [8, 9] who relates the variability in adolescent experience around the world to the specific cultural influences operating to help or hinder the adolescent's integration into adult society. Generally speaking, the kibbutz may be included among those cultural settings in which the adolescent's integration into the social environment takes place from a comparatively early age on and follows structured norms that are well defined with regard to all adolescents. From the age of 15 to 16, kibbutz adolescents usually have their regular place to work where they gradually assume greater responsibility and perform essential functions in the overall work system. They learn at an early age to use sophisticated industrial and agricultural equipment. Most adolescents, particularly the boys, not only have certainty and security with respect to their present occupation but also are aware of their future opportunities for vocational advancement. The kibbutz adolescent gradually receives all the responsibilities and privileges of the adults during the period between graduation from high school and completion of army service. At the age of 20 to 22, the youth of both sexes is basically entitled to the same prerogatives as his parents. At that time the adolescent is admitted to the kibbutz as a member with full and equal rights in all matters concerning the commune. He is given an apartment of his own, a personal budget equal to that received by his parents, and a responsible job comparable to that of the adult kibbutz members. He may conduct his private life, including sex, according to the prevalent norms of his own generation. Hence the kibbutz reduces considerably the noticeable discrepancy present in other societies between the timing of physical, intellectual, and sexual maturation at adolescence and the adolescent's delay in the assumption of socioeconomical responsibility—a discrepancy enforced by the adult world. In the kibbutz, criteria for the assumption of adult roles and responsibilities by the adolescent—marking, in effect, the end of adolescence from a social point of view—appear to be more clearly defined and structured than in the majority of Western societies. Furthermore, kibbutz parents have waived, for ideological reasons associated with the very nature of their society, a large share of their functions regarding their children of all ages in such areas as the provision of basic material needs, commodities, and financial support. All these functions are the responsibility of the community. Although the emotional links between parents and adolescents persist, the lessening of physical dependence reduces the areas of conflict in intergenerational relations. Thus the expected rebellion of the adolescent loses much of its momentum simply because the adolescent in the kibbutz appears to have fewer objective reasons for fighting.

At this point let us stress that we are dealing with hypothetical average situations and reactions that vary in frequency and intensity from one adolescent to another. One must bear in mind that the "typical" kibbutz adolescent exists only in books and articles, not in real life. The kibbutz adolescent does not differ from his counterparts elsewhere in terms of individual variation and ample gamut of personality structures and characteristics of intrafamily functioning. The family scene is not always quiet and harmonious. Most kibbutz parents perceive and have to find their own specific answers to the adolescents' striving toward emotional and intellectual independence. The course of adolescence in the kibbutz, as in other social frameworks in Western civilization, depends to a large extent on the quality of the adolescent's relation with his parents. Here, too, parents' responses to the adolescent's need for independence and their support of or resistiveness to the adolescent's expressions of self-assertive defiance largely determine the modalities and intensity of the intergeneration conflict.

The emotional child-parent relationship in the kibbutz family is no less intensive and complex than outside—even though the child is released from material dependence on his parents. In the kibbutz, as elsewhere, the parents are the most important emotional connection and model of identification for the child, in spite of the obviously important role of the peer group before and during adolescence.

Nowadays, the kibbutz family has ample opportunity of maintaining a close and stable relationship. In obvious contrast with other contemporary cultures [3] the present trend for kibbutz parents, especially in the last decade, is to spend more time with their children and to be much more involved in the child's upbringing. As a result, the specific emotional content and patterns of communication of a family in the kibbutz of today become a paramount factor in the "normal" or "deviant" psychological development of children and adolescents. Six years ago we undertook a survey on prevailing parental attitudes and behavior in the parent-child relationship of about 600 kibbutz parents. The sample consisted of parents of emotionally disturbed children referred to the Kibbutz Child and Family Clinic and a control group of parents of normal children [5]. We found that both extremes in the degree of control exerted by the parent (mother and/or father) over the child—excessive parental dominance, on the one hand, and parental submissiveness, on the other hand—were overrepresented among those families whose teenage children showed sharp disagreements and communication difficulties with their parents. That parental behavior and attitudes affect the nature and strength of the kibbutz adolescent's reactions seems, therefore, beyond doubt. Extreme attitudes in the control-autonomy area of parent-child interaction are liable to produce dysfunctional neurotic syndromes, which may express themselves, among other things, in signs of deviant adolescent rebelliousness.

Indeed, we see that encouraging independence and gradual integration into the adult world, at the social as well as at the family level, reduces signs of storm and stress in the adolescent. That, however, should not lead us to conclude that "uneventful adolescence" is a constant characteristic of kibbutz youth, with the exception of a handful of families with signs of dysfunctional relations. As there are individual differences with regard to the characteristics of adolescent rebellion according to the family context, so too there are differences according to the circumstances and events during the particular period in which the adolescent grows up. The investigators who noted the uneventful transition of the kibbutz adolescent from childhood to adulthood used simple chronological cross-sectional observations. When one traces characteristics of adolescence in the kibbutz from a perspective of 20 years or more, one discerns considerable shifts in the intensity and form in which the process of the adolescent's psychological, ideological, and sociological emancipation expresses itself. The placidity of the 1950s modulated in the 1960s into moderate signs of youth rebelliousness, which exacerbated rather suddenly and culminated in the quinquennium 1970–1975, when signs of "storm and stress" became quite obvious among "normal" kibbutz adolescents. And although today (1976–1978) there are indications that this adolescent rebelliousness may be declining again, the general picture is still very different from the one usually presented of the past.

The Emergence of Intergenerational Behavior Gaps

Expressions of adolescent "revolt" and intergenerational conflict appeared in the 1970s and reached previously unknown proportions among kibbutz adolescents. These changes were expressed, for example, in the increased percentage of adolescents who decided to leave the kibbutz and adopt another social framework. Likewise, a particular idiosyncratic "youth style" emerged—widely different and at times opposed to the adult way of life, from dress and hair styles to new cultural and entertainment fads. In the kibbutz high school there appeared small groups of youngsters who refused to participate in lessons and fulfill any other tasks or obligations in defiance of the teachers' authority. There appeared a more critical approach to the older "establishment," represented by the parental and kibbutz values. A sharp change in attitudes about sexuality during high school years has occurred, a change that has taken the direction of a rapid increase in early, permissive sexual behavior.

Indeed, the need to find an explanation for the lack of "typical" adolescent rebellion in the kibbutz has weakened in recent years. One has to explain instead the significance and underlying causes of the above-mentioned far-reaching changes. Actually, the changing attitudes of the kibbutz youth took place concurrently with changes in the structure, functioning, and value system of the adult society.

The growth of the population and the development of the multigenerational commune ranging from infants to oldsters and the expansion of the kibbutz material needs, tasks, and activities generated the necessity of achieving economic consolidation within the frame of the surrounding capitalist, competitive world. Inevitable gaps have developed between the revolutionary ideology and zealous faith of the original, small kibbutz and the facts of day-to-day life.

The discrepancies between the ideal values and the original set of expectations, on the one hand, and the current conventionalized compromises and norms, on the other hand, appear to be closely related to the index of intergenerational conflict and tension. In the 1950s—following World War II and its sequence of unfulfilled ideals and failing gods, a value crisis appeared and deepened throughout the years, when the founding generation realized that its hopes for the spread of the kibbutz idea in Israel and the rapid expansion of a humanist socialism throughout the world were doomed to disappointment. The upheaval in the doctrinary system resulted in an ideological shock that had an adverse effect on the adult world's ability to serve as an identification model for the younger generation. Parental influence in determining social and political values decreased, and conflicts were more likely to occur when the adolescent's parents lacked the crystallized set of values that had been common in the past.

The truth is that both generations, adults and adolescents alike, have reached the point at which they must come to terms with a whole range of crucial questions, such as the nature of socialism in the contemporary world and the way of life and aim of the kibbutz in its transition from the intimate, idealistic commune to the large and realistic multigenerational commune. Behind the adult generations' general consensus on socialist identity we now find more than a little contradiction and cloudiness of interpretation. Past beliefs sometimes turned into slogans, and a large proportion of the younger generation revolted and abandoned the principles that seemed to them an outdated profession of faith.

Remodeling of Attitudes in a Changing Adult World

This critical attitude to parental beliefs is a sharp departure from the almost absolute conviction of the past that the kibbutz is a militant avant garde that seeks a revolutionary change of the entire society. The corollary of this was the moral duty of the younger generation to remain in the kibbutz and help their parents to complete the task. Today, the younger generation no longer joins the kibbutz automatically, but as the result of free choice between options. The youngster of the 1970s demands recognition of his right to experience other realities, to familiarize himself with other ways of life, and to postpone his decision on whether to join the kibbutz according to considerations of his own. The sociocultural changes and technological progress of the kibbutz have produced a further intergenerational gap in the matter of the relative values and prestige assigned to vocational choices. The founding generation had proclaimed the equality of all occupations, physical or intellectual, and the immediate needs of the kibbutz caused the academic professions and career specialization to be discouraged. The accent was on the image of the "halutz," essentially, a semiskilled worker who dedicatedly performs such manual labor as the needs of the community call for. Unlike the kibbutz pioneers, today's kibbutz adolescent spends a great deal of his time and thought on planning vocational goals. His vocational interests are guided by his own individual aspirations, which have become more reality bound and much more specialized and which at times do not fit in with the needs and demands of the commune. It is clear that the clash between the vocational values of the two generations is not only the result of the youth revolt for recognition of the right to self-realization in the collective community or of the greater complexity of vocational problems in a more diversified and technologically oriented kibbutz society; it is also influenced by changes that have occurred in the adult generation's own value system. Many adults have, as they reach old age and are forced to reduce their physical activity and adjust to new working conditions, gained experience of the realistic disadvantages of having renounced a professional career in their youth and remained semiskilled workers. Actually, the parents' influence on the vocational choice of kibbutz youth is considerable and does not fall behind that in the city [4]. Parental involvement, indubitably, plays a large role in the changes that have occurred in the vocational interests of the youth and the social acceptability of the different kinds of occupations.

Although there are many factors that determine the change in the kibbutz youth's attitudes to their vocational future, the result, whatever the explanation may be, is unmistakably the same: the adolescent is often confused and bewildered by the many possibilities available to him. The certainty of the one clear road, of which the "halutz" used to be the symbol, is no longer.

The obvious impact of the adult social climate on the development of an attitudinal gap between the generations can also be discerned in the failure of the adult generation to achieve peace in the protracted Middle East conflict. The adolescent sees himself forced to accept an undesirable inheritance and to face a seemingly endless succession of cold and hot wars in which he must take part and risk his life. This compulsory situation of threats and tension is a further reason for discarding the ineffective slogans of the past. On the parental side, the long time of ideological disenchantment, wars, and threats of war have undermined the confidence in their ideals and political creed. All these weak points in the positions of the adults have affected the adolescent in his need for a structure of standards, ideas, and models around him. In these conditions the antiestablishment responses of the kibbutz adolescents spread considerably beyond the former smooth type of rebellion. The kibbutz experience, therefore, appears to confirm the postulate that whenever the adult value system is in a stage of transition and becomes an ambiguous model of identification, antiestablishment youth movements are prone to emerge.

Adolescent Peer Culture: Changed Norms

The remarkable identity that had existed between the cultural expression of the adults and the adolescents has steadily diminished in the last few years. For the first time a new style has emerged in the appearance and behavior of the adolescent that is very different from the conventions of the "square" adult society. The parents realized—under protest and with vain attempts to stop the process—that their children have adopted characteristic elements of the style and fads of the outside youth and often have found a common language with the volunteers from abroad who have stayed temporarily on the kibbutz. Kibbutz parents, teachers, and institutions sought ways to put the younger generation back "on the right path" by means of appeals to the traditional values and the old accepted behavior patterns. Moralizing or angry reactions on the part of adults had no impact on the behavior of the rebellious groups and only made it worse. At this stage, attempts were made to change the pattern of ideological education and to avoid the generation-to-generation "transition of values by inheritance and indoctrination." Many of the old teachers left the profession, and their younger replacements attempted to encourage free ideological discussion and self-expression without binding conclusions. Opposition to fashions in clothes, hair style, music, dances, and fads peculiar to adolescents also weakened gradually.

The fight and pressure of high school students for more freedom and new privileges in sexual behavior, mentioned earlier, are additional expressions of adolescent "revolt." The kibbutz young adolescent now rejects the sexual moratorium, part of the adult value system, that requires sexual relations to be postponed till the end of the teenage years. At first the rebellion mainly took the form of change in declared attitudes, without being translated into actual sexual behavior. Gradually, though, an increasing proportion of adolescents have found the way to achieve consonance between their new values and attitudes on sexual relations and their actual sexual behavior [6].

Until the early 1960s educators, parents, and adolescents conjointly adhered to a quite puritanical ideology about sexual relations between adolescents. Actually, sexual intercourse before leaving the secondary school was very rare and was consistently discouraged and criticized by adults and the adolescent group alike. A strong ascetic ideology of self-restraint and the absence of intergenerational conflicts on the subject of sexual values were among the prominent characteristics of the youth mores of those days. Couples who were going steady were expected to refrain from displaying any overt signs of affection and were encouraged to resort to all manner of camouflage tactics in order to keep their special ties a "secret." Only after graduating from high school were young people supposed to be free to engage in premarital sexual relations. Needless to say, promiscuity was strongly condemned by public opinion.

Today, this code of sexual behavior is a matter of past history. Adolescent couples no longer conceal their relationship. They display their affection openly. Today's over-sixteens no longer agree that early sex "hampers or harms the personality." They also do not accept the argument that "preoccupation with sexual matters prevents full concentration on school activities and has a disruptive effect on the peer group." Today's kibbutz adolescents proclaim openly that sexual relations should be considered a personal matter for any couple who have maintained a love relationship for some time. Whether the couple engage in actual sexual intercourse or not is for them alone to decide. Sexual relations should not require the sanction of the social group or be restricted by adult interference.

Surveys undertaken in the seventies on samples of 17- to 18-year-old kibbutz adolescents show that about 90 percent—boys and girls—justify sexual relations while still in secondary school [7]. The present sexual standards set by the adolescents are quite permissive on the subject of early sexual intercourse, though sexual relations are accepted only if they are integrated in the emotional life of both partners. Although there is a considerable degree of personal freedom with regard to sexual behavior, casual or promiscuous sexual relations are still condemned by the prevailing adolescent public opinion.

What is evident by now is that the puritanical attitude on sexual relations in middle adolescence has been abandoned in theory and practice by a considerable part of the kibbutz adolescents. They have demanded and obtained freedom to devise their own rules for sexual behavior. Permissive sexual attitudes and behavior have become the dominant norm for both male and female adolescents in the kibbutz; that this sexual revolution includes both sexes to an equal degree is important for in the kibbutz, the double standard is entirely nonexistent.

Individual Versus Communal Interests

With the disappearance of the intimate framework of the young, small kibbutz, the increase of its economic power, the growth of the family, and the increase of its importance within the kibbutz society, pressure increased for greater individuation, greater privacy, and recognition of the individual's right to achieve personal expression and satisfaction in his life. Terms of the equilibrium between the individual and the commune changed in these new conditions. As Yonina Talmon [13] puts it: "The peculiar character of kibbutz collectivism must be taken into account. It was not inspired by opposition to individualism. In giving priority to the community, collectivists never intended to slight the individual. The underlying assumption is that individual and communal interests are in perfect harmony with each other. Even when the individual dedicates his life to the common good, he does not give up independence. . . . His social activity offers ample opportunities for personal expression. He merely gives up small, transient pleasures for the much more lasting, meaningful satisfaction of knowing that he is working for the common cause." Indeed, according to this ideological approach, which was the accepted one in the kibbutz in its early days, the good of the individual depends in the last resort on the good of the community.

Nowadays there has been a clear turn, particularly among the younger generation, in the direction of increased pressure for recognition of the individual's right to realize his personal aspirations and plans. Thus today a given kibbutz may have a severe manpower shortage in a specific field—child care or industry—while at the same time several members are learning "nonfunctional" professions or working outside the kibbutz context.

The decrease of influence of the collective group on the individual seems to have taken place parallel to an increase in family unity and contacts. Over the past 15 years adolescents' visits to their parents' rooms became more frequent and were sanctioned by all involved. There now appeared an alternative for those adolescents who used to complain about the excessive group life and peer interdependence in the communal children's homes. This change of balance in the youngster's mutual relations with his parents and his peers has worked undoubtedly in the direction of weakening the influence of the group.

Presumably, the revolt against the group's excessive control over the individual is in part due to the parents themselves. The increasing tendency to encourage and satisfy individual aspirations and personal wishes and the growing familistic tendencies are reflected in several trends that are becoming increasingly frequent in the kibbutz movement. Family sleeping arrangements are being adopted in an increasing number of kibbutzim, where children now sleep in their parents' home instead of the customary communal accommodation. In the material sphere there is also a clear trend to expand the personal cash allocation of each kibbutz member so as to include commodities such as clothing, furniture, entertainment, and other consumer goods that used to be within the exclusive province of the communal institutions. The wider availability of "nonfunctional" education programs (nonfunctional in terms of the everyday needs of the collective) such as theoretical academic studies, occupation with art and literature, and the pursuit of all kinds of personal hobbies are further evidence of the change toward individualism and the increase of personal freedom.

It should be borne in mind that the "second generation," the children of the kibbutz founders who grew up in the kibbutz, were educated under conditions of ideological indoctrination that called for priority for communal interests over individual aspirations. Part of this second generation, when they themselves became parents in the kibbutz, sought to use the upbringing of their children as a way of expressing their late rebellion against the monolithic community and lack of privacy. The third generation received the message of their parents, which fitted in with their desire to secure more personal freedom while still remaining within the collective group in a climate of closeness and togetherness.

Youth Leaving the Kibbutz

Additional evidence of increasing intergenerational problems is provided by the increase in the proportion of adolescents who leave the kibbutz. Spiro [12], in field work carried out during 1951–1952, found that almost the entire kibbutz-born generation over the age of 16 viewed the kibbutz as "the best form of societal living not only for them, but for others as well." He also mentioned that although "all the graduates are drafted into the army for at least two years, none have chosen to leave the kibbutz following this experience with the outside world. Moreover, although many of the kibbutz 'sabras' have been abroad, all have returned to the kibbutz, where they prefer to live."

Nowadays, most youngsters struggle for the right to have some experience of a different way of life and an opportunity to explore the world and test their own abilities in a nonkibbutz setting. Under the pressure of the younger generation, it has been decided jointly by the youth and the adult society of most kibbutzim that kibbutz youngsters, after completing their military service and staying in the kibbutz for a short time, are entitled to try city life, to work or study in the city, or to take a trip abroad with the consent and assistance of the commune. The proportion of those who return to the kibbutz after staying outside is still twice that of those who leave, but it is evident that the ratio of those who stay to those who leave diminishes over the years.

The majority of youth who leave the kibbutz view it as a step toward individual emancipation, as an attempt to find "one's real self," to face new emotional relationships and vocational challenges, and to gain desirable rewards hopefully present in the outside world. Generally speaking, the decision to leave the kibbutz reflects no rejection of or alienation from kibbutz society. Mostly, the decision to leave the kibbutz is the result of an inner urge to experiment with personally satisfying alternatives within a culture different from the one the adolescent has known since infancy. Certainly, there is also a reduced minority of maladjusted youth and social dropouts unable to adjust to the kibbutz as well as the nonkibbutz way of life.

Those who in past years were concerned about the lack of a "storm and stress" period (in the idea that it is an essential part of the adolescent's "normative crisis") asked themselves whether this complacent youth could be capable of integrating itself in different frameworks, which called for struggle, competition, initiative, and individual action, without leaning on the group. The answer could only be theoretical, since there were so few who left the kibbutz. But by now the kibbutz movement has been in existence for about 70 years, and there are hundreds of kibbutz youth who have chosen to move to the city, so that an answer on a factual basis becomes possible. Although the subject has not yet been researched systematically, all the indications are that the kibbutz youth is definitively capable of functioning adequately in a new, nonkibbutz framework as an individual, marriage partner, and parent. Youngsters with a kibbutz upbringing are able to continue their education at a university or other educational institution. They engage in a wide range of occupations in town and country: in technical jobs, in academic professions, in agriculture, in the arts, in literature, as officers in the army; some have even become successful businessmen. Thus the large majority seem to integrate well in the social and vocational environment in which they operate outside the kibbutz.

Conclusions

The particular sociocultural conditions of the kibbutz make for fewer areas of conflict between the adolescent, on the one hand, and his parents and the adult society, on the other hand. Generally speaking, the adolescent in the kibbutz has less to rebel against. Nevertheless, observations over a period of years show that there are considerable changes in the way in which kibbutz youth expresses its identification with, or rebellion against, the adult society. Thus in the last decade increasing signs of adolescent rebellion have been discerned in a considerable part of kibbutz youth.

The changing attitudes and signs of rebelliousness of the kibbutz adolescents over the past 10 years have taken place concurrently with changes in the value system of the adult society. No doubt other influences related to the outside world and changes among youth of the Western culture have also made their impact on kibbutz adolescents, but the most influential factors appear to be within the kibbutz itself. Today, the kibbutz adolescent lives in a world with a more flexible and ambiguous value system, which has replaced the former very structured educational, social and political beliefs. The experience of the kibbutz seems to prove that the level of clarity and assurance in definition and realization of the basic values of the adult society is a factor of primordial importance in determining the quality and intensity of adolescent rebelliousness.

References

1. Alon, M. *Adolescence in the Kibbutz* (in Hebrew). Sifriat Hapoalim, Tel Aviv, 1975.
2. Bettelheim, B. *The Children of the Dream*. Macmillan, New York, 1969.
3. Bronfenbrenner, U. (1970): "Two Worlds of Childhood." Russell/Sage Foundation, New York.
   Hesse, H. "Magister Ludi." Bantam Book, New York, 3rd print, p. 69.
4. Horwitz, O. The values and attitudes of the Israeli adolescent (in Hebrew). *Etgar L'Chinuch*, 44 (1975), 12–24.
5. Kaffman, M. Family conflict in the psychopathology of the kibbutz child. *Family Process*, 11 (1972), 171–188.
6. Kaffman, M. (1977): Sexual standards and behavior of the kibbutz adolescent. *Amer. J. Orthopsychiat.*, 47 (1977), 207–217.
7. Nathan, M. and Shenval, A. *Sexual Education in the Kibbutz* (in Hebrew). Bulletin of the Department of Education, Kibbutz Hameuchad, Tel Aviv, 1976.
8. Opler, M. K. *Culture and Social Psychiatry*. Atherton Press, New York, 1967.
9. Opler, M. K. Adolescence in cross-cultural perspective. In *Modern Perspectives in Adolescent Psychiatry* J. G. Howells Ed. Brunner-Mazel, New York, 1971.

10. Rabin, A. I. *Growing Up in the Kibbutz*. Springer, New York, 1965.
11. Rabin, A. I. Some sex differences in the attitudes of kibbutz adolescents. *Israel Ann. Psychiat.*, 6 (1968), 62–69.
12. Spiro, M. E. *Children of the Kibbutz*. Harvard University Press, Cambridge, 1958.
13. Talmon, Y. *Family and Community in the Kibbutz*. Harvard University Press, Cambridge, 1972.

Adolescents' Adjustment to Change as Related to Their Perceived Similarity to Parents and Peers: A Study Within the Kibbutz System

Michaela Lifshitz, Ph.D. (Israel)

Background

THE KIBBUTZ SYSTEM AS A SOCIAL UTOPIA

The birth of the kibbutz at the beginning of the 20th century was embedded within a social ideal [29, 49]. The small communal social structure signified for its pioneers the dream of democracy, equality, and self-regulation through close human contacts. The educational system of the kibbutz has favored upbringing of children in peer-group quarters rather than parents' homes [7]. Total population of the kibbutz has been remarkably small (currently 3 percent of Israel's population of about 3 million). Nevertheless, for youth inside and outside Israel the kibbutz as a concept has remained a social utopia, a rarified answer to their search for meaning in life, for the lost feeling of usefulness and belonging.

Varied studies, which can be arranged in an ascending develop-

* The research was supported by the Oranim Child Guidance Clinic of the Kibbutzim and by a grant from the University of Haifa.

171

mental order, have emphasized that kibbutz youngsters by and large bear little resemblance to institutionalized children in their rate of development (contrary to implications of the findings of several earlier studies, [53, 58, 62]) but more closely resemble children of the urban upper middle class [18, 24, 27, 30, 31, 32, 35, 40]. In reference to social skills, Kaffman [26] reported no autism among kibbutz children and very low incidence of delinquency. Lifshitz [32] and Shapira and Madsen [59] hinted at the high degree of cooperativeness and mutual support up to the beginning of adolescence when a competitive strategy begins to emerge. Adult kibbutz youngsters were reported to show more audacity and a higher sense of social responsibility than urban youngsters by volunteering for dangerous roles and assuming leadership positions in the army [1].

These findings, which were long preceded by the prevalence of favorable impressions, paved the road to the conclusion that the kibbutz could be considered a better alternative than an institution, foster parents, or continuing to live in former conditions for an urban child who suffered from an unfortunate circumstance in the form of a loss of a parent or growing up in a disadvantaged family [48]. Gerson [17] writes that "there are few problems and conflicts of the individual which do not occur in the kibbutz as well; but the *different social system* often provides alleviations and remedies which are not available in the traditional family situation" (p. 56). In actuality, children who survived the Holocaust found a new home within the kibbutz, as did children whose family structure was considered to be problematic or who were problematic themselves. Lifshitz et al. [44] found that kibbutz children who had lost their fathers in war faired better than bereaved urban children in their adjustment to the loss.

POSSIBLE CONTRIBUTING FACTORS

In our times the probability of disruption of family structure increases not only because of wars but also because of changes in family roles [36], higher rates of divorce, lack of the support of the extended family, and shattered social ideals. If we accept the kibbutz as a better alternative to institutions or foster homes, then it would be useful to pinpoint and specify those elements within the system that could be beneficial and contributive to the making of a more socially desired person. Some studies emphasize the element of security the child derives from:

1. The small, relatively stabilized social structure [17, 32, 36].
2. The upbringing within a peer group from very early age, when the concept of sameness is emphasized by the educational authorities [5]; sameness in this respect fosters security in contrast to the feeling of being different and alienated [42].
3. The physical arrangement of the kibbutz, which encourages inspection of surroundings with reduced fear of harm [35].

On the other hand, it was suggested [56] that the better social skills of kibbutz youngsters can be attributed to the higher degree of their perceptual differentiation because as children they interact closely with different socializing agents as well as other children [48, 49, 54]. However, perceptual differentiation was studied only in respect to neutral stimuli [56] and not in the sphere of interpersonal perception.

Lifshitz [33, 39] offered a model (see Figure 1) in which she shows how the need for permanence, sameness, and security, on the one

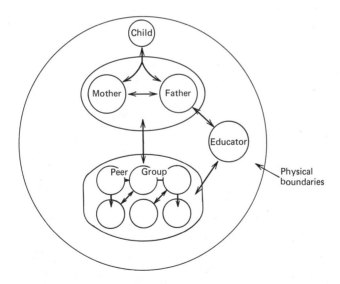

Figure 1. The kibbutz as a multifocal socialization system: physical and perceptual space.

hand, and the need for differentiation and diversity, on the other, are available within the subculture of the kibbutz [28]. Desirable development is viewed as an interplay or an integration between obtaining security and seeking change [16, 43].

PERSON PERCEPTION AND IDENTITY

The psychology of personal constructs is concerned with the ideas and concepts people use when they attempt to impose patterns of meaning on their experience [3, 28]. It is concerned with the way in which human beings construe their world, especially their own behavior and the behavior of other people. Differentiation is regarded as a prerequisite to the development of a coherent cognitive system with which the child organizes and manipulates the world around him, including that of his interpersonal world [38]. The person described with more care and variability than others is considered to be the one whose behavior the child is trying to emulate [45]. Livesley and Bromley [45] contended that between the ages of 8 and 12 years the global evaluative concepts become differentiated into more specific and precise terms, which could be an outcome of a search for useful, predictive psychological concepts. Girls may be more perceptually advanced than boys, that is, more aware of the variety of psychological qualities people possess, perhaps because they have a greater interest and need for persons than do boys [43].

Implicit in the theory of personal constructs [28] is the assumption that an individual's construct system is closely related to his overt behavior (see also [38]). Bannister and Fransella [3] view construing as a fundamental process and regard construct systems as changing strategies for dealing with the person's world.

The multifocal socialization system (see Figure 1) exercised within the relatively stable kibbutz milieu enables the child to inspect, repeatedly, various and different forms of behavior of people who are meaningful to him (e.g., father, mother, peers, caretakers) and to reach around adolescence a feeling of individualized identity. The latter is viewed as an integration of differentiated characteristics the youngster has perceived in his surroundings and can identify as "self" [13]. Lynn [46] considers the perception of sameness to a designed figure to be a necessary step in the development of identification. This perception may help a youngster to withstand the change of moving from a stabilized milieu to one in which he encounters a greater diversity of people and requirements.

QUESTIONS AND HYPOTHESES OF PRESENT STUDY

If we assume that the kibbutz is a milieu which offers both stability and diversity, and that the kibbutz is often the preferable alternative for a child of unfortunate social or family circumstances, several questions are posed in this study with regard to two groups of children—those children who have intact families (both mother and father living together) in the kibbutz and those whose family structure is disrupted (one or both parents are missing or live outside the kibbutz):

1. What are the specific behavioral strategies employed by problematic children from intact and disrupted families as compared to those who are considered to be adjusted?
2. In what way is the interpersonal perceptual structure of adjusted adolescents different from that of children who are considered to be problematic?
3. Is the perceptual structure of children of intact families different from that of children from disrupted families? Do adjusted adolescents from disrupted families employ a different perceptual strategy than adjusted children from intact families? Inversely, is the perception of problematic children from disrupted families different from the perception of problematic children from intact families? How are their perceptual strategies related to their ability to adjust well to drastic environmental changes?
4. Will boys employ different perceptual and behavioral strategies than girls, taking into account their family structure and general adjustment level?

Study I

SUBJECTS

Included in the study were 116 fifth- to eighth-grade children (ages 10–14) raised within the kibbutz. The subjects belonged to nine classes, each class from a different kibbutz. The classes were chosen arbitrarily out of those with which the teacher-supervisors were in touch in the Child Guidance Clinic of the Kibbutzim for the purpose of receiving guidance in treating problematic children in their classes. Excluded were children of known mental or organic deficit. The subjects were composed of 62 boys and 54 girls. Of these 70 were considered to be adjusted children and were not, at the time of the study or shortly before it, under the treatment of the clinic. The other 46 children were considered to be problematic and were either treated by the clinic staff or by a special educator within the kibbutz under the clinic's supervision. Their names were secured through the clinic files and rechecked in an interview with their teachers. Thirty-eight of the problematic children were described by their teachers as social problems (e.g., showing symptoms of aggression, withdrawal, lack of cooperation), and the other eight problematics were considered socially adjusted but lagging in a specific function (e.g., low concentration span). Out of the entire group of subjects, 36 children came from disrupted families (e.g., father died, parents divorced), and at least one of them did not live within the kibbutz.

PROCEDURE

Each subject responded to a task that was presented to the class as a group by the teacher-supervisor. Teachers were naive in regard to the goals of the task or the method of analysis.

Independently, each of the teacher-supervisors (all females) was asked to complete a structured questionnaire, in which she transmitted in detail her impression of the subject.

DEPENDENT MEASURES

Bieri Test of Cognitive Complexity [8].   This test had previously been used with urban adolescents [34, 37]. The test, presented in a 10×10 grid form, assessed the subject's perception of differences in self and among meaningful figures in his social sphere in reference to attributes he commonly uses in describing himself and others. The attributes of kibbutz adolescents were obtained in a pilot study in which the subjects were asked to describe themselves, each of their parents, and a male and a female friend. The 10 most common bipolar attributes were presented to the subjects of this study on the rows of the grid, in conjunction with six-point rating scales. The attributes were good looking–ugly, smart–stupid, popular–unpopular, strong–weak, good/helpful to others–bad, thin–fat, nervous–re-

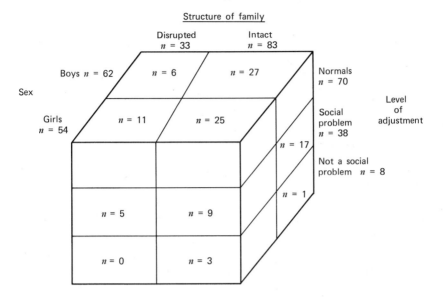

Figure 2. Subjects' distribution according to sex, level of adjustment, and structure of the family.

laxed, old–young, like to work–lazy, and pleasant–unpleasant. The 10 figures, which the subject was asked to rate for their relative "possession" of these attributes, were self, good friend of the same sex, mother, most successful child, father, obnoxious child, good friend of the opposite sex, highly regarded teacher, another loved adult, and brother or sister (or, if lacking, a child who might be regarded as such).

Scoring. Each of the grids was analyzed to yield the following information:

1. The most differentiated figure, that is, the one out of the ten figures whom the child rated more diversely than others.
2. The least differentiated figure, that is, the one rated less diversely than others.
3. The quantity of differences perceived between self-father, self-mother, and mother-father according to a method developed by Osgood et al. [57].
4. The most highly regarded attribute when subject's description of self was compared to that of the most successful child. The

most highly regarded attribute was considered to be that in which the biggest difference was found between the two figures in favor of the "most successful child."

5. The general cognitive complexity score, which is the sum of differences within each of the ten figures.

Teacher's Questionnaire. This was a modified form of a Behavior Check List employed previously [9, 42]. It was aimed at obtaining a detailed description of each child, independent of the fact that he was considered to be a problem child and had been treated by the clinic. The questionnaire included background information about the child (e.g., family status, chronic diseases) and 182 behavioral manifestations arranged randomly. The manifestations belonged to the following clusters: social relations (e.g., intensity of interactions with same-sex peers), aggressive behavior (e.g., curses, interrupts activities of others), self-concept (e.g., expresses negative attitude toward own body: "I am ugly"), extreme affective expressions (e.g., usually sad); fears (e.g., fear of being left alone), learning difficulties (e.g., in reading), and problems with control of bodily functions (e.g., enuresis, hyperactivity). On a three-point scale the teacher was asked to rate each of the specific manifestations on its present frequency and intensity, and also to indicate whether it was present as such in the past.

Scoring. Teacher's ratings were summed within each of the behavioral categories; separately for present and for past behavior.

RESULTS

Each of the obtained scores was analyzed in an analysis of variance for uneven groups. The three independent variables in the $2 \times 3 \times 2$ factorial design were sex (boys and girls), level of adjustment (adjusted, social problems, other problems), and family structure (intact versus disrupted). Intelligence was included as a control variable, since subjects exercised a verbal skill.

A. Teacher's Questionnaire. Tables 1 and 2 display the mean scores ($\bar{X}$) and standard deviations (SD) of those groups that were found to differ significantly in any of the dependent measures and the relevant F values. No main effect for sex or a significant interaction of it with other factors was found.

Table 1: Means and Standard Deviations of Problematic Manifestations on Teacher's Checklist, According to Level of Adjustment

Variable		A_1 n 70	A_2 38	A_3 8	F value df 2/113
			Level of Adjustment		
1. Social relationships	$\bar{x}$	54.43	65.08	62.08	10.18[a]
	SD	11.89	12.69	12.69	
2. Present aggressive	$\bar{x}$	3.34	5.47	6.50	5.09
interactions	SD	3.64	4.27	4.41	
3. Past aggressive	$\bar{x}$	0.27	1.24	1.00	6.22[a]
interactions	SD	0.78	2.02	1.93	
4. Present negative	$\bar{x}$	12.71	21.84	20.00	6.87[a]
self - concept	SD	11.88	13.82	12.54	
5. Present extreme	$\bar{x}$	19.68	36.45	24.38	10.87[a]
affects	SD	17.22	19.82	12.66	
6. Present fears	$\bar{x}$	9.64	17.24	40.00	10.68[a]
	SD	31.84	20.02	31.84	
7. Present learning	$\bar{x}$	11.57	35.40	36.88	18.62[a]
problems	SD	15.58	28.81	27.89	
8. Present control of	$\bar{x}$	2.69	8.08	25.25	13.36[a]
bodily functions	SD	8.45	15.68	18.75	
9. Past control of	$\bar{x}$	0.36	1.37	1.00	5.46[a]
bodily functions	SD	1.02	2.21	1.14	

[a] $p < .01$.
A_1—Adjusted; A_2—Social problem; A_3—Not a social problem.

Those who were generally considered to be social problematics when compared to the adjusted subjects were also reported by the teachers to have a higher rate of past and present aggressive behavior, learning problems, characteristics indicative of negative self-concept, and difficulties in controlling affective expression. Fears and difficulties in controlling body functions and movements were especially prevalent among the not-social problematics (see Table 1).

Also, significant interactions of level of adjustment with family structure were found (see Table 2) for:

1. Social relationships. Subjects from disrupted families, whether being considered adjusted or socially problematic, were viewed as being far less aggressive than children from intact homes, in the past ($p < .01$) as well as in the present ($p < .05$).

Table 2: Means and Standard Deviations of Problematic Manifestations on Teacher's Checklist, According to Interaction of Adjustment and Structure of Family

Variable		SA_1 n 53	SA_2 17	SA_3 26	SA_4 12	SA_5 4	SA_6 4	F value df 5/110
				Structure of Family and Adjustment				
1. Social relationships	$\bar{x}$	54.43	54.41	64.65	66.00	62.50	61.50	3.99[a]
	SD	12.21	11.19	14.17	9.22	6.86	8.74	
2. Present aggressive	$\bar{x}$	3.42	3.12	6.00	4.33	6.00	7.00	2.35[a]
interactions	SD	3.81	3.14	4.55	3.47	2.83	6.05	
3. Past aggressive	$\bar{x}$	0.28	0.24	1.65	0.33	0.75	1.25	4.20[a]
interactions	SD	0.84	0.56	2.31	0.49	1.50	2.50	
4. Present negative	$\bar{x}$	12.93	12.06	22.50	20.42	12.50	27.50	3.38[a]
self-concept	SD	11.62	12.99	13.73	14.53	6.15	13.22	
5. Present extreme	$\bar{x}$	17.76	25.89	37.31	34.58	20.00	28.75	4.98[a]
affects	SD	14.96	22.42	21.46	16.44	4.08	17.50	
6. Present fears	$\bar{x}$	7.55	16.18	22.31	6.25	46.25	33.75	6.74[a]
	SD	12.31	20.81	21.78	8.82	22.50	41.91	
7. Present learning	$\bar{x}$	11.04	13.24	35.19	35.83	26.25	47.50	7.84[a]
problems	SD	13.31	14.68	25.39	36.42	19.31	33.78	
8. Present control of	$\bar{x}$	1.64	5.94	.0127	3.33	40.00	10.50	9.78[a]
bodily functions	SD	1.56	16.89	18.51	3.47	8.16	13.18	
9. Past control of	$\bar{x}$	0.36	0.35	1.73	0.58	1.50	0.50	3.34[a]
bodily functions	SD	1.07	0.86	2.52	0.99	1.73	1.00	

[a] $p < .01$.
Structure adjustment: SA_1—adjusted from intact home; SA_2—adjusted from disrupted home; SA_3—social problem from intact home; SA_4—social problem from disrupted home; SA_5—not a social problem from intact home; SA_6—not a social problem from disrupted home.

2. Negative self-concept. It was especially prevalent among those children from disrupted families who were not social problematic ($p < .01$).

3. Extreme affective expression. Among the adjusted subjects the frequency of extreme affective expressions was remarkably higher for those from disrupted families compared with those from intact families ($p < .01$).

3. Fears. The adjusted subjects from disrupted families showed far more fears than those from intact families. The situation is reversed within the group of social problematics: there, the children from intact families showed more fears than those from

disrupted families. The social problematics from disrupted families were reported to show fewer fears than any of the other groups ($p < .01$).
4. Bodily control. The problematic subjects from intact families were reported to show in the past more difficulties than the adjusted subjects from intact or disrupted families ($p < .01$). In reference to the present time the adjusted subjects from disrupted families were reported to show far more difficulties in bodily control than adjusted subjects from intact families ($p < .01$).

B. Bieri Test of Cognitive Complexity. Tables 3 and 4 display the mean scores ($\bar{X}$) and standard deviations (SD) of those groups that were found to differ significantly in any of the dependent measures (Table 3) and its interactions (Table 4). No main effect for sex was found; also, an interaction of the sex variable with other variables was not found to be significant in any of the measures. The following were noted:

Table 3: Adolescents' Responses to Bieri's Test—Means and Standard Deviations of Groups in Respect to Structure of the Family and Level of Adjustment

Variable		Structure of Family			Level of Adjustment			
		S_1 n 83	S_2 33	F value df 1/114	A_1 70	A_2 38	A_3 8	F value df 2/113
1. Most differentiated figure: same-sex friend	$\bar{x}$ SD	0.43 1.59	1.58 3.41	4.85[a]				NS
2. Most differentiated figure: successful child	$\bar{x}$ SD	0.30 1.63	1.30 3.32	4.74[a]				NS
3. Least differentiated figure: father	$\bar{x}$ SD	0.52 2.03	2.12 4.14	8.74[b]				NS
4. Quantity of differences: self-father	$\bar{x}$ SD	4.85 1.56	4.09 1.75	5.15[a]				NS
5. Quantity of differences: self-mother	$\bar{x}$ SD			NS	4.16 1.34	5.25 1.85	4.85 2.41	5.73[b]

[a] $p < .05$.
[b] $P < .01$.
Structure of family: S_1—intact families; S_2—disrupted families; level of adjustment: A_1—adjusted; A_2—social problem; A_3—not a social problem.

Table 4: Adolescents' Responses to Bieri's Test—Means and Standard Deviations of Groups in Respect to Interaction of Structure of Family and Level of Adjustment

Variable		SA_1 n 53	SA_2 17	SA_3 26	SA_4 12	SA_5 4	SA_6 4	F value df 5/110
1. Least differentiated	$\bar{x}$	0.66	2.94	0.31	1.03	0.0	2.50	2.26^a
	SD	2.40	4.69	1.12	2.93	0.0	5.00	
2. Quantity of differ-	$\bar{x}$	4.57	3.65	5.30	4.64	5.55	4.33	2.52^a
ences: self-father	SD	1.35	1.99	1.93	1.36	0.66	1.51	
3. Quantity of differ-	$\bar{x}$	4.19	4.05	5.37	4.97	5.55	4.15	2.70^a
ences: self-mother	SD	1.44	0.98	1.98	1.59	2.78	3.41	
								NS
4. Preferred construct:	$\bar{x}$	0.76	1.77	2.89	0.67	0	0	2.35^a
relaxation, not	SD	2.43	3.40	4.21	1.61	0	0	
nervous								

$^a p < .05$.
Structure adjustment: SA_1—adjusted from intact home; SA_2—adjusted from disrupted home; SA_3—social problem from intact home; SA_4—social problem from disrupted home; SA_5—not a social problem from intact home; SA_6—not a social problem from disrupted home.

1. The most differentiated figure. For subjects of disrupted families, the figures of a good friend of the same sex and the most successfully personally known child were more differentiated than for the children of intact families ($p < .05$).
2. The least differentiated figure. For subjects of disrupted families the father was significantly more frequently the least differentiated figure ($p < .01$) compared to subjects from intact homes. Additionally, a significant interaction between the level of adjustment and the family structure was found; the father was found to be the least differentiated among those children from disrupted families who were considered to be well adjusted ($p < .05$).
3. Perceived differences between self–father–mother. Differences between self and father were found to be significantly lower among children of disrupted families compared to children of intact families ($p < .05$). Also, a significant interaction was found between level of adjustment and family structure ($p < .05$): the adjusted subject of a disrupted family perceived

differences between self and father to be much smaller than did other groups, whereas the largest perceived difference between self and father was found among the groups of problematic children from intact families. For self and mother the smallest perceived difference was found among adjusted children, whereas the largest difference between self and mother was found among the social-problem subjects ($p < .01$). The significant interaction between the level of adjustment and the structure of the family ($p < .05$) indicates that the adjusted subjects of disrupted families, as well as those of intact families, perceived the difference between themselves and their mothers to be the smallest. The biggest perceived difference between self and mother appeared among the groups of problematic children of intact families. Perceived difference between mother and father was not found to differentiate significantly among the groups.

4. The most highly regarded attribute. A significant interaction between the level of adjustment and the structure of the family was found for the attribute of "relaxed, not nervous" ($p < .05$). The social problematics from intact families, especially, regarded the most successful child as superior to them in "relaxation," but this attribute was also found to be highly desired among the adjusted children of disrupted families.

5. General cognitive complexity scores. Subjects' groups were not found to differ significantly from each other on this measure.

Study II

SUBJECTS

One year after the completion of Study I, a follow-up study was conducted on 42 of the 116 subjects. These 42 subjects were sixth graders at the time of Study I. On graduation, they moved to a regional school, away from their home kibbutz. The subjects in the present study (now seventh graders, aged 12–13), were situated in eight classes at four regional schools. The children were originally from four different kibbutzim.

The sample consisted of 25 boys and 17 girls. Of them 26 came from intact homes, and 16 were from broken homes. Prior to the move 17 of the children were considered by their teachers to be adjusted; 17 were considered to be social problematics, and 8 were considered to have other problems.

The move to the regional school, which is a complete live-in social-educational setting, constituted a major change in the children's lives, because

1. The small, tight-knit peer group is broken down; the children are dispersed to different classes and intermingle with children from different kibbutzim. The children have to reestablish their social position within a new hierarchy.
2. In contrast to the home-kibbutz, where children were taught by the same teacher, a member of that kibbutz, the children are now exposed to an array of teachers who are not necessarily members of the kibbutz.
3. The children are, literally, away from their parents most of the week.

Experimenter.   All testing and scorings were carried out by one experimenter.[1]

Measures.   The group administered Bieri Test of Cognitive Complexity (discussed in Study I) was used. The test was given to entire classes, in order not to single out the subjects. However, only the responses of the 42 subjects were later scored. The scores obtained were (1) the degree of differentiation for each of the 10 significant figures where each rating was successively compared with all other ratings for that figure [37], (2) the general score of cognitive complexity, which is the sum of differences within each of the 10 figures, and (3) the quantity of differences between pairs of figures (e.g., self and mother, self and most successful child, self and father, mother and father).

The teacher-supervisor of each new class was interviewed individually to find out which students they considered to be adaptive or to have a social or other kind of problem (e.g., a specific learning disability). The teachers were also presented with a grid, in which the 10 rows pertained to the same attributes given to the children (e.g., smart–stupid, popular–unpopular). Each column represented a student in the class. The teacher was asked to rate each student according to his/her position on each of the attributes-rating scales. Only col-

1 Thanks go to Mrs. Shulla Tubin, from the Oranim Child Guidance Clinic, for so effectively conducting the work.

umns pertaining to the 42 subjects were scored. The degree of differentiation within each subject's column was then measured.

RESULTS

The childrens' past and present grid scores as well as the present teacher's grid score with regard to degree of differentiation of each subject were analyzed for the main effects of sex, family structure (intact versus disrupted), and past and present adjustment (according to teacher's report). Also included was a score comparing past and present adjustment according to four categories: adjusted today and in the past, problematic today and in the past, problematic in the past but not today, and problematic today but not in the past. Means and standard deviations (SD) of significant main effects are shown in Tables 5, 6, and 7.

Table 5: Analysis According to Subjects' Present Adjustment:
Means and SD of Significant Grid Scores

Variable	F df 2/41	Group 1, n = 30 Normals	Group 2, n = 7 Social Problems	Group 3, n = 5 Other Problems
How differentially	5.11[a]			
present teacher perceives	$\bar{x}$	30.53[c]	36.29[d]	35.20[c, d]
subject	SD	5.39	2.14	3.96
Child's *present* degree	3.59[a]			
of differentiation of	$\bar{x}$	31.43[c]	35.29[d]	37.20[d]
another child he dislikes	SD	7.16	3.86	2.68
Past degree of dif-	3.33[a]			
ferentiation of the	$\bar{x}$	30.60[c]	40.14[d]	30.60[c, d]
"mother" figure	SD	5.28	14.83	6.58
Child's perception of differ-	5.58[b]			
ences between self and	$\bar{x}$	37.50[c]	52.00[d]	54.00[d]
mother (*past* grid)	SD	11.48	16.80	19.81
Child's perception of differ-	3.57[a]			
ences: self and successful	$\bar{x}$	37.83[c]	55.86[d]	43.00[c, d]
child (*past* grid)	SD	16.47	17.88	9.46

[a] $p < .05$.
[b] $p < .01$.
[c] Subset 1 in Scheffe procedure for .05 level.
[d] Subset 2 in Scheffe procedure for .05 level.

Table 6: **Analysis for the Main Effect of Differences between Subjects' Past and Present Adjustment: Means and SD of Significant Grid Scores**

Variable	*F* df 3/41	Group 1, n = 16 Adjusted: Past and Present	Group 2, n = 2 Problematic: Present Adjusted: Past	Group 3, n = 14 Problematic: Past Adjusted: Present	Group 4, n = 10 Problematic: Past and Present
How differentially the subject is perceived by present teacher	4.10[a]				
	$\bar{x}$	31.69[b]	36.50[c]	29.21[b]	35.70[c]
	SD	6.09	0.71	4.28	3.19
Subject's degree of differentiation of another child he dislikes (present grid)	2.98[a]				
	$\bar{x}$	33.56[b]	37.00[b]	29.00[c]	35.90[b]
	SD	6.03	0.00	7.77	3.76
Subject's perception of differences between self and mother (past grid)	3.79[a]				
	$\bar{x}$	36.06[b]	50.50[c]	39.14[b]	53.30[c]
	SD	10.47	9.19	12.73	18.79

[a] $p < .05$.
[b] Subset 1 in Scheffe procedure for .05 level.
[c] Subset 2 in Scheffe procedure for .05 level.

Table 7: Analysis according to Subjects' Family Structure:
Means and SD of Significant Grid Scores

Variable	F 1/41	Intact Homes $n = 26$	Broken Homes $n = 16$
Present grid:	6.37^a		
Differentiation of	$\bar{x}$	29.12	32.81
most-successful	SD	5.48	3.49
child			
Past grid:	4.34^a		
Differentiation	$\bar{x}$	34.04	29.18
of "mother"	SD	11.14	4.51
Past grid:	4.03^a		
Differentiation	$\bar{x}$	31.65	27.88
of "father"	SD	4.45	7.29

$^a p < .05$.

According to the present teacher's report, 30 of the children (17 boys and 13 girls) were considered to be adjusted; 7 were considered to be social problematics (5 boys and 2 girls), and 5 were considered to have a special problem (3 boys and 2 girls). It seems that, generally, regardless of the children's sex and their family structure, children were presently regarded more positively than prior to the change. Subjects who, following the change, were considered by the teacher and also by the children (in reference to a child they dislike) to behave in an adaptive way were perceived to be significantly ($p < .05$) less differentiated than children who were regarded as problematics (see Tables 5 and 6).

Past grid score pertaining to the subject's perception of difference between himself and his mother, as well as degree of differentiation within the "mother" figure, distinguished significantly between children who adjusted well to the change and those who did not ($p < .05$). This result also pertained to the child's past perception of the degree of differences between himself and the most successful child he knows personally ($p < .05$). Subjects who adjusted well to the new situation, whether they were considered in the past to be normal or problematic (see Table 5) perceived significantly less difference between themselves and the mother, on the one hand ($p < .01$), and themselves and the most successful child, on the other hand ($p < .05$).

The subjects from broken homes (see Table 7) were found, after the change, to differentiate the most successful child they know personally significantly more than did the children from intact homes ($p < .05$). In their past grid the 42 subjects differentiated their mother and father to a significantly less extent than did children from intact homes ($p < .05$).

Discussion

The findings throw light on the ways in which adolescents—going through a transient period in their lives with more or less immediate parental support, but who at the same time are exposed to the stable, yet diversified, kibbutz environment—adjust to their milieu in terms of overt behavioral manifestations and in terms of integration of their perceptual field.

To adjust well to the environment, kibbutz children from disrupted families, relying less on the combined support of both parents [34, 37, 61], must employ perceptual and behavioral strategies that are somewhat different from those of children who have both parents interacting as an intact unit.

BEHAVIORAL MANIFESTATIONS

Problem kibbutz children from intact families manifested the prevalent array of undesired characteristics [9]. At the same time, children (both problematic and adjusted) from disrupted families, were regarded as less aggressive in their social interactions than were children from intact homes. Studies on urban population [23, 51, 60] discussed responses of open aggression and acting-out behavior among maladjusted fatherless adolescents. It could be that the kibbutz children from disrupted families internalized their aggression (see also [28, 23, 42]) out of fear that they might, during the stressful period of adolescence, lose the remaining supporting ties within their family and the closed social group. In the present study those children from disrupted families who were considered to be well adjusted were those who, although restrained in their interpersonal relationships, overtly expressed their anxiety by showing extreme affects, fears, and restlessness. By their own account, the adjusted children from disrupted families saw themselves as far more inferior to their ideal peer in level of nervousness and lack of relaxation. It seemed as if these children were in a kind of an agitated state, actively trying, in a process similar to an adult type of mourning response [50, 60], to reconstrue their lost family ties, thereby undergoing a process of change and adaptation [44]. On the other hand, those children from disrupted families who were regarded as problematic were characterized by their attempt to restrain the expression of intrapsychic concerns. By not giving any overt manifestation of their possible anxiety and fears due to change and loss of family support, it is probably that those children actually did not go through the process that could enable them to restructure the change and adapt to new circumstances.

INTERPERSONAL PERCEPTUAL DIFFERENTIATION

Results of the present study indicate that the degree of differentiation of self and meaningful others may hint at adaptive mechanisms. The degree of differentiation could also predict future adjustment to drastic environmental changes, regardless of the adolescent's actual family structure or his/her sex (see also [67]).

Perception of Parents. Children from disrupted families, especially those who were adjusted, reported the least amount of differences between themselves and the oft-absent father, who was perceived in very global and undifferentiated terms; whereas problematic children from intact families reported the greatest difference. Also, in reference to differentiation of self and mother, adjusted children from disrupted families, who in most cases had a direct access to the mother, reported fewer differences than did problematic children. The largest difference between self and mother was reported by problematics from intact homes (see also [17]). Those children who, before moving to the mixed regional school away from their home base, reported less differences between themselves and the mother and made a better adjustment to the new situation than those who perceived fewer similarities between themselves and their mother, regardless of whether they had been formerly considered to be problematic or not.

Livesley and Bromley [45], who studied urban English children aged 7 to 15, found global undifferentiated perception of parents and differentiated and articulated perceptions of friends. These researchers explained their findings by noting the children's close and frequent contact with peers, out of the children's own choice, compared to the often forced and limited contacts with adults. Their finding that mothers were often described in global undifferentiated form was attributed to the notion that the mother represented the less-preferred sex. However, the findings of the present study, along with others [34, 44], show that the relative lack of differentiation of parental figures is associated with good adjustment to environmental disruption. The more the child's reality is disrupted, the more he, in order to adjust well to broader environmental demands, tends to perceive himself as close and similar to the mother.

Other studies, conducted on the social schemata of preadolescents and adults [12, 14, 15, 65, 66], have shown that the disturbed individual places greater distance between figures than did normals. The latter placed themselves closer to mother than to father or peer figures. Distance from mother tended to decrease following psychotherapy [20, 64]. Parkes [55] noted, while studying 2 year olds, that the mother is a mobile base from which forays can be made into a semifamiliar world. To the young toddler, mother is a haven of safety, and it is from this personal bond between child and mother that all subsequent relationships develop. Later on in life, when encountered with the necessity of adapting to seminovel circumstances, the child derives a feeling of security from the perception of similarity to the mother, just as the young child derives a feeling of security from close physical and affective contacts with the mother.

In reference to the father, perception of him as a solidified (global) figure and perception of similarity to him may further act to strengthen for the child of a disrupted home the base from which he can embark to inspect his outer surroundings (see [5, 10, 47]). It is the mother, however, who seems to provide the adolescent with an anchor or stability necessary to counteract feelings of disintegration. Thus focusing on the child's perception of differentiation of self from mother would seem to be useful for predicting future positive adjustment to stress caused by leaving home (and thus losing direct contact with parents).

It seems that in the kibbutz social system, with its emphasis on communal rearing of children, a strong parent-child tie exists [11, 17, 46, 47], and the child's perception of his nuclear family extends its influence on the child's behavior in a wide range of social areas. Though kibbutz parents are assumed to share equally in nurturing and directing the child, the importance of the mother figure stands out, as it does in many other Westernized and industrialized cultures [22, 25, 38]. This is especially apparent when the child is confronted with the need to test out seminew surroundings and opportunities [6, 21, 58].

Bannister [2], while elaborating on Kelly's [28] notion of transition, makes the point that "while a person's interpretation of himself and his world is probably constantly changing to some degree, there are times when his experiences of varying validational fortunes make change, or resistance to change, a matter of major concern. At such times we try to nail down our psychological furniture to avoid change or we try to lunge forward . . ." Narrowing of the perceptual field, as seen here by the adolescents' decrease of perceptual distances to parents, is perceived as an adaptive function vis-a-vis disruptive circumstances. It is in accord with Kelly's [28] concept of tightening as a defense against anxiety [4, 37]. It is "a kind of protective behavior" ([28], p. 498). Perception of similarity to parents acts as a security ring. Only when it is present can the adolescent interact satisfactorily with the multitude of stimuli and figures that he encounters on his way to adulthood. Tightening within the family system may be a prerequisite to the process of loosening and for an attempt at reconstruction within the broader social sphere, including that of the peer group.

Perception of Peers. McNelly [52] expressed his impression that during adolescence it is the individual's social roles and achievements with respect to his relationships with peers that are of major relevance to his feeling of identity and self-worth.

The kibbutz, with its multifocal socialization agents and its continued emphasis on peer-group upbringing, provides conditions for person differentiation that supplement the family structure. The reciprocal interaction among peers seems to be an indispensable condition for the formation of logical grouping structures in middle childhood. The concept of self is developed by contrasting oneself with other meaningful figures [4]. Vis-a-vis the relatively undifferentiated form of adjusted-adolescents' perception of parental figures and their close similarity to them, particularly to the mother, the best same sex friend and the most successful child known personally become the most meaningful stimulus persons (as contrasting points) in the differentiation process [45, 63]. As a matter of fact, it seems that in predicting adolescents' adjustment to change it is the perception, before the change, of similarity to the most successful child that is important, in addition to similarity to mother figure.

Findings of the present study suggest that an intervention strategy of focusing on the child's or adolescent's perceived similarities and differences to key people in his life would be beneficial for those undergoing stress related to leaving home and the adjustment which this entails.

References

1. Amir, Y. The effectiveness of kibbutz-born soldiers in the Israel Defense Forces. *Hum. Relat.*, 22 (1969) , 333.
2. Bannister, D. The logic of passion. In *Perspectives in Personal Construct Theory*, D. Bannister, Ed. Academic, London, 1977.
3. Bannister, D. and Fransella, F. *Inquiring Man: The Theory of Personal Constructs*. Penguin, Hardmonsworth, England, 1971.
4. Bannister, D. and Agnew, J. The child's construction of self. In *Enquiries into Personal Construct Theory* (report to the Nebraska Symposium on P.C.T. 1975). Lincoln, University of Nebraska Press, 1976.
5. Becker, J. and McArdle, J. Nonlexical speech similarities as an index of intrafamilial identifications. *J. Abnorm. Psychol.* 72 (1967), 408.
6. Bernard, J. *Women, Wives, Mothers*. London, Aldine, 1975.
7. Bettelheim, B. *The Children of the Dream*. New York, Macmillan, 1969.
8. Bieri, J., Atkins, A. L., Briar, S., Leaman, R. L., Miller, H., and Tripoli, T. *Clinical and Social Judgment: The Discrimination of Behavioral Information*. New York, Wiley, 1966.
9. Borgatta, E. F., and Fanshel, D. The child behavior characteristic (CBC) form: Revised age-specific forms. *Multivariate Behav. Res.*, 5 (1970), 49.
10. Cowan, P. A. Two measures of "inferred identification" in normal and emotionally disturbed children. Paper read at the Society for Research in Child Development meeting at Pennsylvania State University, March 1961.
11. Devereux, E. X., Shouval, R., Bronfenbrenner, U., Rodgers, R. R., Kav-Venaki, S., Kiely, E., and Karson, E. Socialization practices of parents, teachers, and peers in Israel: The kibbutz versus the city. *Child Dev.*, 45 (1974), 269.
12. DeHamel, T. R., and Jarmon, H. Social schemata of emotionally disturbed boys and their male siblings. *J. Consul. Clin. Psychol.*, 36 (1971), 281.
13. Erikson, E. H. *Childhood and Society*. New York, Norton, 1950.

14. Evans, G. W., and Howard, R. B. Personal space. *Psychol. Bull.* 80 (1973), 334.
15. Fisher, R. L. Social schema of normal and disturbed school children. *J. Educ. Psychol.*, 58 (1967), 88.
16. Fromm, E. *Escape from Freedom*. New York, Holt, Rinehart and Winston, 1941.
17. Gerson, M. The family in the kibbutz. *J. Child Psychol. Psychiat.*, 15:47; 1974.
18. Gewirtz, J. L. The course of smiling by groups of Israeli infants in the first 18 months of life. *Scripta Hierrosolymitanna*, 14 (1965), 9.
19. Gewirtz, H. B., and Gweirtz, J. L. Visiting and caretaking patterns for kibbutz infants: Age and sex trends. *Amer. J. Orthopsychiat.*, 38 (1968), 427.
20. Gottheil, E., and Paredes, A. Parental schemata in emotionally disturbed women. *J. Abnorm. Psychol.*, 73 (1968), 416.
21. Gould, J. (Ed.). *The Prevention of Damaging Stress in Children.* J. and A. Churchill, London, 1968.
22. Green, M. *Goodbye Father.* Routledge and Kegan Paul, London, 1976.
23. Hartup, W. W., & Zook, E. A. Sex-role preferences in three- and four-year-old children. *J. Consult. Psychol.*, 24 (1960), 420.
24. Holdstein, I. A Comparative Study of Children's Syntactic and Articulatory Abilities in Two Different Israeli Societies. M.A. thesis. Tel-Aviv University, 1974.
25. Hsu, F. L. K. (Ed.). *Kinship and Culture.* Aldine, Chicago, 1971.
26. Kaffman, M. A comparison of psychopathology: Israeli children from kibbutz and from urban surroundings. *Amer. J. Orthopsychiat.*, 35 (1965), 508.
27. Kaffman, M. Toilet-training by multiple caretakers: Enuresis among kibbutz children. *Israel Ann. Psychiat.*, 10 (1972), 341.
28. Kelly, G. A. *The Psychology of Personal Constructs.* (2 vols.) Norton, New York, 1955.
29. Kerem, M. The child and his family in the kibbutz—The environment. In *Children and Families in Israel,* Janis, A. et al. Eds. New York: Gordon & Breach, 1970.
30. Kohen-Raz, R. Mental and motor development of kibbutz, institutionalized and home-reared infants in Israel. *Child. Dev.*, 39 (1968), 489.
31. Landau, R., and Greenbaum, D. The emotional reactions of the mother during the first year of life in three sub-cultures. Paper presented at the International Conference on the Effects of the Environment on Cognitive Functioning in Children, Israeli Scientific Research Conferences, Arad, Israel, October 1974.
32. Lifshitz, M. Internal-external locus of control dimension as a function of age and the socialization milieu. *Child Dev.*, 44 (1973), 533.
33. Lifshitz, M. Is there any impact of the socialization milieu (kibbutz) on children's development? An invited paper, The International Conference on the Effects of the Environment on Cognitive Functioning in Children, Israeli Scientific Research Conferences, Arad, Israel, October 1974.
34. Lifshitz, M. Social differentiation and organization of the Rorschach in fatherless and two-parented children. *J. Clin. Psychol.*, 31 (1975), 126.
35. Lifshitz, M. Psychological and psychomotor tests. In *Follow-Up Study of High-Risk Children for Schizophrenia,* D. Rosenthal, Ed. National Institute of Mental Health, Bethesda, in press.
36. Lifshitz, M. Toward obliterating sex-role dichotomy: An alternative conception. *Israel Ann. Psychiat.*, 14 (1976), 74.

37. Lifshitz, M. Long range effects of father's loss. The cognitive complexity of bereaved children and their school adjustment. *Brit. J. Med. Psychol.,* 49 (1976) , 189.
38. Lifshitz, M. Person perception and social interaction of Jewish and Druze kindergarten children in Israel. *Ann. N. Y. Acad. Sci.* (in press), 1977.
39. Lifshitz, M. Girls' identity formation as related to perceptual development of family structure. *J. Marriage Family,* (in press).
40. Lifshitz, M., and Chovers, A. Encopresis among Kibbutz children. *Israel Ann. Psychiat.,* 10 (1972), 326.
41. Lifshitz, M., and Gerson, N. Stuttering among kibbutz children. *Kibbutz Educ.,* 76 (1972), 23 (in Hebrew).
42. Lifshitz, M., Baum, R., Balgur, I., and Cohen, D. The impact of the social milieu upon the nature of adoptees' emotional difficulties. *J. Marriage Family,* 37 (1975), 221.
43. Lifshitz, M., Reznikov, R., and Aran, M. Perceived similarities versus contrast between kibbutz parents and their preadolescent children's adjustment. *Child Psychiat. Human Dev.,* 5 (1975), 150.
44. Lifshitz, M., Berman, D., Gilad, D., and Galili, A. Bereaved children: The effect of mother's perception and social system organization on their short-range adjustment. *J. Amer. Asso. Child Psychiat.,* in press.
45. Livesley, W. J., and Bromley, D. B. *Person Perception in Children and Adolescents.* Wiley, New York, 1973.
46. Lynn, D. B. *Parental and Sex-Role Identification: A Theoretical Formulation.* McCutchan, Berkeley, Calif., 1969.
47. Lynn, D. B. *The Father: His Role in Child Development.* Brooks/Cole, Monterey, Calif., 1974.
48. Marcus, J. Early child development in kibbutz group care. *Early Child Dev. Care,* 1 (1971), 67.
49. Marcus, J., Thomas, A., & Chess, S. Behavioral individuality in kibbutz children. *Israel Ann. Psychiat.,* 7 (1969) , 43.
50. McConville, B. J., Boag, L. C., and Purohit, A. P. Three types of childhood depression. *Canad. Psychiat. Asso. J.,* 18 (1973), 133.
51. McCord, J., McCord, W., and Thurber, E. Some effects of paternal absence on male children. *J. Abnorm. Soc. Psychol.,* 64 (1964), 361.
52. McNelly, F. W. Jr. Development of the self concept in childhood: A brief historical review and an investigation of the effects of manipulating leadership position within a structured role system upon self concept, perception of locus of control, and performance. *Diss. Abstr.,* 34 (1974), 4024-B.
53. Nagler, S. Mental Health. In *Children and Families in Israel,* A. Janis, J. Marcus, G. Oren, and C. Rapaport, Eds. Gordon and Breach, New York, 1970.
54. Newbauer, P., Ed. *Children in Collectives.* Charles C. Thomas, Springfield, Ill., 1965.
55. Parkes, C. M. *Bereavement: Studies of Grief in Adult Life.* International Universities Press, New York, 1972.
56. Preale, I., Amir, Y., and Sharan, S. Perceptual articulation and task effectiveness in several Israeli sub-cultures. *J. Personal. Soc. Psychol.,* 15 (1970), 180.
57. Osgood, C. E., Suci., G. J., and Tannenbaum, P. H. *The Measurement of Meaning.* University of Illinois Press, Urbana, 1957.
58. Rabin, A. I. *Growing Up in the Kibbutz.* Springer, New York, 1965.

59. Shapira, A., and Madsen, M. C. Cooperative and competitive behavior of kibbutz and urban children in Israel. *Child Dev.*, 40 (1969), 609.
60. Shoor, M. and Speed, M. H. Death, delinquency, and the mourning process. *Psychiat. Quart.*, 37 (1963), 540.
61. Simmons, R. K. and Lamberth, E. L. Q Sort Technique as a means of determining the relation of family structure to self-concept. *Marriage Family Living*, 23 (1961), 183.
62. Spiro, M. *Children of the Kibbutz*. Harvard University Press, Cambridge, 1958.
63. Sullivan, H. S. *The Interpersonal Theory of Psychiatry*. Norton, New York, 1953.
64. Tolor, A. Psychological distance in disturbed and normal adults. *J. Clin. Psychol.*, 26 (1970), 160.
65. Tolor, A., and Orange, S. An attempt to measure psychological distance in advantaged and disadvantaged children. *Child Dev.*, 40 (1969), 407.
66. Weinstein, I. Social schemata of emotionally disturbed boys. *J. Abnorm. Psychol.*, 70 (1965), 457.
67. Wilde, J. E. A descriptive analysis of children's cognitive styles: Conceptual tempo and preferred mode of perceptual organization and conceptual categorization. *Diss. Abstr.* 1974, 34, 4013-A.

Modifiability During Adolescence: Theoretical Aspects and Empirical Data

Reuven Feuerstein, Ph.D., David Krasilowsky, and Yaacov Rand (Israel)

The theoretical framework for modifiability at the age of adolescence, presented in this chapter, is supported by empirical data from a variety of sources. Most of the data pertain to the cognitive area because it is, in many cases, the most important avenue for environmental intervention as well as the most accessible for systematic measurement.

Modifiability is herein defined as a structural modification in the functioning of the individual that reflects a change in the expected course of his development. Cognitive modifiability refers to such transformations in the structure of intellect of the individual that are essential for better adjustment to life requirements and situations. *Thus defined, "modifiability" differs from "change" in that change is produced by developmental and maturational processes, whereas modifiability represents a noticeable departure from the normal developmental course of the individual as determined by his genetic and/or neurophysiological and/or experiential educational background.*

Such structural modification, even when it is in the desired direction, is considered by many behavioral scientists as an aberration of the organism and, as such, not to be conceived of as a phenomenon that can be produced at will and relied on. Our report on significant changes obtained by the Treatment Group Technique (TGT) [8], with deeply disturbed, severely deficient-functioning adolescents provoked skepticism among some psychotherapists.

Reasons for the strong resistance to the concept of modifiability, particularly at adolescence, are numerous. Some of them are theoretical, and others are more practical. But as a result of this resistance, very few attempts have been made to create appropriate conditions for modifiability in adolescence; this, in turn, has also limited opportunities to analyze reported phenomena in an adequate theoretical perspective. The reliability of reports that indicate significant modifications is questioned or their theoretical implications are denied. There is, therefore, a strong need for a theory of the modifiability concept, not only as a basis for understanding the phenomenon, but also as the sole means of controlling it and producing it at will for the benefit of those in need. The outcome of a successful effort to validate such a theory would change considerably the current approach toward the adolescent segment of the population. Educational efforts would be geared to the active modification of the retarded-performing adolescent so as to make him more adaptable to life [7].

CASE STUDY

Martin is a 15-year-old severely retarded youngster with an IQ in the 35–40 range who was referred to the author 11 years ago by the welfare department of a European country for lifelong placement in custodial care. His transfer to Israel was in response to the last wishes of his Jewish mother.

The second of three brothers, Martin was born into a pathogenic family. His father was a schizophrenic, alcoholic, poorly adjusted,[1] Foreign Legion soldier who had met and married the mother during his service in North Africa. The mother, a primitive, illiterate, and cognitively retarded[1] woman died as a hospitalized, diagnosed psychotic.[1] Heredity had affected Martin and one of his brothers. In addition, Martin suffered brain damage,[1] produced by prematurity.[1] His low birth weight of 2½ lbs necessitated prolonged incubator care.[1] Martin's infancy and childhood were marked by nutritional deficits[1] and by repetitive and prolonged separations[1] from his family, with placements[1] in creches and

---

[1] All these factors would put Martin in a very high risk category.

foster families. His early adolescence was largely spent in socially and education-ally restrictive environments.

When first seen, Martin manifested a level of functioning even lower than that which could have been anticipated from his IQ. He showed an almost total lack of constituted language with a count of 40–50 words on the expressive level and severe impairment of spatiotemporal orientation, imitation, retention, and social behavior. Echolalia, echopraxia and echomimy were observed, but no psychotic-autistic signs were detected. With very poor prognosis for trainability, custodial care seemed unavoidable.

Dynamic assessment of Martin with the Learning Potential Assessment Device (LPAD) *provided an index of modifiability which gave rise to unexpected hopes for radically changing his destiny.* Based on the assessment, Martin was placed in a foster home, group-care treatment program for the redevelopment of severely disturbed and low-functioning adolescents [6]. The program included a variety of strategies of mediating the world to Martin by selecting stimuli, framing them for him, providing them with meaning and reinforcing them, and equipping him with learning sets of which he was initially totally devoid.

A concerted effort over 11 years has resulted in the development of an inde-pendently functioning individual, oriented in time and space, with a fully and richly constituted language (Hebrew), humor and social skills, and goal-oriented needs. Martin is now almost completely self-subsistent as the man responsible for the upkeep of a huge public indoor swimming pool. Although he still has diffi-culties in mathematics, he reads, writes, and uses complex inferential and con-ceptual levels of thinking. Surprisingly, following his mastery of Hebrew, he has learned to speak French and some German.

Despite adverse pathogenic conditions, heredity, organicity, early separation, hospitalization, traumata, and continuous stimulus and social deprivation, modi-fiability proved possible through powerful and systematic intervention. This has radically changed the course of development from that of anticipated placement in lifelong custodial care to that of an autonomous, independent, contributing, socially adaptive young man, looking forward to building his own family.

Cases such as Martin are much more numerous than one would tend to believe. Clarke and Clarke [4] summarize a great wealth of relatively little-known research, surveys, and follow-up studies that provide solid evidence of modifiability in cases in which intervention started at the latency period. *They conclude that the ill effects of many kinds of adverse early experience can be wiped out simply by the discontinuation of the depriving conditions and, even more so, by the establishment of the necessary intervention for the redevelop-ment process to occur. In fact, they found that "the worse the early history of social deprivation, the better the prognosis for change"* (p. 72).

Hypothesized Determinants of Differential
Cognitive Development

Three etiological categories of variables are usually considered as the basis for differential cognitive development and the production of quite stable, immutable characteristics of the individual:

GENETIC HYPOTHESIS

The *genetic hypothesis* attempts to explain differential cognitive development in large masses of individuals from a variety of ethnic groups, socioeconomic levels, cultures, and so on. It leaves little, if any, hope for significant changes in those who, by virtue of their hypothetically established genetic endowment, are afflicted with a low level of cognitive functioning. Prevention is considered to be difficult and limited to eugenic means.

What remains possible, as suggested by Jensen [14], is *to accept the limits* set by the individual's genetic endowment and orient him towards low-level educational goals, determined by "Level I" type of cognitive functioning.

Jensen's dichotomous model of intelligence divides humanity genetically into two different species: the true *homo sapiens* who functions at Level II, who is creative, and who makes use of extensive transformational, operational, and abstract thinking; and the limited Level I type whose intelligence is characterized by simple mental acts of an imitative, reproductive nature and who does not differ in quality from the type of mental activity found in subhuman species. This kind of dichotomy is dangerous on both theoretical and practical grounds and gives rise to the question: can one and should one derive an approximation of hereditability from data that, at best, represents a *manifest* level of functioning, reflected by static "inventory" types of data produced by conventional IQ tests? Would it not be more appropriate to consider the genetic factor as producing variations in the level of *responsiveness* of the organism to learning situations requiring corresponding variations in the quantity and quality of investment necessary for the production of growth? Formulated in this way, the nature-nurture controversy may be resolved by restating the relationship as a ratio of investment/outcome rather than as setting limits on the future development of the organism.

The model of mastery learning, suggested by Bloom and Caron [3], postulates differences in capacity that are matched with variations in the amount and quantity of investment so as to bring about equality in achievement, and seems to be a more adequate paradigm to analyze differential levels of human performance.

NEUROPHYSIOLOGICAL HYPOTHESIS

The neurophysiological hypothesis includes a very wide variety of factors ranging from basic elements controlling the chemistry of the central nervous system to the very minor and almost imperceptible differences implied in the often vaguely used term minimal brain dysfunction (MBD).

In their thorough review, Sameroff and Chandler [17] point out the very limited links between incidents at the pre-, para- and postnatal stages and the negative outcomes they are supposed to determine once a *prospective* rather than a *retrospective* research methodology is applied. Retrospective studies often give the impression of having established a clear, causal relationship between pregnancy and delivery complications and later deviance. Prospective studies of the same variables have, however, not succeeded in demonstrating the predictive efficiency of these supposed risk factors. Most infants who suffer perinatal problems go on to normal development.

This category, in contradistinction to the genetic one, is considered to be accessible to preventive measures, such as the provision of adequate nutrition, a propitious emotional climate, and safe conditions during the pre-, para-, and post-natal periods. However, once the organic or neurophysiological condition has occurred, there is *little belief* that its ill effects can be modified. A passive-acceptant approach characterizes the educational, remedial, and vocational goals for those suffering from genetic or neurophysiological handicaps.

This hesitancy in approaching the cognitive and mental processes of the "organic" child in an active, modifying way is anchored in the belief that whatever is determined by the central nervous system cannot be changed. This, however, raises the question as to the extent to which there is a direct, causal relationship between the organic condition and the retarded performance. There is considerable variation in the levels of functioning of children said to be suffering from brain damage. This and the fact that many children are diagnosed as minimally brain damaged solely on the criterion of their inefficient functioning in one or another area of cognitive processes make the relationship between brain damage and its outcome far from satisfying the criteria of causality. Youngsters, diagnosed and treated as suffering from neurophysiological impairments, have shown a high level of modifiability even in those areas of functioning said to be typical and symptomatic of their condition. Such evidence militates against the irreversibility of the effects of organicity, thereby making the constancy of this causal relationship highly questionable.

ENVIRONMENTAL FACTORS

This category of etiological variables is usually considered less pessimistically. Environmental determinants can be efficient for prophylactic purposes and for remediation of existing deficient levels of manifest functioning. But, even so, efficiency of the environmental intervention is admitted only if it occurs within the hypothesized limits of critical periods of development.

The concept of "critical period" was borrowed from embryology and has been used by developmental psychology in a rather confusing way. In embryology critical period is defined as the temporal condition for given stimuli to affect the organism efficiently. It is an optimal period, but this does not imply that the temporal dimension acts in a restrictive way. It says rather that at certain times the appearance of stimuli is more efficient than at other times.

The Hebbian conception of the role of stimulation in the development of cell assemblies has introduced a neurophysiological basis to the environmental determination of differential cognitive development and has used the concept of critical period in the *restrictive* sense of the word rather than as an optimal period of stimulation [12].

This is a basic reason for the notion of irreversibility of the ill effects of early adverse experiences, once the critical period has passed, on the cognitive development of the individual. To this one may add other areas affected by adverse early experiences (such as emotional attachment and social behavior) which have been elaborated by psychoanalytic and other psychological schools dealing with early development.

The great benefit resulting from the critical-period concept consists of the large number of projects such as preschool programs

(Head Start)[2] established to prevent and remediate within the limits of time set by the critical period. The negative aspects of this concept center on two basic effects: (1) Although optimistic toward prevention and remediation at the early ages, it is pessimistic as to the possibility of remediation at *later* stages of development, such as adolescence and early adulthood. This has resulted in an almost complete neglect of adolescents as a target population for intervention and investment for meaningful improvement of their levels of cognitive functioning. (2) The above-mentioned pessimism has also negatively affected the early remediational programs themselves by turning them into a one-shot type of intervention, perceived almost as a strategy for producing immunity in the organism.

A number of theoretically and experimentally derived conclusions adhering to this approach were drawn by Hunt [13], Deutsch [5], Yarrow [20], and others. An effort was made, especially by Wolf [19] and Schoggen and Schoggen [18] to define better the role of environment in the development of specific characteristics—cognitive, emotional, behavioral, and motivational—of the growing child. However, the relationship found between the dependent and the independent variables which were considered has always left significant, unexplained residuals.

Another problem concerning the environmental determinants of differential cognitive development is that many of the outlined processes cannot be perceived as universally explanatory. Thus the hypothesis of poverty of stimulation to explain the low cognitive functioning of children living in slum areas is not in accord with the facts. According to Riessman [16], slum children, instead of lacking stimulation, are actually overexposed to stimuli impinging on them at a greater rate, higher intensity, and greater variability than is the case for the middle-class child for whom child-rearing practices produce highly controlled, overscheduled incoming stimuli. And yet, this overexposure to stimuli from a very early age does not result in more adequate levels of functioning. The same is true for many other dimensions of interaction between the child and his environ-

---

2 One of the explanations offered for the supposed failure of the Head Start program was that it intervened too late, that is, beyond the supposed critical period. This became a justification for earlier intervention with infancy programs such as The Parent and Child Centers.

ment. Early interaction between the child and his mother is often marked by a much greater degree of dependency and strong mutual attachment in these slum families than is observable in the middle-class families. Can one then attribute to this very dimension the inadequate cognitive and emotional development observed at later stages in the development of these children?

Jensen's argument [14] against environmental as opposed to genetic determinants is partially justified in the sense that the stimulus deprivation which has been invoked to explain the low cognitive functioning of this segment of the population is never as severe nor as massive as in the conditions that produce lasting deleterious effects found in the laboratory animal studies.

A recent paper by Konrad and Melzack [15] has a very different interpretation of the outcome of stimulus deprivation in isolated animals than the one offered by Hebb. This new interpretation has a very strong bearing on both the concept of critical period and the prognosis for modifiability of the affected organism.

The authors point out that what was considered to be a permanent deficit of the central nervous system, produced by stimulus deprivation and reflected in the inefficiency of the organism to master certain basic tasks is, in fact, a highly modifiable condition once the deprived animal is subjected to stimulation. The observed period of inefficient behavior on the part of the deprived animal, as compared to normal controls, is interpreted as resulting from excessive exploration of novel stimuli ("novelty enhancement") by animals that had remained "naive" by virtue of their experienced isolation.

The novelty-enhancement effect of isolation-rearing implies that many aspects of most testing environments will be experienced as more novel by isolation-reared subjects than by normally reared subjects. Novelty is presumed to be enhanced for isolates because of the experience-restricted nature of their earlier life. This can be demonstrated by showing that after habituation to novelty, isolates come to behave like normal animals and that in extreme cases of object-situation novelty, normals can display the behaviors of isolates ([15], p. 254).

The fact that this inefficiency is temporary, as Konrad and Melzack support with evidence from a variety of studies, casts doubt on the hypothesized neurophysiological substrata of sensory deprivation.

Having discussed the various hypothesized determinants of differential cognitive development, one must pose the questions: In what way do these determinants produce the final outcome of retarded performance? What are the mechanics by which genetic endowment, organic conditions, or environmental deprivation affect the capacity of the individual to use representational, abstract thinking? The fact that we find such great variability in the outcomes within various populations, despite the relative uniformity of the etiological factors, makes the relationship between them highly questionable.

In an attempt to answer the above questions, two categories of etiological factors, distal and proximal, are considered:

1. Distal etiologies comprise those determinants that do not lead directly and invariably to certain specific outcomes but have, rather, a trigger effect (genetic factors, organicity, poverty of stimuli, disturbance in child or parent, socioeconomic disadvantages, etc.).

2. Proximal etiologies comprise those determinants that when triggered by the distal factor lead directly and almost invariably to specific outcomes. When the distal factor triggers the proximal determinant, then the specific outcome will appear. However, when for certain reasons the distal determinant does not succeed in or is prevented from triggering the proximal one, the expected end product may not necessarily appear. The most important proximal factor is the mediated learning experience, conceptualized by Feuerstein and Rand [10] under the acronym MLE, or a lack of it.

The living organism develops by the maturational and growth processes built into the system of the organism itself and by the interaction between the organism and its environment. For the latter source of development, two main modalities for change can be distinguished:

1. Change brought about by direct exposure to stimuli impinging on the organism from the very beginning of life that transforms its reactions and elicits new responses that change its behavioral patterns. This process is equated with learning because it produces lasting effects on the behavioral repertoire of the organism. Such learning is continued throughout life, provided that new stimuli are offered to the receptive organism. This modality also includes the activities and manipulations that the organism

imposes on the stimuli, a process subsumed in Skinner's S-R and Piaget's S-O-R paradigm.

2. Change brought about when an experienced, well-intentioned and active human being is interposed between the individual and the sources of stimuli and mediates them to the individual. In this mediation, each stimulus is transformed as it reaches the organism. Thus the experienced and well-intentioned adult selects certain stimuli, frames them, orders them in a given sequence of "before and after" (representing causal as well as teleological systems), schedules them both on temporal and spatial dimensions, provokes anticipatory behaviors, provides meaning to certain stimuli by emphasizing them through repetition, wipes out others by discontinuing their appearance, produces categories of behavior by associating certain stimuli, and eliminates certain associations between others. This mediation occurs at a very early stage in the development of the child, at the preverbal level, and continues into early childhood on verbal levels in those areas which are novel to the organism.

The MLE, as an alternative modality through which the organism is transformed, is typical of the human species, even though certain rudiments of mediation are observable in animals. Humans transmit their culture to their offspring as a part of their need to ensure their continuity beyond the biological limits of life.

It is our contention that MLE provides the organism with instruments of adaptation and learning in such a way as to enable the individual to use the direct-exposure modality for learning more efficiently and thus become modified. The more an individual is subjected to MLE, the greater is his capacity to use the wealth of stimuli impinging on him and be constantly modified by them. On the other hand, the individual lacking MLE remains a passive recipient of information and is limited in his capacity for modification, change, and further learning through direct exposure to perceptual, motor, emotional, or intellectual experience. Each event is grasped in an isolated way without any attempt to establish a relationship between it and its antecedents and consequents. This passivity is reflected in a failure to organize the stimulus world through deficiencies in the input, elaborational, and output levels of the mental act.

Two explanations have been offered for the lack of MLE:

1. A failure on the part of the environment to mediate the world to the child, reasons for which include poverty, parental disinterest, and defective or disturbed parent-child ties.
2. A failure stemming from the individual himself because of factors obstructing mediation by parents and other mediators, rendering it temporarily or permanently difficult to effect.

The barrier may have resulted from genetic factors, but the child's limited responsiveness may in turn dampen the mediation effort of the parents instead of increasing it. The same may be true for the "organic" child whose hyperkineses or other impairments may make him inaccessible to MLE. With him, there is no lack of stimuli but rather a lack of MLE that reduces his capacity to organize the stimulus world actively.

Retarded performance will be elicited whenever the lack of MLE is caused by one of the distal determinants. However, if in spite of heredity and/or organicity, the child is provided with MLE, when the barriers obstructing mediation are overcome and bypassed by special strategies or by increasing the intensity of exposure, then the expected deficiency may not necessarily occur.

If the viewpoint is accepted, it would follow that many of the so-called retarded children who manifest low mental functioning do so not necessarily because of a particular distal etiology but because of the lack of MLE, caused either by a failure of the environment to offer it or because of a permanently or temporarily limited penetrability in the child to the MLE.

The deficiency produced by lack of MLE is mainly in the areas of attitude, orientation, habits, and cognitive strategies of the individual toward the world and toward himself. A detailed inventory of deficient functions resulting from a lack of MLE have been catalogued [9].

In summary:

1. Lack of MLE is an obstruction to the process of transmitting cultural values, habits, and behavioral repertoires to the child and results in cultural deprivation.
2. MLE, being environmental in nature, carries the assumption that deficits produced by its absence or insufficiency are reversible by environmental intervention.
3. This model does not set time limits to remediational and rede-

velopmental processes and, as such, does not imply critical periods of development with its supposition that intervention at later stages is impossible or very difficult. Although early childhood can be considered as an *optimal* period for MLE, a great deal can be achieved by providing MLE at later stages of development.

4. The findings of cognitive modifiability in deprived adolescents and adults, both as a result of spontaneous remission and of systematic intervention, seems to be best explained by this model.

These conclusions are also based on four sources of empirical data derived from clinical and experimental work:

1. The Learning Potential Assessment Device (LPAD) by means of which we have studied modifiability *in vitro* [9].
2. Follow-up studies of high-risk adolescents 25 years after intervention [9, 10].
3. The Treatment Group Technique (TGT) by which we have studied cognitive emotional and social therapeutic interventions on the modifiability of severely disturbed and extremely low-functioning adolescents [8].
4. The study of the effects of an intervention program aimed at producing meaningful modification in the cognitive structure of the retarded performing adolescent by Instrumental Enrichment (IE) [10].

The major source of empirical evidence for the modifiability of the culturally deprived and culturally different adolescent is based on work with populations of children of the Youth Aliyah, a department of the nongovernmental Jewish Agency charged with the ingathering of large numbers of high-risk children and adolescents from the Diaspora into Israel and providing them with total care programs until the age of 18 or 19, when they are integrated into the Israeli army or society.

During its 43 years of existence, Youth Aliyah has cared for approximately 140,000 children and adolescents, the majority of whom had been exposed to extreme conditions of deprivation, danger, and trauma during the Holocaust or in countries where they suffered as an oppressed minority. For many of them coming to Israel meant separation from family, encounter with a new language and culture and pressure for socialization. For those children from both culturally different and deprived backgrounds, there was also the requirement for acculturation and the redevelopment of cognitive functions.

Many of the children manifested extremely low levels of functioning, as reflected by psychometric measurements; they displayed gaps ranging between 3 and 5 years in mental age and no less in terms of school performance. Others were handicapped by their illiteracy and emotional disturbance, which cast grave doubts as to their capacity to integrate into normal life conditions as well as to adapt to the new educational framework with its scholastic and social requirements. Their educators were very pessimistic after their initial encounters with some of these children whom they found inaccessible to educational attempts.

Children were usually placed in kibbutzim, agricultural schools, youth villages, and religious institutions, but some children were placed in foster homes or institutions for the disturbed.

What was common to all Youth Aliyah programs was the great emphasis on three goals:

1. The active participation of the individual in the life of the large community in which he was living.
2. Academic studies with the goal of personal development through cognitive enrichment and identification with value systems.
3. Cooperative social life with the group as mediator for the transmission of values, attitudes, and cognitive skills.

The Learning Potential Assessment Device

The first source of support for the theory of modifiability is to be found in the theory, practice and data derived from the LPAD study [9]. The LPAD is a method of assessment that produces processes of change *in vitro* during the assessment procedure. These changes can be provoked in a variety of modalities and measured both in terms of their psychological meaning as well as in the amount of investment required in order to produce them. Preferential modalities by which a change is produced can be isolated, conceptualized, and defined for prescriptive treatment and teaching methods. Furthermore, since this method includes a test-teaching-test sequence which allows the examiner to uncover the intimate cognitive processes of the examinee, it enables identification of those cognitive components that are responsible for the success or failure of the examinee on a specific task.

The LPAD differs from the conventional tests used for intellectual assessment because its goal is to assess the cognitive modifiability of the individual rather than to establish an inventory of existing functions that the individual can mobilize efficiently and use at the request of the examiner; because process rather than product is the main assessment target, offering a wider variety of possibilities to direct specific and systematic interventions; and because the criteria for prediction, linked as they are to the index of modifiability, preserve a dynamic character and allow continuous adjustments to be made apropos of the modifications that have already occurred because of developmental or environmental factors.

Through the LPAD the alleged incapacity of retarded immigrants to handle abstract thinking was changed very easily when appropriate orientation equipped them with the learning sets necessary for problem-solving behavior. The results obtained with this population point to the cultural nature of the observed deficiencies and the relative ease by which such a cultural barrier may be overcome once the necessity emerges and the prerequisites for such a change are provided.

Follow-Up Studies [9, 11]

Youth Aliyah graduates were tested by the recruitment branch of the Israeli army prior to their entrance into the regular army. Measures included the Dapar (a nonverbal intelligence measure), Hebrew knowledge (reading comprehension and writing), Tziun Derekh (personality variables) and Kaba, a combined score used by the army authorities in order to determine the prospective army assignment of the new recruit. The data reported in the study mentioned above compare the Youth Aliyah subjects to their siblings closest in age, not referred to the Youth Aliyah educational settings because they were considered to be functioning normally and were of lower risk.

The main findings of these studies were that although the Youth Aliyah graduates had been considered initially as high-risk in function of a great number of variables including low intellectual functioning, they outperformed their initially more-normal-functioning siblings in most of the above-mentioned army measures as shown in Table 1.

Table 1. **Means, Standard Deviations, and *t* Values for Significance on Army Criterion Measures—Youth Aliyah versus Non-youth Aliyah Groups ($N = 182$)**

Variables	Youth Aliyah			Non-Youth Aliyah			
	N	Mean	SD	*N*	Mean	SD	*t*
Dapar	83	5.12	2.55	92	4.80	1.72	n.s.
Hebrew	89	7.80	1.25	69	6.85	2.04	3.55[a]
Tz. Derekh	25	25.48	3.86	39	23.33	4.30	2.14[b]
Kaba	76	49.04	2.98	95	47.66	3.37	2.76[b]

[a] Significant at the .01 level or better.
[b] Significant at the .05 level.

These results demonstrate that the adolescent is highly modifiable despite adverse basic conditions, provided that intervention is systematically geared toward obtaining a meaningful departure from the expected course of development, predicted by the individual's low level of functioning at a given stage.

Treatment Group Technique (TGT)

The TGT provides another source of evidence for the modifiability of the adolescent. In addition to cognitive redevelopment, the TGT involves the emotional and social adaptation necessary in cases where severe emotional problems are the primary cause for nonadaptation.

In practice, 25 deeply disturbed youngsters are placed as a group unit into a youth village containing five or six group units of so-called normal children. In the last 20 years six treatment groups have been established. The positive results obtained through this technique have been confirmed by follow-up studies on these children over a prolonged period of time [6, 8]. The application of three basic treatment conditions was considered necessary for the meaningful redevelopment and social integration of high-risk, severely disturbed, and behaviorally inadapted adolescents:

1. The TGT attempts to disrupt the vicious circle of disturbance-rejection-disturbance by an unconditional acceptance of the youngster on his own terms. This generates an atmosphere that is continuously subject to fine readjustments by the educational environment. It may be exploited by the adolescent but, with time, brings a higher level of adaptation.
2. The TGT calls for living with normally functioning children, and this integration leads initially to an increase in the level of anxiety because of poorer scholastic performance. A special, separate program offered the disturbed youngsters the option of rejecting school achievement as the sole criterion for being measured and valued while gradually improving their performances in limited and specific areas, partially academic and partially nonacademic. Special tutoring as well as other methods more adequate to their special needs, capacities, and ways of working served as ego-strengthening, supportive, and anxiety-reducing means.
3. The TGT allows for regression in the service of readaptation. Regression can be induced [1, 2] by well-planned manipulations designed to bring about meaningful relations with highly responsive staff members; by keeping the group at a slow pace of development by periodically introducing less adapted newcomers; by creating a variety of compensatory experiences; and by enhancing group identifications.

The special environmental setting was the subject of an extensive follow-up study [8]. The results clearly show significant and meaningful reversibility for this group on dimensions pertaining to intellectual and scholastic functioning, adaptations to social frameworks previously inaccessible, better emotional adjustment, almost complete alleviation of known delinquency, and acceptance into the Army. The data highlight what is the most important in the lives of these youngsters: the opportunity to become integrated into their social environment. These changes are even more dramatic when compared with the initial level of functioning: the high level of illiteracy (only 1 out of 43 could read fluently), low level of writing skills (only 6 out of 43 were satisfactory in writing), and poor elementary arithmetic (only 2 out of 43 could perform four basic operations on a rudimentary level).

In the Army follow-up [11], the TGT subjects performed on a level close to normal on all criteria independently measured by the Army authorities (see Table 2).

Table 2

Variables	TGT Group			General Youth Aliyah			P
	N	Mean	SD	N	Mean	SD	
Dapar (IQ)	34	5.27	1.52	83	5.12	2.55	n.s.
Hebrew	34	7.00	1.31	76	7.80	1.25	3.08[a]
Personality measures	24	24.71	4.60	25	25.48	3.86	n.s.
Kaba (quality group)	34	48.35	2.95	76	49.04	2.98	n.s.

[a] Significant at the .01 level.

As can be observed, despite their initial low level on all relevant criteria measures, there were no significant differences between this group and their counterparts in the general Youth Aliyah population (except for Hebrew), demonstrating the impact of environmental variables in the modifying process of the human being.

The Instrumental Enrichment (IE) Program

The IE program aims at the modification of the cognitive structure of the retarded performer so as to render him sensitive to, and therefore modifiable by, direct exposure to stimuli in his encounters with life situations as well as in formal learning situations.

The student and his teacher work together (400 hours of paper-and-pencil exercises spread over 2 or more years, together with individual tutoring) to modify the low-functioning adolescent by direct exposure to an intensive, systematic, age-specific substitute for MLE. The subgoals include remediation and redevelopment of the deficient cognitive functions that are characteristic of the retarded performer, such as blurred perception, unsystematic exploratory behavior and lack of spatial and temporal orientation at the input level, a disregard of the need for logical evidence, and a poor capacity for synthesis and conceptualization at the elaborational level; impulsivity and inaccuracy; the provision of concepts, skills, operations and strategies necessary to master such complex tasks as comparative behavior, analytic perception, and syllogistic thinking; the development and cultivation of intrinsic motivation through habit formation (repeated creative exposure to the same principles in new and varied situations, and continuous rediscovery of the learned principle); an orientation of the learner toward reflective thinking, toward insight into the mental act, into the reasons for his success and failure, and into other interactional processes taking place while solving problems; the creation of a strong task-oriented motivation by making tasks accessible to mastery and challenging by being age-specific and difficult enough even for adults as a result of which a greater equity in the student-teacher-task relationship is obtained and motivation enhanced; and the modification of the individual's perception of himself as a passive recipient of information to that of an active generator of information.

A research was undertaken over a period of 2 years to evaluate the efficiency of the IE program in residential centers providing a total-care program that included scholastic, work, and social activities; shared living facilities and sports and other group activities; and day centers where students attend during the day but continue to live with their families. Social contacts are mainly outside of the day center.

Both settings are oriented to low-functioning students, school dropouts for a variety of reasons, and the severe culturally and socially deprived. The results [11] can be summarized as follows:

1. Systematic intervention in order to provide MLE at adolescence has proven to be highly effective for a large number of cognitive and intellectual functions in both types of settings.
2. The IE program was most effective in the intellectual area. Groups in the IE program have overtaken their comparison counterparts on the total score of the Primary Mental Abilities (PMA) test, as well as on four out of eight subtests of the same test. Those results were obtained on a Matched Pairs sample

($N = 114$) where groups were matched at the prelevel on the same total score of the PMA, as well as on other matching variables such as age, sex, and ethnic origin. In addition to this main finding, the IE groups outperformed the comparison groups on the following intelligence measures: Terman nonverbal intelligence test, D-48 (measuring the G factor), and the Kuhlman-Finch Postures test, which is highly loaded on the spatial primary mental ability.

3. Although the IE groups had 300 hours less of regular scholastic studies, their results in achievement tests were either equal or superior to those of the control groups.

4. IE groups were shown to have a more analytic cognitive style as compared to the control groups when measured by the Embedded Figures Test (EFT), by the Human Figure Drawing (HFD), and on a test measuring the complex of Precision-Rapidity.

5. Significant differences in favor of the IE groups were also found in some nonintellective variables such as classroom behavior as measured by teacher ratings.

6. Settings themselves, especially the residential centers, have also been shown to have a significant effect on the level of performance of the students, albeit to a lesser degree than the more systematic and intensive strategy of the IE program.

Summary

In conclusion, we feel that the four sources of data to which we have briefly referred are supportive of a concept of modifiability and offer empirical evidence that may be considered highly conclusive. They demonstrate that significant and meaningful modifications are possible and achievable through environmental intervention. These modifications can be obtained at ages beyond the so-called critical periods of development and with very low levels of intellectual functioning.

Further research should address itself to the discovery of the most adequate intervention systems and to the creation of the optimal environmental conditions for making interventions even more efficient and of longer duration. There is a Hebrew proverb that says, "He who struggles unremittingly will find what he seeks."

References

1. Alpert, A. A special therapeutic technique for certain developmental disorders in prelatency children. *Amer. J. Ortho.* 27 (2) (1975), 256–270.
2. Alpert, A. Reversibility of pathological fixations associated with maternal deprivation in infancy. *The Psychoanalytic Study of the Child,* Vol. 14. New York, International Universities Press, 1959, pp. 169–185.
3. Bloom and Caron. In *Mastery Learning: Theory and Practice,* J. H. Block, Ed. New York, Holt, Rinehart and Winston, 1971.
4. Clarke, A. M. and Clarke, A. D. B. *Early Experiences, Myth and Evidence.* London, Open Books, 1976.
5. Deutsch, C. P. Environment and perception. In *Social Class, Race and Psychological Development.* M. Deutch, I. Katz, and A. Jensen. Eds. New York, Holt, Rinehart and Winston, 1968.
6. Feuerstein, R. and Krasilowsky, D. Treatment group technique. *Israel Ann. Psychiat. Related Disc.,* 5 (1), Spring (1967), p. 69–90.
7. Feuerstein, R. *The Instrumental Enrichment Method: An Outline of Theory and Technique.* Laboratory report of Hadassah-Wizo-Canada Research Institute, 1968.
8. Feuerstein, R. and Krasilowsky, D. The treatment group technique. In *Group Care: An Israeli Approach.* M. Wollins and M. Gottesman, Eds. New York and London, Gordon and Breach, 1971.
9. Feuerstein, R. et al. The learning potential assessment device, theory instruments and techniques. *Studies in Cognitive Modifiability, Report No. 1.* Hadassah-Wizo-Canada Research Institute, Jerusalem, 1972.
10. Feuerstein, R. and Rand, Y. Mediated learning experiences: An outline of the proximal etiology for differential development of cognitive functions. *Int. Understanding,* 9/10 (1974), 7–37.
11. Feuerstein, R. et al. Instrumental enrichment. *Studies in Cognitive Modifiability.* Hadassah-Wizo-Canada Research Institute, Jerusalem, 1976.
12. Hebb, D. O. *The Organization of Behavior.* Wiley, New York, 1949.
13. Hunt, J. McV. *Intelligence and Experience.* Ronald, New York, 1961.
14. Jensen, A. How can we boost I.Q. and scholastic achievement? *Harv. Edu. Rev.,* 39 (1969), 1–123.
15. Konrad, K. and Melzack, R. Novelty enhancement effects associated with early sensory-social isolation. In *The Developmental Neurophysiology,* Academic, New York, 1975.
16. Riessman, F. *The Culturally Deprived Child.* Harper, New York, 1962.
17. Sameroff, A. J. and Chandler, M. J. Reproductive risk and the continuum of caretaking casualty. In *Child Development Research,* Vol. 4. D. F. Horowitz, Ed. University of Chicago Press, Chicago, 1975.
18. Schoggen, P. H. and Schoggen, M. F. Behavior units in observational research. In *Methodological Issues in Observational Research.* W. Hartup, Ed. Symposium at meeting of American Psychological Association, San Francisco, 1968.
19. Wolf, R. M. The identification and measurement of environmental process variables related to intelligence. Unpublished doctoral dissertation, University of Chicago, 1964.
20. Yarrow, L. Y. Mother-infant interaction and development in infancy. *Child Dev.,* 43 (1972), 31–41.

Changing Family Life in an Arab Village

Helen Antonovsky, Ph.D.,
Mahmoud Meari, M.A., and
Judith Blanc, M.A. (Israel)

The central focus of this study was description and analysis of changes that have occurred over the past 50 years in certain aspects of village and family life in a small Moslem Arab village. We investigated certain aspects of the sociodemographic structure of village (educational level, occupational structure, and family structure) and certain areas of family relationships (authority patterns, discipline, emotional support).

The village in which the study was carried out is located a few kilometers south of Bethlehem. This village was chosen not because it was assumed to be representative of small Moslem villages in the area but because it was the location of a study done almost 50 years ago by the Finnish anthropologist, Hilma Granqvist [5, 6, 7]. Granqvist was interested mainly in problems of childbirth, child care, and the role and status of women. Although her methods of study and data analysis are very different from our own, her research provides us with background material and the opportunity to measure change over time in a number of areas of life in the village.

Our findings about changes over two generations in the aspects of life noted above are presented in the context of Granqvist's data. The discussion focuses on an analysis of how changes in different aspects of life influence one another. An attempt is made to predict the kinds of changes we would expect to occur in the near future.

Methodology

THE SAMPLE

The village had a population of 1045 people in 1967, the last census for which records are available. There are about 240 households in the village.

The plan was to include all families having children between the ages of 10 and 16 in the sample. Because of a lack of precision in birth records, we are not sure the sample includes all these families. The interviewers visited every house in the village and inquired as to whether there were children of the age group in which we were interested.

The sample chosen was made up of 89 families. These included 100 boys, 53 girls, 81 fathers, and 94 mothers.[1] For some of the analyses we used all these families. For the analyses of the data on family relationships only the 77 monogamous nuclear families for whom we had data on both parents and the children were used. For these analyses we chose one child at random from each family if there was more than one child per family in the sample. Thus for the analyses on family relationships the sample consists of 77 fathers, 77 mothers, and 77 children (51 boys and 26 girls). For all other analyses the sample consists of 81 fathers, 94 mothers, and 153 children (100 boys and 53 girls).

DATA COLLECTION

Both qualitative and quantitative data were collected. The qualitative data were collected by means of open-ended anthropological type interviews and participant observation. The quantitative data were collected by means of personal interviews, with all respondents based on closed questionnaires. All respondents were interviewed by same-sex interviewers. All interviewers were Arabs who had at least completed high school. None of them were from the village. The field work was conducted in 1973.

[1] See Appendix for comment.

DATA ANALYSIS

The quantitative data were analyzed in terms of differences by family, sex, age, and generation.

Findings

SOCIODEMOGRAPHIC STRUCTURE

Granqvist [5, 6, 7] notes that in the 1920s there was less Western influence noticeable in this village than in many other places in the general area of Palestine during that period. It seems reasonable to assume that since 1948 and especially since the Israeli occupation in 1967 certain changes in village life can be noted and measured. One of the most obvious of these is the type of work engaged in by the adult males in the village. Another area is the level of formal education.

Changes in these areas are related mainly to the operation of factors outside of the village itself, factors that set the frameworks, opportunities, and pressures for change. The existence of these new conditions may or may not influence the behavior of the villagers, but without the operation of these external factors there is less likelihood that behavior of the villagers would change. The interesting question is whether changes in level of education and occupational structure have influenced modifications in traditional patterns of family structure and relationships. Studies such as that of Rosenfeld [10] have pointed up the influence of change in occupational structure on the break-up of the extended family in some Israeli Arab villages. Clear changes have occurred in the village since the time of Granqvist's study in the three sociodemographic areas with which we are concerned: (1) rise in level of education, (2) changes in types of occupation, and (3) tendency toward living in nuclear-family households. The data from our interviews with parents and children permit us to measure and specify the degree to which change has occurred over the last two generations.

LEVEL OF EDUCATION

Formal schooling at any level is to a large extent a phenomenon of the last 20 years. In the 1920s, lessons for boys alone were given by one teacher on the roof of the mosque when weather, work, and other social obligations did not interfere. Except for occasional sewing classes offered by the convent (located in the village), girls had no possibility of formal instruction [6]. One gets the clear impression from her writings that little importance was attached to school attendance. She was there during the early years of the British Mandate. Some time during the period of the Jordanian occupation (1948–1967), an organized compulsory school system was set up in the area of the West Bank. The present school for boys was established sometime in the early 1960s and the school for girls a few years later. Mosque schools were in existence for many years. The establishment of the schools with a formal curriculum and the hiring of teachers to work in the village has clearly had an impact on school attendance.

In 1973 there were two elementary schools in the village, one for boys and one for girls, each covering the first six grades. There were 130 boys and 99 girls attending school at that time. Of these 18 boys and 6 girls were in the 6th grade. An additional 11 boys and 3 girls were in mission schools in Bethlehem and Hebron. Preparatory grades (seventh through ninth years) are located in government schools in a neighboring village. There were 21 boys and 2 girls from Artas enrolled in these schools. Approximately a dozen children are in high school or trade school in Bethlehem and Bet Jala.

Sixty-two percent of the fathers who were interviewed attended some type of school. Fifty-two percent reported that they could read and write. Of the mothers, 20 percent said they had attended school and 17 percent reported that they could read and write.

Since there is a clear sex difference in the level of education in both the parent generation and the child generation, comparisons are made between fathers and boys and between mothers and girls. Only 1 percent of the boys as compared with 38 percent of the fathers never attended school. Whereas only 6 percent of the fathers studied beyond the sixth grade, only 6 percent of the sons stopped going to school in the sixth grade or earlier. Thirty-eight percent of the boys are already studying beyond the sixth grade, and the rest are planning to do so. A similar pattern is found when mothers and girls are compared. Eighty percent of the mothers never attended school, as compared with 6 percent of the daughters. Only 5 percent of the mothers attended school beyond the fourth grade. Only 20 percent of the daughters stopped going to school at the fourth-grade level or earlier.

These data show that there has been a real change in the last generation in school attendance. This has probably been influenced both by the setting up of a system of compulsory education and the fact that two elementary schools (grades 1–6) are situated in the village. There is little evidence that the compulsory education law of 8 years of schooling is enforced. A majority of girls drop out before the sixth grade, and very few continue beyond the sixth grade. From conversations with the area superintendent of schools one gets impression that school attendance is encouraged but not enforced. Nevertheless, school has become an accepted part of the daily routine of life in childhood. In this context it is interesting to note that over 60 percent of the husbands said that they would agree that their wives learn to read and write if classes were held in the village. A similar percentage of wives said they would like to attend such classes.

OCCUPATIONAL STRUCTURE

During the years Granqvist spent in the village (1925–1930) almost all the men were engaged in agricultural work as their main source of livelihood. Our interview data on types of occupations of the fathers before the Israeli occupation in 1967 indicate that a change had occurred since Granqvist's time. Fifty-one percent of the fathers stated that their main source of livelihood before 1967 had been from agriculture. Another 30 percent reported that they worked as unskilled laborers. A further shift away from agriculture has taken place since 1967. In 1973, at the time this study was done, 35 percent of the fathers were engaged in agricultural work as their main source of livelihood, 42 percent worked as unskilled laborers, 12 percent worked as skilled laborers, and 11 percent had low-level white collar occupations.

There is a clear trend away from agriculture to work in an industrialized economy. Although someone in every household still works in the fields, income from agriculture is not the only or major source of income for most families.

A generation comparison (1973) of occupations of fathers and sons who are working (older siblings of the children in the sample) shows that very few sons work in agriculture (9 percent) as compared with fathers (35 percent). Many more of the sons work in skilled occupations (33 percent) than do fathers (12 percent). It should be noted that 22 percent of the working sons ($N = 38$) are working abroad. When the occupational aspirations of the sons in the sample are compared with occupations of both their fathers and older brothers, a strong shift is evident in the direction of aspirations for professional occupations requiring higher education (60 percent). Only 7 percent of the boys in the study want to work in agriculture, and 28 percent say they would like to be skilled laborers (the remaining 5 percent gave a variety of answers). These data, then, indicate a shift away from the traditional village occupation of farming toward skilled work in an industrialized economy and toward aspirations for professional work. This trend probably reflects both greater opportunities for work outside the village and the influence of the level of education. Although it is unreasonable to assume that anywhere near the percentage of younger boys who aspire to professional occupations requiring higher education will indeed work in these professions, it does seem reasonable to assume that as long as the opportunities for skilled work outside the village remain available more and more younger people will engage in these occupations than will engage in the traditional occupation of agriculture.

FAMILY STRUCTURE

Granqvist reported that the household of parents, unmarried children, and married sons with their wives and children was the norm, ideally and in fact. However, few families met the demographic prerequisite for full extended families. In the majority of cases the father was dead by the time his sons were married, and in about half of these cases the married sons set up separate households. If we add to this the number of families of only sons of dead fathers, approximately 40 percent of households consisted of nuclear families, with the occasional addition of a widowed mother or unmarried sibling.

According to Granqvist [5], the father—or after his death, the eldest son—controlled the family purse, receiving the income of all males in the household and dispensing funds at his discretion. Although there is some evidence that the eldest brother could keep control over the fixed property of his brothers, some sets of brothers divided at least some of their inheritance and probably constituted completely independent domestic units [5]. Interviews with village elders now indicate that most of the family patrimony was kept intact, so that major expenditures like paying out bride price still required the consent of the eldest brother. In other words, many nuclear family households were not independent in important respects.

The pattern of family structure at the present time does not fit the traditional pattern described above. Of the 81 families in the sample on which we have data from the father interviews, 50 (60 percent) live as independent nuclear families. Of the 31 families in which other relatives live in the household, only 18 fit the description of the traditional extended family of three generations, which includes the parents, their married sons, and their sons' children. However, of these 18, only half of the sons have children. This means that they are newly married and may move out as soon as they have the opportunity.

Thus we may conclude that only 18 (or 22 percent) of the families live in extended-family households. If a more strict definition of an extended family is used, the percentage is much smaller.

To learn whether there had been a change in residence patterns over the last generation the respondents (fathers) were asked where they had lived in the first year after marriage and where their married sons and daughters had lived in the first year of marriage. The data show no change between the parent's and child's generations. Just over 60 percent of the fathers and sons lived in their father's house in their first year of marriage, and 72 percent of the daughters as compared with 61 percent of the mothers lived in their husband's father's house in the first year of their marriage.

The unmarried boys and girls in the sample were asked where they would *like* to live during the first year after their marriage. Only about one-third (34 percent of the boys and 32 percent of the girls) said they would like to live in the home of the husband's father. Seemingly, this is a change when compared to their parents and married siblings. However, in addition, 48 percent of the boys and 25 percent of the girls stated that they would like to live in a house adjacent to that of the husband's parents. During the course of our visits to the village it became clear that there is a tendency for young couples to live in their own room within the husband's father's house. In this way they are living in the paternal residence but also have their privacy. This arrangement could be described both as living in the father's house or adjacent to it. No data are available on how long the young couple continues to live in or adjacent to the father's house. There is a tendency, however, for close paternal kin to live near or adjacent to one another.

In summarizing our findings thus far, it is clear that there have been notable changes in the level of education, types of occupations, and the form of the family over the past half century, especially over the last generation. Forces external to the village have clearly influenced the rise in level of education and the change from a primarily agricultural to a wage-labor economy. Changes in family structure have been less dramatic and more gradual and less directly influenced by outside forces. These have probably been influenced to some extent by the changes in the occupational structure.

The next question to be dealt with is the extent to which the changes in the direction of nuclear-family structure have influenced or are reflected in changes in patterns of family relationships.

FAMILY RELATIONSHIPS

The traditional Arab village family is described in the literature [4] as an authoritarian extended family in which the proper roles of family members are clearly laid out. The father exercises great authority, and other family members are expected to show him respect by words and deeds. Granqvist [6] describes the village as a strictly patriarchal community. The father is very strict, and children are expected to obey their parents. The children must behave in accordance with the demands and expectations of their elders [7]. She states also that though the father is strict, the mother shows tenderness to the children and can always be depended on to give them support. Ammar [1], in his study of child-rearing customs in a village in Egypt, stresses the point that parent-child relations (especially father-child relations) can be characterized as a pattern of dominance—submission induced by fear. The child's devotion to and respect for parents is absolute.

The mother is subordinate to the father but wields power through being solely responsible for the rearing of the young children and functioning as guardian of household finances [4]. Parents are described as being fairly permissive in early childhood. Later childhood and adolescence are characterized by restrictions and limits on freedom, especially for girls. In adolescence boys are less restrained, but girls are kept under strict surveillance [1]. Granqvist [6] says that the fathers train the boys and the mothers train the girls. The father may discipline his daughters if they do not obey their mother.

We concentrated in three aspects of family relationships—authority or control, techniques of discipline, and emotional support—to investigate to what extent the patterns described above are characteristic of the village at the present time.

AUTHORITY

The Arab village family is characterized as being patriarchal, authority within the family being invested almost exclusively in the father. Authority may be defined as the power to control that has been legitimized by those being controlled. That is, those being controlled accept the control for reasons other than the fact that the one who controls has the power to do so. Among these reasons are respect for the authority figure and acceptance of his authority as right and proper.

Other dimensions of authority are its pervasiveness and exclusiveness. Pervasiveness refers to the number of different areas of life—in our context, family life—over which the authority figure has control. Exclusiveness refers to the degree to which only one figure—in this case the father—perceives and is perceived by others (those being controlled) as the one who is in control.

We can say, then, that the extent to which the Arab village family can be considered a patriarchal family is a function of the degree to which the father:

1. Controls resources for and makes decisions about many areas of life affecting members of the family.
2. Perceives himself and is perceived by other members of the family as being the person in control.
3. Is respected by members of his family.

Six areas of control or decision making were investigated. They were chosen as a sampling of a wide range of decisions made in any family both in terms of husband-wife relationships and parent-child relationships. Two of the areas—control of money and decisions about large expenditures—are relevant mainly to husband-wife relationships. The other four areas—decisions about continued attendance at school, permission to go out of the house, permission to go out of the village, and choice of marriage partner—are important areas of control in parent-child relationships in the Arab village. We investigated who makes the decisions as perceived by fathers, mothers, and children.

It seems reasonable to assume that agreement by all parties involved on who is in control reflects acceptance and legitimation of this control. Thus if most of the fathers, mothers, and children perceive the father as the one who makes the decisions, the father can be considered the figure of authority. Where there is disagreement among fathers, mothers, and children, the father cannot be considered the clear authority figure. If we follow this line of reasoning, an authoritarian father would be one who perceives himself and is perceived by other members of the family as in control of most aspects of family life.

In response to a series of questions about control or decision making an interesting pattern emerged. We discuss these results in terms of specific areas of control, number of areas of control, and extent of agreement between husband-wife pairs.

First of all, the father does not perceive himself nor is he perceived by the other family members as the authoritarian father defined above. Only the sons tend to see their fathers in this role. For three of the four areas of decision making about which the children were asked, a very high percentage of the sons responded that their fathers were the source of authority (money, permission to go out of the house, and permission to go out of the village). The typical pattern of response for both husbands and wives was to perceive either the husband or both husband and wife together as the source of authority (see Table 1). The percentage of husbands who reported that they made the decisions ranged from 29 percent (permission for girls to go out of the house) to 57 percent (permission for boys to go out of the village). The only area in which the mother was perceived as in control was permission for daughters to go out of the house. This is probably because there is a greater likelihood for mothers and daughters to be in the house together than fathers and daughters, so

Table 1. Source of Authority for Decision Making as Perceived by Fathers, Mothers, Sons, and Daughters in Six Different Areas of Famly Life

Area	Father Says (N = 77)			Mother Says (N = 77)			Sons Say (N = 51)			Daughters Say (N = 26)		
	Father	Mother	Both	Father	Mother	Both	Father	Mother	Other	Father	Mother	Other
1. Control of money	49	18	33	24	16	60	82	8	10[a]	73	23	4[a]
2. Large expenditures[b]	40	10	50	40	12	48	—	—	—	—	—	—
3. School attendance:												
Sons	44	9	47	43	13	44	48	2	36[c,d]			
Daughters	41	9	50	36	16	48				35	35	23[c,e]
4. Out of house:												
Sons	56	6	38	41	9	50	72	11	17[f]			
Daughters	29	33	38	10	57	33				20	68	12[f]
5. Out of Village:												
Sons	57	7	36	57	4	39	68	20	12[f]			
Daughters	33	11	56	41	24	35				55	45	—
6. Choice of marriage partner[g]	50	10	17[h]	33	17	30[i]						

[a] Other refers to other relative.
[b] Children were not asked this question.
[c] Child himself decided.
[d] Older siblings 14%.
[e] Older siblings 7%.
[f] Doesn't ask permission.
[g] Based on 30 sons who are already married.
[h] Sons decided themselves 23%.
[i] Sons decided themselves 30%.

that if a girl wants to go out she asks permission from her mother. In general, more daughters perceive their mothers as the source of authority than do sons. Over one-third of the sons and almost one-fourth of the daughters said that they themselves had made the decision about whether to continue attending school. It is worth noting also that 23 percent of the fathers and 30 percent of the mothers reported that their married sons had made the decision about their partner.

It should be noted that in response to the question about permission to go out of the village, a high percentage of sons (47 percent) and daughters (57 percent) reported that they never go out of the village. The percentages appearing in Table 1 refer only to those who do get permission to go out.

There tends to be agreement between husbands and wives with regard to the number of areas over which fathers, mothers or both have control. There is a slight tendency for more wives than husbands to respond that both husbands and wives make decisions in a greater number of areas. More husbands than wives tend to say that they make decisions in a greater number of areas (see Table 2). However, only three fathers said they make the decisions in all areas.

Table 2. Number of Areas in which Each Parent Makes Decisions as Perceived by Fathers and Mothers (%)

Number of Areas	Husband Says (N = 77)			Wife Says (N = 77)		
	Husband	Wife	Both	Husband	Wife	Both
0	17	65	26	25	56	19
1–3	51	30	45	48	36	47
4–6	32	5	29	27	8	34
	100%	100%	100%	100%	100%	100%
Mean no. of areas	2.7	0.7	2.3	2.2	0.9	2.6

The children tend to perceive the situation somewhat differently from their parents. They were not given the opportunity to answer "both," but had to choose between "father" and "mother." Sons perceive their fathers as the source of authority in more areas than daughters do. Daughters tend to perceive their mothers much more often as a source of authority than the sons do (see Table 3). This would seem to indicate that fathers have more responsibility for sons and mothers for daughters. However, it is also clear that mothers have less control over sons than fathers have over daughters.

Table 3. Number of Areas in which Each Parent Makes Decisions as Perceived by Sons and Daughters (%)

Number of Areas	Son Says (N = 51)		Daughter Says (N = 26)	
	Father	Mother	Father	Mother
0	6	80	23	27
1	16	12	27	19
2	31	6	31	42
3	33	2	15	12
4	14	0	4	0
	100%	100%	100%	100%
Mean no. of areas	2.3	0.3	1.5	1.4

When husband-wife pairs are matched we find a relatively high degree of agreement in their responses. Over 60 percent of the husbands and wives agree on who makes the decisions in matters of money and large expenditures, whether it is husband, wife, or both (see Table 4). The lowest percentage of agreement is with regard to who gives permission to girls to go out of the house (24 percent). This is the one area in which a high proportion of wives say they make the decision (57 percent), whereas only 33 percent of the husbands say that their wives do. It should be noted, however, that this is the one area in which such a high proportion of husbands say their wives make the decision. The percentage of agreement in the other areas ranges from 40 to 60.

Thus we can say that although a high proportion of sons tend to perceive their fathers as the main source of authority for most of the areas of control that were investigated, neither husbands, wives, nor

**Table 4. Percentage of Husband-Wife Agreements about Who Makes
Decisions in Six Areas of Family Life**

Area	Husband	Wife	Both	Other	Total Agreements
1. Money	23	8	30	—	61
2. Large expenditures	26	4	31	—	61
3. School: sons	22	3	22	—	47
daughters	17	3	24	—	44
4. Out of house: sons	29	0	23	—	52
daughters	0	12	4	8	24
5. Out of village: sons	33	2	21	4	60
daughters	12	0	4	24	40
6. Marriage partner	24	3	14	10	51

daughters do. Rather than an authoritarian patriarchal pattern of
control, there are many areas in which decisions are made by both
husbands and wives. Both husbands and wives agree that they make
decisions together.

Since there are no similar data on the previous generation, one
cannot say that these data indicate a change. They do present a different picture of husband-wife relations than most previous studies
on family life in the Arab village do [7, 1, 3]. The data from these
studies were more global and impressionistic and may refer to the
"ideal" pattern, whereas the data from the present study may be
closer to the "real" pattern. One factor that would tend to support
the hypothesis of a change over time in husband-wife relationships
is the change in family structure and residence patterns. As indicated
previously, there are few traditional extended family households in
the village. Young couples who live in the husband's father's home
during the first year after marriage have a room of their own. These
two conditions would tend to provide the opportunity and indeed
pressure toward discussions between husbands and wives on issues
about which decisions have to be made. This does not necessarily
mean that the husband does not make the decision himself. He is,
however, more likely to take his wife's opinions into consideration
under these circumstances than would be the case if he were living
in an extended family in which there would be more opportunity to
discuss these same issues with his father and brothers. If this is the

case, these findings have implications for change in the traditional pattern of husband-wife relationships.

The data on decision-making patterns indicate that there has been considerable modification of the authoritarian, patriarchal patterns of control (though least of all in the eyes of the sons). The responses to several other items round out this picture. Obedience is one of the components of authority. The children were asked whom in the family they most obey. The alternatives from which they could choose were father, mother, grandmother, grandfather, or older siblings. Although a majority of both sons and daughters said they most obey their father (55 and 54 percent), a rather high percentage (33 and 42 percent) answered mother. A parallel question asked whom they respected most, respect being viewed as a further indication of the acknowledgement of authority. Fathers are more often cited than mothers by both sons and daughters (47 and 58 percent and 22 and 19 percent). Thus in forced-choice questions, the father is indeed more often perceived as the authority figure. But it is, we believe, far more significant that this is not an absolute norm. The picture, then, is fairly consistent, though it should be noted that the sons do not differ from the daughters on these items.

If, however, there has been some change in the authority role of the father—assuming the literature on past family relationships to be accurate—one further item may suggest a note of caution. Although respect and obedience are crucial elements of the relationship to authority, fear may or may not be, but it is surely related to power. Asked whom they feared most in the family (with alternatives as above), the responses are clear-cut: 80 percent of the sons and 69 percent of the daughters cited their fathers, and no sons and almost no daughters (8 percent) cited their mothers. It seems crucial to note that the question made sense to the children. None replied that he did not fear anyone. The great majority, particularly among the sons, perceive fear to be part of their relationship with their fathers but not with their mothers.

TECHNIQUES OF DISCIPLINE

Discipline is one method of maintaining authority and control, especially in the area of parent-child relationships. Granqvist, in addition to characterizing the village family as an authoritarian patriarchal family, reported that the main techniques of discipline were beating and shaming. We have already shown that the patriarchal authoritarian system has changed in the direction of a more diversified pattern of authority relations. To what extent has there been a change also in techniques of discipline used by the parents? Do most parents now use physical punishment and shaming as a way of disciplining their children?

In order to investigate this problem each parent was asked what he did when his child disobeyed his father and what he did when his child disobeyed his mother. They could choose among four alternative responses: physical punishment, threats and shaming, persuasion, and ignoring. These types of discipline were assumed to represent a descending degree of severity.[2] The sons and daughters were asked a parallel set of questions about what each parent did when they disobeyed their father and when they disobeyed their mother. In this way we were able to measure not only the relative frequency of use of the different techniques but also the degree of correspondence or discrepancy between the responses of fathers and mothers and between parents and children. Since the responses to disobedience to fathers and disobedience to mothers showed a very similar pattern for both parents and children, only the data on disobedience to fathers are presented here.

The responses to these questions (see Table 5) indicate that the techniques of discipline used by most parents are persuasion and physical punishment. There is little consensus about the use of the different techniques among the four groups (fathers to sons and daughters and mothers to sons and daughters). Most of the fathers say they use persuasion. More mothers say they beat their children than do fathers. Mothers use persuasion and physical punishment about equally but differentially for sons and daughters. They use much more persuasion than physical punishment with daughters. They use slightly more physical punishment than persuasion with their sons.

It is clear from these data that few parents report that they threaten and shame their children as a technique of discipline. The

---

[2] For purposes of calculating the mean severity of discipline (see Table 5) the different techniques were assigned the following values: physical punishment = 4, threats and shaming = 3, persuasion = 2, ignoring = 1.

use of persuasion is rather widely used by the parents, especially the fathers. These data tend to corroborate our previous contention that the Arab village father is not an authoritarian figure demanding strict obedience and submission from his children as described, for example, by Ammar [1]. Whether the behavior he reports corresponds with what he actually does is not particularly relevant to this issue. He does not perceive himself (or does not want to appear to the outsider) as a severe disciplinary figure. This would indicate that at the very least the norms are changing even if the behavior is not.

The next question to be asked is to what extent do the parents discipline their sons and daughters differently. More mothers and fathers say they beat their sons more than they beat their daughters. More mothers report using physical punishment with both their sons and daughters than do fathers. We can offer no adequate explanation

Table 5. Techniques of Discipline for Disobedience Reported by Parents and Children (%)

Type of Discipline	Fathers for		Fathers as Seen by		Mothers for		Mothers as Seen by	
	Son	Daughter	Son	Daughter	Son	Daughter	Son	Daughter
Physical punishment	30	19	49	28	41	32	50	18
Threats and shaming	8	5	16	24	18	14	18	23
Persuasion	62	71	32	43	35	50	29	45
Ignoring	0	5	3	5	6	4	3	14
	100	100	100	100	100	100	100	100
Mean severity of discipline	2.7	2.4	3.1	2.8	2.9	2.7	3.1	2.4

for this finding. Perhaps since the boys tend to perceive their father as the main source of authority in the family, a word from the father is sufficient, whereas the mother who is seen less as a figure of authority has to use severe punishment to achieve obedience.

What degree of correspondence or consensus is there between the perception of the children and their parents about disciplinary techniques? Sons tend to see their fathers and mothers as equally severe in their punishment. However, only half the boys say their parents beat them when they disobey. There is slightly more correspondence between the responses of mothers and sons than between fathers and sons. More sons say their fathers use physical punishment than fathers say they do. More girls report that both mothers and fathers use threats and shaming than the parents report. In addition, girls tend to see fathers as more severe and mothers as less severe than their parents say they are.

What becomes clear from these data is that there is no clear consensus about techniques of discipline. The techniques used depend both on the giver of the punishment (father or mother) and the receiver of the punishment (sons or daughters). Boys see both parents as more severe disciplinarians than do girls. Mothers and fathers say they are more severe with sons than daughters. These data indicate a change from the situation reported by Granqvist in techniques of discipline used and their severity.

The last question to be dealt with in this section is whether the children perceive their same-sex parent as the chief agent of punishment. Granqvist reported that fathers are responsible for the discipline of their sons and mothers for the discipline of their daughters. In the findings reported here on areas of control and decision making, the sons clearly tended to perceive their fathers as the source of authority, and the daughters saw both fathers and mothers as sources of authority. As reported above, both mothers and fathers punish their children for disobedience, girls less severely than boys. We asked the children one more question in the area of punishment, "Who punishes you most?" The same pattern emerges here. Over half of the boys (58 percent) answered father and almost none (6 percent) answered mother. An almost equal percentage of girls answered father and mother (28 and 20 percent). What is of equal interest is that 28 percent of the boys and 36 percent of the girls answered that they are hardly ever punished. This again indicates a change from the traditional pattern of the father as a very strict disciplinarian demanding absolute obedience.

EMOTIONAL SUPPORT

Thus far we have dealt with the controlling and disciplinary aspects of family relationships. Another very important aspect of parent-child relationships is the area of closeness and emotional support from which the child derives his feelings of security and belonging. In the descriptions of the traditional Arab village family the roles of the parents have been portrayed as clearly differentiated. The father has the role of the strict disciplinarian demanding absolute obedience and the mother plays the loving, supportive role to her children. She is the source of comfort and security for her children. Our data have shown that the father is not perceived by his wife and children as the authoritarian patriarch at the present time. Has there been any change in the perception of the mother as the sole or main source of emotional support?

We asked a series of questions to find out to what extent the mother is perceived as the giving, loving, comforting figure as compared with the father. The questions and distribution of answers are shown in Table 6. The general pattern that emerges is that sons feel closer to their fathers and daughters feel closer to their mothers. Two specific points are worth noting. First of all, neither boys nor girls, but especially boys, tend to turn to either parent when they feel sad. Almost two-thirds of the boys and more than one-third of the girls said they did not turn to anyone when they feel sad. This may be part of a more general cultural pattern that one does not show when one is sad (especially males) or that one just does not talk about it. The second point, related to the first, is concerned with the responses to the question about with whom one talks. The fact that a substantially higher proportion of daughters than of sons talk with the same-sex parent may reflect sex differences in the way a relationship is expressed. Sons and fathers may not talk to each other but express emotional closeness by just being together, whereas daughters and mothers tend to talk to each other more. From casual observation in the village one gets the impression that men talk mainly with their peers, whereas mothers, who do not get out much, spend a lot of time talking with their daughters.

These data indicate again that the role of the father has changed in this area. He is a very important figure for his sons not only as a source of authority but as a source of emotional support as well. Again, there is not a high degree of consensus. Relatively more boys choose their fathers than choose their mothers. Among girls the difference between the number choosing mother and father as a source

Table 6. Parents as Sources of Emotional Support as Perceived by Children (%)

| | Sons Say | | | | | Daughters Say | | | | |
| | | Older | | | | | Older | | | |
Question	Father	Mother	Sibs	Other	Total	Father	Mother	Sibs	Other	Total
Who is nicer to you?	39	35	18	8	100	27	62	8	3	100
Who spoils you more?	47	33	6	14	100	38	46	12	4	100
With whom do you talk more?	25	18	43	14	100	4	58	27	11	100
To whom do you turn when you are sad?	6	6	25	63[a]	100	12	23	30	35[a]	100
To whom do you feel closer?	41	33	18	8	100	31	42	19	8	100

[a] The other in this case is *no one.*

236

of emotional support is greater than that for the sons choosing father and mother. The most important point, perhaps, is that just as the father is not the sole source of authority in the family, the mother is not the sole source of emotional support for children of this age.

SUMMARY AND DISCUSSION

We have attempted to describe a number of changes that have occurred in the Arab village family over the period of the last 50 years. Changes in such sociodemographic characteristics as level of education, occupational structure, and family structure are clear, observable, and objective. There has been a clear rise in the level of education. School attendance is part of the daily routine of most children, whereas 50 years ago only boys went to school, and then largely when weather and work permitted. School for girls was practically unheard of. Most families at the present time receive their major source of income from work in a wage-labor economy rather than from agriculture. Most of the men work outside the village as unskilled or semiskilled laborers. Most households include only parents and children. There are few families of the traditional extended-family type.

The changes in patterns of family relationships are less easy to document in an objective way, mainly because of the nature of the subject matter under investigation and partly because of the methods available for study. The information was obtained from interviews with our respondents, and we were limited by what they chose to tell us. Since our findings are so different from the characterizations of the Arab village family in the literature, a few words of caution and explanation are relevant here.

A number of writers (e.g., [4] who have done research in the Middle East have pointed out that what a person says does not necessarily correspond with the "fact." There is no necessary connection between what is said and reality. People tend to get carried away with words. This would lead one to question the validity of some of our findings.

There are, however, a number of reasons why we believe that our findings are valid. First of all, we interviewed fathers, mothers, and children separately about the same set of topics. There was a certain degree of correspondence in their answers. If there had been complete correspondence or no correspondence at all, one might question the validity and reliability of the data. This, however, was not the case. Second, unlike most other anthropological studies in which the investigator essentially gathers all his data from a few good informants in depth, we had a large number of respondents. We asked each of them to respond to a similar set of questions and to tell us what he thinks. Thus we learned how each respondent perceived a given situation. These data should correspond more to the "real" pattern than the "ideal" pattern because we obtain a wide range of individual answers. Third, our findings point up certain patterns that have an internal logic and can be explained in terms of more objective factors operating in the environment.

What are the main patterns of family relationships which we found? One very important finding is that the Arab village family is not an authoritarian, patriarchal family in terms of the kinds of decisions that have to be made within the family. Neither the fathers, mothers, nor children perceive the father as the exclusive source of authority. This is the case whether one is concerned with specific areas of decision making, the number of areas of control, respect and obedience, or techniques of discipline. In all cases there was a range of responses. The only group who tended to see the father in the patriarchal role were the sons. This does not mean, however, that the mother is perceived as equal with the father in this sense. There is rather a tendency toward joint decision making on the part of husbands and wives with regard to family matters.

There are a number of factors that seem to be pushing toward greater sharing of decision-making power between husbands and wives: the nuclear family structure, the practice of giving a newly married couple a room of their own, increased verbal contact between future marriage partners, the increase in level of education, and the changing occupational structure.

Factors that are working in the opposite direction are the different expectations from boys and girls in terms of freedom of movement, the level of education, and the importance of female modesty, which is expressed in terms of early age of marriage and restriction of freedom of movement. We noted a clear tendency for the like-sex parent to be an important image for the child, not only as a source of authority and control but as a source of emotional support. This differential responsibility of fathers and mothers for sons and daughters has not changed much. The traditionally different roles for boys and girls are reflected in this pattern. Thus although the level of education for girls has risen from no schooling to an average of 4 to 6 years of school, most boys attend school now through the eighth or ninth grades. There is still more restriction as noted above in freedom of movement for girls than for boys.

Despite the clear differentiation in expectations for boys and girls, it would seem that one of the most important factors that will push in the direction of greater sharing by the wife in decision making in the Arab family is the increasing level of education. School attendance is important not only for what is learned in school but also because it allows greater freedom of movement and exposure to alternative expectations and aspirations. There are data [4] which indicate that urban highly educated girls delay marriage, want fewer children, and are interested in careers. Although this is a very different situation from that which exists in the village at the present time, the more girls who finish six grades and the few who continue beyond this may be enough of a catalyst to lead to change in this direction over a period of years. If opportunities for work outside the village continue at the present rate, these, too, will influence the expectations of the girls for their future.

Appendix

The sample of 89, including 94 wives and 81 husbands, can be broken down as follows:

	No. of Families	No. of Husbands	No. of Wives
77	monogamous families	77	77
3	polygamous families with 2 wives	3	6
1	polygamous family with 3 wives	1	3
3	families—husband not interviewed	—	3
5	families—husband dead	—	5
89		81	94

The preponderance of boys in the sample (100 boys, 53 girls) was due to a variety of reasons. Birth records are not accurate. The most reliable data available were school records. Since there were more boys attending school than girls in the age group in which we were interested, we were more likely to pick them up. A number of girls were already married by the age of 14 or 15. They were not included, and we have no way of knowing how many there are. All population statistics since 1927 have shown a larger number of males than females. One of the possible explanations for this phenomenon is that the villagers show greater concern about the health of male children than female children. Since chronological age is of no particular importance in the village, even though the interviewers visited every house asking if there were children in the 10 to 16 age group, they may have been given a negative answer either because the parents' estimate of their child's age was wrong or because they did not want to be interviewed.

References

1. Ammar, H. *Growing up in an Egyptian Village.* Routledge and Kegan Paul, London, 1954.
2. Baldensberger, P. *The Immoveable East.* Pitman and Sons, London, 1913.
3. Beck, D. F. (1957). "The Changing Moslem Family of the Middle East" *Marriage Family Living* 19 (1957), 340–350.
4. Berger, M. *The Arab World Today.* Anchor Books, New York, 1964.
5. Granqvist, H. *Marriage Conditions in a Palestinian Village,* Vols. I and II. Academic Bookstore, Helsingfors, 1931, 1935.
6. Granqvist, H. *Birth and Childhood among the Arabs.* Soderstrom, Helsingfors, 1947.
7. Granqvist, H. *Child Problems among the Arabs.* Soderstrom, Helsingfors, 1950.
8. Kressel, G. Realization of agnatic endogamy in Jawarish: Maintenance of cultural objectives. *HaMizrah Hehadash* 20 (1970), 20–52 (in Hebrew).
9. Parsons, T. and Bales, F. *Family, Socialization and the Interaction Process.* The Free Press, Glencoe, Ill., 1955.
10. Rosenfeld, H. Change, barriers to change, and contradictions in the Arab village family *Amer. Anthropol.* 70 (1968), 732–752.
11. Yerushalmi, M. Artas—seminar paper, Tel Aviv University (mimeographed, Hebrew), 1973.

A Two-Step Change of Role in the Emancipation of the War-Bereaved Widow from the Traditional Family

Karen Moses, B.S.W. and Rafael Moses, M.D. (Israel)

Preamble

> *"I don't even know how to do the shopping."*
>
> (Zvia, 25-year-old mother of three children under three years of age, 2 months after her husband was killed in the Yom Kippur War.)

> *"I am a complete nothing."*
>
> (Giselle, 26-year-old mother of two children under 6 years of age, shortly after her husband was killed in action.)

> *"I don't even know how to write a check."*
>
> (Nora, another war widow.)

> *"God damn you, you help me yet!"*
>
> (Claire, 28-year-old widow of a regular army paratroop officer, meaning that she needed help to get out from under her past and present life situation.)

Claire knew the function, obligations, and resources of the Rehabilitation Service because her husband was in the regular army, whereas

Zvia, Giselle, and Nora had no inkling of their rights and felt completely lost now that they were deprived of the link between themselves and the outside world—their husbands. Nora, although belonging to the upper-middle professional class, had grown up in and continued to live in a very religiously orthodox environment. The other three were of a low socioeconomic status and of Middle Eastern or North African origin.

The Rehabilitation Wing of the Israeli Ministry of Defense functions under a law that lays down the state's responsibility for meeting the basic needs of families when the father has been killed while in the service. These needs include an income *above* the national average, complete health care, complete educational and vocational training for the widows and children, and good public housing according to the needs of the individual family.

The philosophy of the Rehabilitation Service vis-a-vis the widow is to supply her with as many resources as possible—economic, supportive, and therapeutic—and make available the most suitable rehabilitation program to enable her to achieve a fuller life and be a better mother and thus fulfill both an instrumental and expressive role in relation to the outside world and to her family.

Every bereaved family is assigned a caseworker who acts as the link between them and the Rehabilitation Service. The economic resources are centrally administered, whereas the supportive casework or occasionally therapy is carried out by the caseworker, by local health agencies, or by private therapists. This is only one facet of a network of resources available to the bereaved family, but it is one with a declared philosophy of assistance.

The goals set by the service are achieved by what can be viewed as a two-phase intervention. The first is crisis intervention when a family is helped to reorganize and return to an optimal level of functioning under the existing circumstances; the second involves an effort to make use of the crisis as the foundation for growth and development.

The Traditional Background in Its Shaping Aspect

The opening remarks given reveal some of the desperation experienced by young women from traditional families following the death of their husbands, constricted by the shock of bereavement, by the traditionalism that had dictated their lives until this crisis, by class and economic determinants, but mainly by the lack of awareness of the potentials dormant within them.

All these widows came from families with a traditional outlook in which the man's role was to fulfill all instrumental tasks relating to the outside world, while the woman was the homemaker and the physical caretaker of the family. Thus the paterfamilias was the breadwinner and, as such, determined the social status of the family. It was he who paid the bills and did the weekly shopping at the city market. It was he who decided if and when they would visit friends, go to the movies, or go dancing. Although all social activities were based on the unit of the couple or on family ties, there was hardly any individual independent social activity for the women. The education of the children also fell within the father's domain. It was he who disciplined them, he who helped them with their homework, and even he—alone or with his wife—who would go to parents' meetings or talk to the teacher at school. These were upwardly mobile families who strove intensively to better themselves. This was demonstrated, among other things, by their having moved recently from substandard housing to modern, three-room apartments, a first step on the socioeconomic way up. Many more such upward steps were in their sights, yet after the death of their husbands, they appeared to have lost all momentum and push and felt ignorant and incapable of fulfilling the instrumental functions required for the family.

This, roughly, was the setting in which the woman faced her husband's death. True, these families were exposed to and formed part of the wider social network in Israel, with its pressures on changing the status for both men and women: the former were in the process of losing their exclusive positions, and the latter were coming into some of the rights and duties of women in modern Western society.

The Aftermath of Bereavement

One of the interesting impressions obtained in working with the widows was that they seemed to regress to a lower stage of emancipation in response to the trauma of the husband's violent death. Subsequently, they reached new heights of freedom not yet visible to them before. This naturally created a revolutionary change for the family unit as a whole—widow and children.

One of the more conspicuous economic resources placed at the disposal of widows with children by the Rehabilitation Wing was a car which they could purchase without the usual 150 percent tax and with a loan of £10,000. They were also allocated a sum to pay for about 20 driving lessons, and the annual car license was paid for them. The car thus became a symbol of being taken care of by the state, of a marked increase in socioeconomic status, and of a newly felt sense of power. It also acted as a catalyst for mobilizing hidden strengths. None of the widows regarded the car as a mere mode of transport; for each it was invested with intense ideas and ambivalent feelings. But this was equally true for other new activities such as the buying of clothes or the furnishing of apartments, all of which inevitably developed symbolic value on the way to freedom.

Illustrations

GISELLE

Giselle's husband was missing in action for 6 months. She was shocked and dazed and regressed to patterns of behavior that dated back to her Morrocan origins in this situation of acute and terrible uncertainty; she visited a variety of fortune-tellers, crystal gazers, coffee readers, and other such in an attempt to learn about her husband's fate. During this period of acute distress she completely neglected her house and children and moved over to her mother's home. At the same time she began taking driving lessons, and after only 25 half-hour lessons she passed her test on the first try. It was striking to see Giselle, who felt "a nothing," who behaved confusedly and erratically, and who reverted at times to previously discarded earlier patterns of behavior, sitting at the wheel of her own car—relaxed, competent, and self-assured. It was as if the world of the new and the world of the old were represented in her quite incompatibly side by side.

NORA

Nora, who worked as a professional while her husband was a Yeshiva student, did equally well in passing her driving test about 4 months after her husband was killed. She began to experience a marvelous sense of freedom while driving and would, when feeling tense, take off in the car to work off her feelings. She was soon able to drive out of town to visit parents and friends and thus achieved a new geographical mobility. At the wheel she felt "like the queen of the road" and relished the sense of physical power that came when the car responded to the pressure of her foot on the accelerator almost as if it were a living part of her. At the same time, her hands transmitted a physical sense of well-being as she felt herself in control of the powerful machine (a small Volkswagen). The traditional walls that had enclosed her for so long had seemingly become elastic and expandable. The "Queen of the road," in Israeli lore, was also a whore, and Nora felt that she had acquired the car in exchange for her husband's dead body. She even experienced strong guilt feelings at times as if she were betraying her husband by enjoying the car.

CLAIRE

Claire began taking driving lessons 2 months after her husband's death in a jeep accident. Although confused and disorganized in many areas following the loss, she had been able to maintain her home minimally. After only 20 half-hour lessons, she passed the driving test on her first try. Her brothers-in-law induced her to buy the car while she was still in a state of shock, picking it out for her and closing the deal. She signed a large check that was not covered in part; she was functioning "like a robot in a complete fog." The car stood in front of her house for 2 months after she had passed her driving test. She would clean it religiously twice a week but not drive it. Finally her 8-year-old daughter said: "Mummy, if you don't drive the car, I will!" But she could only begin driving when she herself felt ready. To this day Claire feels that the car belongs not to her but to the Ministry of Defense. Every now and then she hands her caseworker the keys and says: "Take them, it's your car," adding that if it had not been for her husband's violent death, she would never have had a car for herself. "Take the keys and give me back my husband."

In all these instances, the car became a psychological instrument for increasing the self-esteem, the competence, the self-confidence and the socio-economic status of the widow as a first step toward her emancipation as a woman.

MARGOT

The provision of an education and a vocation for the widow serves a similar role as an instrument for change but adds an important factor to her growth and development by helping to bring a change in her status within the family.

Margot is the mother of six sons, the oldest of whom was 9 years old when his father was killed; the youngest was born 7 months after the father's death. She came from an underprivileged Kurdish family and had to start earning money as a cleaner at the age of 11. She was illiterate and could barely sign her name when her husband was killed on the Sinai front, a day after the cease-fire. Her father-in-law was an unskilled building laborer who spent all his free time learning the scriptures. Her husband had been an unskilled worker in a supermarket but had also laid great store on learning: in addition to religious studies he acquired encyclopedias and consistently encouraged his sons to read books of all kinds. After working late most evenings, he would help his children do their homework, would tell them stories, read to them and read with them. The first question Margot posed to the social worker only 2 days after her husband's death was, "How will I raise five sons to the scriptures and to good deeds?"

Margot was certainly capable of raising her sons to good deeds, and she also slowly, very, very slowly, began to read the scriptures. With the help of a private teacher she started out to master "the three R's." When the caseworker first suggested this in the presence of the children, her 11-year-old son said: "What, this one (pointing at his mother) will learn? She is a mere woman!" But now her oldest children help her do her work and are very proud of her progress.

THE OTHERS

Nora, the professional, went back to study to widen her knowledge of religious studies. Giselle is entering the fashion world, a dream of many years fulfilled but a dream she had very gladly given up as a girl when the right man came along—her now-dead husband. Zvia is going to secretarial school, and Claire is working toward the high school finals that she had barely finished 7 years before her marriage.

The Two-Step Change of Role

Beginning with the phase of crisis, concrete economic benefits are made available to these widows that lead to a radical change in socio-economic status. Along with this marked shift from external benefits, the widow is helped by the social worker through casework to perform a series of instrumental tasks that were previously the sole domain of the husband. This represents the first step.

The second step comes after the widow has learned to cope with the daily exigencies of her new life situation. It consists of a working through on a deeper level of her past patterns of adjustment. This takes place under the protective shield of a casework or therapy relationship. It is only after these patterns have been worked through to some extent that the widow is able appropriately to utilize another set of benefits offered her—further education and vocational training—that consolidate her increased sense of freedom and self-reliance.

The result at the present time, 2½ years after the Yom Kippur War, is a considerable change for the whole family, visible both in the external appurtenances of living and in the increased internal sense of well-being and self-esteem on the part of the widow as well as in the improved functioning of both her instrumental and expressive roles within the family.

A constant preoccupation of the widows, naturally enough, is the subject of a new relationship with a man and ultimately the question of remarriage. Clearly, it takes time for the widow to feel both ready for such a relationship and to deem it permissible. Just as clearly, the timing for this is quite individual and has a wide range. An interesting phase—for many widows presumably an interim phase —is an enjoyment of her freedom both from and with men. The widow enjoys her lack of accountability and her freedom to move and act without the limitations imposed through marriage. At this point she feels that she neither wants nor needs marriage. She may be concerned, as was one widow, whether relationships with men are an escape from something or a road leading to something more positive. The conflict around this is accentuated by economic considerations. Many of her benefits will cease on remarriage. On the other hand, there is also an economic incentive for marriage—a one-time allotment of £100,000. Some of the Six Day War widows apparently have settled for the freedom of not being married. Also to be taken into consideration is the fact that some of the children react intensively and ambivalently to the mother's ties to a new man. At this time— 2½ years after the Yom Kippur War—there is much interest in the subject of remarriage amongst widows of that period.

Changes in the Children of Bereavement

Most of the children show some symptoms: enuresis, learning difficulties, sleep disturbances, and eating difficulties. In most families there is an increased mutual dependency (shown most often by the mother's taking one of the children regularly into her bed). As the children grow older, one of the most noticeable difficulties is with discipline—in many cases, they are overdisciplined.

Both widows and children react ambivalently to the marked improvements, both external and internal. They are all delighted with the increase in their economic status and competence, but at the same time they all feel strongly that their considerable gains have come about at the expense of the death of the father-husband. (This aspect is further complicated by the prevailing emotional climate of the national debt to bereaved families.) The feelings of guilt can be worked through in the casework relationship with the widows but not directly with the children. There is also the problem of projection. The Ministry of Defense (and its representative, the caseworker) is somehow held accountable for the death of the husband-father, in the first place by the mother but then transmitted, through her bitterness, resentment, and hostility, to the children. Surprisingly, these mixed feelings related to the death of the husband-father vary little with the *cause* of death, whether it be in action, through accident, or from illness. From a preliminary survey done on children under the age of 4, the fact that the father was *killed while in service* is of major importance. The child takes it from there, identifying with a heroic father and elaborating stories of his heroism.

Are these children of bereavement overtly sad? There is no doubt that they are troubled and that many of them express repeated wishes to die and rejoin the lost father. Some refuse to join in neighborhood children's groups because of their sensitivity to tactless references to their bereaved state. Many of the younger ones have great difficulty in separating from the mother on entry to kindergarten. *Yet it is quite rare to find a young child who is overtly and persistently sad.* In fact, mothers report with an admixture of pleasure and resentment on the cheerfulness of their children. And if a mother does talk of a child's sadness, it soon transpires that she is really talking about her own feelings and using the child as her medium of expression.

The newly acquired emancipation and freedom that have entered the lives of these young widows so unexpectedly is best verbalized by one of them: "You know," said Claire, "all the roads used to be one-way streets. And now we can choose to go either way."

Report of Site Visitors on Changing Conditions in Israel, July, 1976

Jon Lange, M.D. (Norway)
Luis E. Prego-Silva, M.D. (Uruguay)

The purpose of these visits was to introduce the International Study Group and its invited experts to the way in which in a rapidly growing society like Israel the traditional and modern often continue to exist side by side, so that it is not uncommon to see a train of camels walking with studied dignity past a convoy of mechanized tractors. Yet, there is no shock of incompatibility: change and changelessness have become common bedfellows in this young country. The program that was organized proved very successful in demonstrating the contrasts.

The first day's visit was to Rosh Ha-Ayn, a village east of Petah Tikwa with a population of about 15,000 of whom 90 percent were of Yemenite origin. There was a Family Health Center dealing tactfully and comfortably with representatives from both the old and the new. The visitors were invited into the homes of two families who both occupied modern four-room apartments but lived quite different lives. The traditional family had accumulated nine children in 12 years, with the prospect of continuing at the same rate. The traditional father worked at handwriting the Holy Scriptures, and this necessitated a ritual bath every time that he wrote the name of God. The modern family had four children and lived in a thoroughly

Westernized way. There was seemingly no enmity in relation to the striking differences.

The next visit was to Amishav, a suburb of Petah Tikwa with a population of about 8000 mostly of North African origin. This was a community with considerable social problems, among them a high rate of delinquency. Once again, there was a chance to observe the juxtaposition of a traditional and modern family. The former was an extended-family group in which recently a child had been born simultaneously to mothers of three generations. Six adults and nine children lived an overcrowded existence in a two-room apartment where little privacy was available. On the other hand, the modern family had only one child and led a much less spartan existence than their traditional counterpart. The visitors also had an opportunity to see a day camp for *mothers* who had five or more children. While the mothers are away, the youngest children are taken to day-care centers, the middle-aged ones are accommodated with relatives or friends and the adolescents either go off to a camp or take care of themselves with the help of the father during the week of mother's absence. The idea of giving mothers, ranging from the 20s to the 40s, a rest from family activities seemed both novel and therapeutic. New conditions, to which a rapidly developing society is exposed every day, called for new measures.

The next stop was at the Kibbutz Horeshim with 200 inhabitants, 73 children, no members over the age of 40, and a history of 20 years. It was an exclusively agricultural society whose products helped to feed the rest of the nation.

The last stop was at an Arab village, Kfar Kassem, of about 10,000 mostly Moslem Arabs who had been citizens of Israel since the founding of the state. Their leaders were clearly proud of the fact that their community was well-adjusted and satisfied with the situation. There had been no manifestations of unrest recently prevalent among Israel's Arab population. It was impressed on the visitors that as far as Israel was concerned, there were three kinds of Arabs: those who have lived in Israel since its foundation, those who belong to the territories acquired by Israel after the Six Day War, and those who live in Arab countries. The Family Health Center in this village was run by an Arabic-speaking Jewish nurse of Iraqi origin whose warmth and friendliness had made her a favorite with both parents and children. Kfar Kassem had been the scene of a massacre performed by Israeli police under conditions of high tension. The case at the time had been thoroughly investigated, and the guilty policemen were sentenced to imprisonment. Yet here, 15 years later, the villagers were proud of their good relations with the larger Israeli society.

Despite the exposure to many different exotic aspects of this country, the most striking impression was made by the Kibbutz Horeshim. This tiny community was able to offer comprehensive care to its members at a level that has never been reached in any free-enterprise society. Child care was an integral part of the kibbutz activities, and contented adults and children were everywhere in evidence. In other communities the Family Health Center appeared to generate trust and confidence in its clientele who came to it for all its physical health needs. As yet, mental health facilities were not as available as in the kibbutz, but this development was anticipated in the near future.

The impact of change was more obvious in the physical environment, where it was clear that sometimes change was a two-edged weapon. For example, the change from wells and time-consuming water transportation to a modern water-supply system with running water in each house had created enormous problems with epidemics, because the old sewage system was unable to cope with the increased flow of water.

What the psychological effect of airlifting 400 families to Yemen in 1954 can only be a matter of speculation, but it seemed fair to assume that "going home" must have been a very spiritual experience. They had been brought from an ancient setting to live in the paradoxically modern Israel, a state with a religious *raison d'être,* but with a largely secularized, European-type society. The great flight brought to their religious minds the words of the Lord to Moses (Exodus 19, 4–6): "Ye have seen what I did unto the Egyptians, and how I bare you on eagles' wings, and brought you unto myself. Now therefore, if ye will obey my voice indeed, and keep my covenant, then ye shall be a peculiar treasure unto me above all people: for all the earth is mine: and ye shall be unto me a kingdom of priests, and an holy nation." In these words, one could detect the wellsprings of the feelings of confidence and competence and the ability to deal

with change as it came that was very much in evidence wherever we
went.

Anna Potamianou, Ph.D. (Greece)

Those of us belonging to the group that visited the Beit-Shemesh
area had the opportunity to see a developing industrial town with an
extremely diversified range of industries (coffee, bicycles, clothing,
cement, airplanes). In this area poor and deprived families of immigrants have been established since 1956, coming from Italy, Spain,
Russia, Rumania, and some parts of North Africa. Their establishment determined multiform problems in terms of adaptation to the
life of an industrial town, training, communication between groups
coming from very different backgrounds, the necessity to establish
hygiene, education and community facilities that would not rebut
the people they were supposed to serve, and so on. An additional difficulty seemed to stem from the fact that plans for the establishment
of the immigrants had to be made under the pressures caused by
the precarious conditions existing in the country. The network of
nurses and social workers intended to cover this area, as well as the
area of Beit-Sheba which we visited in the south on the frontier of
the Negev desert, seems to have been successful in establishing relationships with the various groups of immigrants as well as with the
Arab groups that have remained in Israeli territory.

The "open door" policy of the mother and children clinics, each
one of which is serving 300 to 500 families, and the home visits by
the nurses encourage personal contacts and facilitate exchanges between mothers and children in the various groups. This factor certainly keeps up the old neighborhood spirit many of those families
were accustomed to, while helping to introduce new techniques of
child rearing and hygiene in the home. The prominence of the role
of the nurses compared to that of other professionals certainly has to
do with the planning of the location of the different clinics with their
availability for daily consultations and their community-oriented
training.

The process of change may be slow and hesitant where families of
very conservative background are concerned or where the proposed

changes are too demanding—for example, from tent to apartment houses for Bedouin families. Yet, we saw no family wanting to go back to the prerefrigerator, pretelevision era. For many the old ways have been abandoned for good. In the Arab families women of three generations (grandmother, mother, and daughter) received us in the absence of their men and were unveiled. Also, the fact that Arab women are allowed to leave home for the day programs of the "summer camps" further induces the image of change in a spectacular way.

In the summer camps women who had never before left their houses, who had never had a day free from housework, and who had never been exposed to the experience of being treated as persons in their own rights, are taught how to plan housework, how to take care of their appearance, how to appreciate and plan their leisure time.

Our team was invited to a farewell party given by a group of mothers who had completed their 3-week stay in the vacation camp. The presence of strangers did not seem to inhibit their activities. Those women, with very little or no education at all, made speeches, participated in presenting a wedding according to the old Yemenite tradition, laughed, and sang quite freely. Of course, our home visits left us with the impression, as was to be expected, that some of the families adapt better to the new ways of life and are better able to take advantage of what is offered to them than others. Also, even in traditional families the pattern of expectations and wishes for the children is changing. Young girls want to go to a university to study, and very often the parents do not stand in their way.

The same pattern of change can be discerned in the policy followed by the kibbutz. Life in the collective is changing toward more flexibility in the schedule and regulations, more liberal attitudes as regards the right of young individuals to leave the kibbutz or of kibbutz members to lead a more family-oriented type of life. This may explain why young people seem, nowadays, more contented to share the kibbutz life than they were several years ago. Also, one can detect a tendency of young people who have left the kibbutz to come back. This trend should be evaluated not only in relation to the growing stresses and demands of city life but also in terms of the exasperation of dependency needs of individuals living in a country where too much is expected from them too soon. Of course, one cannot help viewing the attraction exercised by collective life on the Jewish population involved also in the light of a repetitive experience.

One last comment: undoubtedly, it is the Israeli people who take the initiative and responsibility for the implementation of programs leading to new modes of life for the polymorphous population inhabiting the land of Israel. But the inevitable stresses those changes are bringing about, as well as the impact of the country's living conditions, are absorbed and felt by all. If it can be said that such a climate engenders tensions, it can also be said that common experiences favor the interpenetration of the systems of the various population groups. One could express the fear that this may lead to a confusion of identities. But one could also express the hope that if the right channels of communication are established, this could lead to the shaping of a common social conscience based on the recognition of what each group is contributing to the formation of common ideals and aims.

Before concluding these remarks, which certainly cannot convey the richness of the impressions left with us after our site visits, our most grateful thoughts go out to all those who helped to bring to life the sign—spelt out with flowers—which awaits the foreigner entering the city of Jerusalem: "Welcome."

General Discussion

J. Noshpitz, M.D. (U.S.A.)

Relatively little attention has been directed to the nature, the definition of change. Dr. Anthony did refer to its protean character, and Dr. Hersch spoke of it as "becoming different," but in no case was the definitional issue explored in depth. Most of the participants seemed content to accept it at face value, to view it as something flowing, directional, or transformational. I propose to discuss the notion of change making use of two ancient models.

The first, or Heraclitean model, involves a conception of reality based on dynamic flux: everything flows; one never steps twice into the same stream; like the proverbial shuttle, reality is in a state of continuous motion. Such a model of change underlies the thinking of functional social work, the interpersonal therapists, and the transactional analysts. The focus of therapy is directed toward the work of the shuttle and not to the pattern it weaves, to the back and forth of the interactive process and communication rather than to unyielding internal dynamics. Such a model is excellent for family communication disorders but does rather less well with the structured internalized neuroses.

A contrasting model was constructed by Parmenides. His vision of reality was static and changeless; all apparent variations are superficial. They may be ignorantly confused with reality but merely represent appearance. This type of model underlies the geneticist's viewpoint comprising the stable genotype covered over by the variable and less-meaningful phenotype or a personality theory that sees the conflictual experiences of earliest childhood as the basic templates or blueprints upon which the character structure is erected. All the variations of everyday behavior, if carefully analyzed, are seen to be recapitulations of such stable, underlying themes. These continue unchanged and are, indeed, not easily changeable throughout most experience. Such a model is suitable for understanding and treating chronic character problems, but in turn, it has trouble accounting for interactive and certain kinds of action-oriented disorders.

My purpose in this discussion is to emphasize that the nature of change is not simple and can rapidly lead us into complexities and contradictions unless and until we can develop a true psychology of change. To even begin to do this we must first decide on the type of model upon which we wish to build, and then begin to observe what in any situation changes and what remains unchanged.

Since we are only at the beginning of a scientific study of the nature of change as it affects our work as clinicians, it may seem premature to raise questions about its form in our daily encounters with it. Sooner or later, however, we will need to inquire to what extent clinical change is linear, curvilinear, cyclical, or pendular, carrying our patients (and ourserves) forward, spiraling upward, or backward and forward between such poles as passivity and activity, dependence and autonomy, giving and getting. It now appears that biologically (and perhaps psychologically) we are governed by profound inner rhythms that themselves are susceptible to change under stress. Since we, the observers, are also undergoing change along with the environment around us, the study of change becomes even more problematical. How can we contrive a fixed point from which to conduct our investigations? How do we decide what is fixed and what moves? As in Heisenberg's dilemma, the observer of change is himself caught up in both its effects and its begetting.

This kind of thinking should permeate the formulations of change theorists. It is not enough to adapt theory developed for other purposes and call it change theory. Thus Caplan's work on support structures was not originally designed as a part of a theory of change. It grew out of other considerations, although in this presentation he showed how it might be so adapted.

We need to ask ourselves some fundamental questions: Are we talking or dealing with change that is expectable and the very stuff of existence or with change that is special and unpredictable, meriting a psychology, and perhaps even a psychopathology of its own? Are we focusing on change that is largely external (as evident in Anthony's presentation) or on change that is within the individual or within his family?

In keeping with this, three well-known concepts might prove useful in clarifying this new psychology: first, Escalona's notion of state —the prevailing dynamic equilibrium or homeostasis and the vectors associated with this; second, Lewin's notion of field or living space and the vectors associated with that; and, third, Durkheim's notion of anomie that concerns itself with the psychological dislocation brought about by environmental change. (Anthony refers to this but does not elaborate on it.) This kind of change is symbolic rather than material; it involves meaning and not geography.

In addition to an overall theory or model incorporating a number of sound concepts of change, we also need an operational approach— some measure of the extent to which we can or should become change agents in the service of making things better. This brings up difficult and disturbing questions concerning values. Do we know enough to manipulate changes in children's lives? In therapy we assume that we do, as in custody cases, but our more skeptical selves remind us that clinical work is rife with ambiguities and unknowns. It is important to know what and when we do not know and not to be ashamed of our not knowing. We should keep in mind that all our helping methods are two-edged—helpful in one instance and harmful in another—

and so we should prescribe change with caution and circumspection and be wary of the wild and the dramatic.

If the notion of change is to become the new wave of the future on many clinical fronts, it behooves us to pay special attention to the groundwork in theory, conceptualizations, modes of implementation, values, and the study of the dynamics and methodology of change. With this in mind, the work can proceed both safely and scientifically.

Jon Lange, M.D. (Norway)

The Moses' chapter has many interesting aspects to it. One aspect is the way in which Israel copes with a special kind of mass disaster that it has experienced four times during its short 28 years of existence as a state. On the family level this is *change* at its most dramatic. A particularly impressive feature is the massive support offered to the widows of soldiers, both in the form of economic aid and of professional help. I have been told that even bringing the news of the death of the husband/father is usually done by a mental health professional. However, the main focus of the presentation is on the impact of the disaster—and of the help offered—on the nonemancipated widow, and the aim of the helping process is clearly to increase her freedom and assist her in becoming a more instrumental person.

Bereavement, however, is a universal experience. The sudden death of a breadwinner is always with us, but it is not only war that claims him. Even in more peaceful corners of the world death may strike *en masse,* as for instance when a Norwegian fishing boat is shipwrecked, and a little coastal community, through one blow of fate, loses seven of its adult males, all husbands and fathers. Death may be a part of life for every one of us but a part that we are often ill prepared for. One of the questions provoked by this thoughtful chapter is whether the liberated, emancipated women of today are better equipped and better prepared for withstanding the stresses of widowhood. To illustrate my question I refer to a personal experience. In 1970 two brothers I knew well died. Both had been in German concentration camps during World War II. The younger brother suffered from a KZ syndrome that had forced him some years previously to leave a leading position in education, and the older brother died following a second apoplexy at the age of 67 (the first attack some few years earlier had left only negligible residual signs). The younger brother drowned while swimming, possibly precipitated by a heart attack, at age 63. My "cases" are the two wives, at that time aged 58 and 62, respectively. Both wives had a professional training before marriage, one as a teacher and the other as a painter. Both had for years after the war been forced by external circumstances connected with the work of their husbands to live primarily as their husbands' wives and not as professional people in their own right. Following her bereavement, the younger of the two, the former teacher and wife of the older brother, continued to live her life "through her husband." The other, in the later years of her married life, decided that she, for her own sake, had to create a life of her own. As a painter, she felt she had "dried up," so she trained to become a weaver, and this became the new profession she was practicing when the death occurred. The extent to which these two women have been able to live through their loss and retain a "wholeness" has been strikingly different, and the difference has corresponded closely to the different levels of emancipation achieved before the bereavement. Thus one aspect of emancipation for the women may be that it acts as a preventive measure in this kind of life crisis.

Colette Chiland, M.D., Ph.D. (France)

There is a reality of change, but there is also an ideology of change. Change can have both a negative (retrogressive) or positive (progressive) value—at least as seen from the Western point of view.

In every society, in every epoch, there is simultaneously continuity and change, but at times one is more manifest than the other. Formerly, in Western society continuity and tradition were more visible; today it is change that catches the eye.

Some changes involve all or almost all members of a society, while other changes, as striking and as spectacular, reach only a small circle: thus there are islets of change or marginal changes.

One must take into consideration a scale of change that is not the same for all societies and for all phenomena that, understandably, follows if one considers the millennia of human evolution.

Actually, we are observing an obliteration of differences between cultures as anthropologists, such as Levi-Strauss, regard as a likely danger. Man has need of his differences; how else can he develop a self-concept.

In the human psychic organization there are two contradictory factors at work:

1. Resistance to change, compulsion to repetition, the search for sameness;
2. An appetite for change without which growth cannot occur.

* * *

[These comments were made about Dr. Caplan's chapter.] It has been known for some time that grandparents can exert a pathogenic role, which has been subsumed in the theory that it takes three generations to produce a psychotic child.

We have been struck at the Day Hospital of the 13th zone in Paris by the number of psychotic school children who were living in families in which three generations were present in the same home. One of my students has carried out an investigation on these families as part of her doctoral thesis. It could have been postulated that the role of the grandparents, more often that of the grandmother, was related to setting up conditions for the emergence of childhood psychosis and the necessary type of child care, but, in fact, it became apparent that each generation was disturbed. Moreover, the grandparents were more often observed in a negative way as interfering with the treatment than as a positive support for their children and grandchildren.

In cases of neurosis and minor character disorders, it was discovered that disturbances during development tended to occur when the children were raised during certain critical periods, for instance during the first 6 years of life, by grandparents, even though the parental function was taken back later by the natural parents. This arrangement was not conducive to helping the parents themselves to cope with the problems and educational tasks of the early years. It should be added that these findings occurred with equal frequency in school children referred for consultation and those taken at random, during the study, from the general population.

* * *

I am not sure that I am the right person to comment on Dr. Lifshitz's communication, which is based on results obtained through the use of two instruments (the Beery Test of Complexity and Witkin's Embedded Figures Test) with which I am not familiar. However, while reading the text provided by the author, I wondered about the possible relationship that might exist between the findings furnished by these methods and what we know from our own clinical experience. What might be the significance for our daily practice of the fact that the father or mother demonstrated this or that pair of contrasting characteristics located at the same or different points on a six-point scale?

In talking about her paper, Dr. Lifshitz has displayed a rich and factual knowledge of the kibbutz adolescent that she does not make use of in her written text. Currently, the kibbutz system is of great interest to the French. One of the best sellers on this subject is the book by Bettelheim, for the reason perhaps that it has been translated. Even the left-wing critics of Israel, who consider it a bastion of American imperialism, make frequent references to the experience of the collective socialist education of the kibbutzim (without apparently feeling that they are contradicting themselves).

For us, the central topic that has brought us together for this international study group relates to the changes and the interaction between external and internal changes. It is from this point of view that I wish to ask Dr. Lifshitz two questions.

The first question refers to the educational changes that have taken place in the collectives. One kibbutz that we visited yesterday had remained relatively faithful to its standards, and we were told only about 15 percent of the kibbutzim had altered the rule that after the newborn had slept in the parental house for the first few weeks, it was transferred to the infants' home. Whatever changes have occurred have stemmed from the pressures of the new generation who were born and brought up in the kibbutz; they have become parents who are demanding easier and less restricted access to their infants. Another change that has taken place in the past 2 years has been that the adolescents are being sent outside to high school and not completing their total education within the kibbutz system as previously. These changes are leading to a tightening of the bonds between parent and child as occurs in the nuclear family. Under such conditions, is the kibbutz perhaps less able than before to protect the child who has lost one of its parents or is otherwise deprived? This is my first question.

My second question has to do with the return (perhaps no more than a tendency) toward a more traditional role for the woman, even though the kibbutz ideology has always been basically equalitarian. What impact would such a development have on the child's differential attitude and approach to his parents? One would so like to have access to material of some depth allowing one to compare the manner in which first- and second-generation kibbutzniks experience their relationship with their parents. One would like also to know what happens in the case of separation or divorce when the child loses contact with the mother as compared with the father. The situation cannot be regarded as symmetrical (even for research purposes). This is simply not possible. Moreover, in the kibbutz a particular problem arises from the fact that the children have relations with several "mothers"—the natural mother, the metapélet, the house parents—while there is only a single father. Is the idealization of the absent parent encountered as frequently with these children as with children brought up under ordinary conditions?

Another intriguing detail caught my attention: according to Dr. Lifshitz, the kibbutz children without fathers tend to show less aggressiveness. Such a finding would be in opposition to what we know today about the psychology of aggression and clinically about the higher rates of delinquency among fatherless children.

Finally, the experience that we had yesterday on the site visit gave us an idea of the importance of the children to the kibbutz community and the investment of time, concern, and protection lavished on them, particularly on orphaned children. At the kibbutz we visited we had a language problem. At one point we understood a mother to say that she had four children. She had said to us: "One of our sons died during the Yom Kippur War." We also heard of another son who had suffered from combat neurosis. We talked about this and were moved by the suffering this particular mother had experienced. Gradually, in the course of the day, we were made aware of the meaning of the phrase "one of our sons." It related to a son of the kibbutz and not to the actual son of our host.

Some General Remarks on
the Israeli Experience

Reginald S. Lourie, M.D. (U.S.A.)

When the human or anthropos, as the Greeks called them to bypass calling them men, first appeared on this earth in the present form it was the result of change. It is only recently that it has become clearer how this process takes place as defined by Nobelist Jacques Monad in his book *Chance and Necessity*. I can summarize all this by pointing out that we can no longer ask "which came first, the chicken or the egg?" It had to be the egg, because the chicken cannot change, but the egg can, particularly in its earliest phases of development. But through natural selection the changes, the mutations created by chance or necessity that allowed anthropos to survive and then progress to an advanced condition and then become perpetuated, took literally millions of years. In turn, anthropos has produced changes in the earth and the environment that are taking place rapidly and are challenging us as responsible humans to deal with the changes. However, the basic structure of the human cannot change as fast. Rapid physical adaptations cannot be expected if we look at the history of how many millennia were necessary to evolve appropriate changes in body structure. For example, the human male evolved into a usually larger, stronger, and more active person than the female in order to be the hunter and the fighter, the provider and the protector. Technology and industrialization are changing the

need for those male roles, in many parts of the world, but male structure can be expected to take at least thousands of years to change.

The impact of environmental changes on the man's ability to function is most dramatic in the developing countries. At the International Study Group meeting in Senegal it was seen that many men
from the bush villages go to work in the cities or the mines and the
women grow the food and protect as well as raise the children alone.
At the same time, from biblical reports onward and currently on an
accelerated rate in the industrial parts of the world, men have taken
a more active part in bringing up the children.

Since change in basic body structure and its associated biological
tasks and roles cannot be expected to keep pace with the need to
function to deal with the changing conditions created by anthropos,
we have to look at the other major capacity made available through
chance and necessity that is involved in the makeup of human beings.
Anthropos has the capacity to shape or prepare the individual from
birth to fit into the role necessitated by the conditions to be faced
in order to survive. Survival is the most basic concern of the individual, the family, and the society. The cultural patterns of the
community and the larger society grew out of the survival needs, and
only then did the pleasurable needs of all of the individuals become
involved.

The family in almost every society has the responsibility for the
process of "shaping" the child. There is hardly a variation in the
type of family that anyone can think of that has not been tried somewhere on this planet. Even the most bizarre arrangements have been
found, such as that prohibiting a married man who was head of a
family to do any manual work, which meant that a man could not
formally marry until he had sons old enough to assume responsibility
for the household. There are societies where men only visit their
wives in the middle of the night and do not stay for breakfast. Yet
the essentials are there: the children's place and the children's unquestioned right to be cherished and cared for and the couple's relationship to their children. Over and over again, throughout history,
there have been attempts to destroy this family unit. Mythological
past happenings have been used to justify contemporary social experiments, such as the assertion that in earlier times there was no
family and human beings practiced "group marriage." So far in
human history, however, societies have not found a way to rear chil-

dren without the ties of parents to children and children to parents.

Just a brief look at the tremendous variety of solutions in the past should reassure us that a society can devise new systems of economic sanctions for human effort within which new viable family forms can be developed and cultivated. A glance at the changing styles of expectation among young people in the United States in the last 50 years, in response to changing conditions from the small family of the 1930s to the over-domestication of the 1950s to the irresponsibility of the early 1970s, should reassure us of our capacity to react to change and to change rapidly.

We inevitably get back to the individuals involved as we try to assess how children and families respond to change and what can be done to help them. But the basic question remains: Who changes easily, who changes with more difficulty, and who cannot change? Who in the Arab village that Helen Antonovski reported on moved away to attempt to establish independence and a new way of life in conformity with the majority society? Who moved only a little distance away or did not change at all? Which of the fathers are able to help their sons and daughters change from traditional patterns? Which fathers were helpless and which were left floundering, or depressed, and which were left with the loss of face in their own extended families or in the community?

From the kibbutz visits and Michaela Lifshitz's report we found we had to read between the lines to find that again the same questions come up. Which are the individuals who cannot fit into the philosophy of the individual kibbutz? Who from the kibbutz become the best officers in the army and air force and which ones remain privates and have a harder time adjusting to change from the relatively protected environment in which they were raised? From this unique environment in which every baby is known, and I mean really known, we heard that from the first months on there are observant and wise metapelets who can tell which of their babies are at risk for optimal development. The slower ones and the ones who have trouble in dealing with even expectable stresses and anxieties are known early. Can we then say that they are therefore suspect of being the ones who would have more difficulty in dealing with or accepting change?

In other words, we come back to consideration of the individual when we look at the statistics of successes in dealing with change.

Just as important, if not more important, we must look at those who turn up in a different kind of statistics. These are the statistics of those individuals who cope poorly in response to change and are then found in the welfare programs: the unemployed, the delinquents, the retarded, the mentally ill. These are the ones who tax our treasuries and overwhelm the capacities of our service systems.

As mental health professionals, along with the very special metapelets, we have learned a great deal about individual differences in the earliest years of life. We begin to know how to identify at least some of the factors that can lead to poor coping skills. Anna Freud and Dorothy Burlingame described three kinds of babies in the Hampstead Nurseries set up during the London Blitz, with not enough mothering people available. There were those who found out how to become the favorites. Others needed closeness and attachment so much that when adults were not available they turned to other children. Then there was the third group, who had poor coping equipment and were then left out.

Solnit spelled out for us the principles of development that must be our guidelines in prevention of disabilities in personality development. If we do not apply them, we are fostering a form of deprivation we can prevent. Most often in our welfare and mental health services we have to deal with the casualties of such deprivation.

Our field visits and anthropological reports highlight a truism, the importance of the functioning family and its cultural and religious values, both in child rearing and dealing with societal, economic, and technological change. Where these breakdown and parents have been weakened, Gerald Caplan has provided us with innovative strategies of intervention. But what should we look for in the families successful in dealing with change? I suggest that from what we heard and saw this week we can set up a classification in broad terms which can fit both families and individuals:

1. Those who can accept, facilitate, and even initiate change
2. Those who have to be prepared for change
3. Those who have to be carried, supported into change.

This last group is what Dr. and Mrs. Moses have talked to us about in the development of the women's camps, that is, providing a break in the pattern of life the individual or family is locked into.

But when we look at which capacities to deal with change we must look for, enhance, or even stimulate (encourage) in their development, two have been repeated here at least a few times, namely, flexibility and the capacity to fantasy. We still do not know enough about these to be able to establish criteria and techniques for a curriculum in infant education, if you will, to foster their development. We are particularly aware here in Israel of what can be done with the fantasy and the dream if it is combined with the flexibility to change them into reality.

I have one comment about Solnit's pointing to a difference between a psychology of survival versus a psychology of development is not always a dichotomy. We have heard here of a latency-age boy who not only survived the Nazi Holocaust but also became a leader and contributor. Dozens of other case histories can be quoted. Looking at it also in terms of one complaint we heard in one of the kibbutzim about a lack of motivation in many of their young people, we can learn from it that perhaps we are misusing the latency period of development by protecting school-age children too much from participation in societies' needs and problems. Can the stimulus of participating in the tasks needed for survival enhance personality development if properly dosed and applied in the 6- to 12-year-old children? Have the child labor laws that were established to correct abuses and stultifying or development gone too far?

I suggest, therefore, that we dare look again at the tasks we have assigned to middle-aged children. They are in the period of development that is unique to human beings— unlike any other mammal — who after the phase of growing up completely in the "family" are pushed out to leave the nest, the cave, or the lair. The human child, at the point of reaching outside the nurturing family, is without the physical or mental equipment to take a place in the world. The tasks of this phase should be looked at again in terms of a world of change. Should we begin to look at the value of including, along with school, properly dosed and appropriately structured work—which can have many implications for development of the value systems of our children and prepare them to better be able to deal with change? We would then also be dealing with part of the problem of the millions who run away, turn off, become alienated, and the like, as Dr. Hersh brought to our attention. Another of Dr. Hersh's contribution points to a phenomenon of change that is reversing nature's law of survival of the fittest—those who used to die, from birth on, we now can keep alive. We must learn how to accommodate to these changes, or else our world could end up with a significant portion of its population as the handicapped. We must learn how to deal with this problem, too, or we must face Einstein's offhand comment on one of his morning walks in Princeton when he was confronted by an angry student. The student said, "How can you be so calm when you have made possible the means to eliminate all people from the earth?" Einstein replied, "Maybe that wouldn't be too bad, because the fishes would come out of the sea and maybe they would do a better job than we did." We can be reassured from what we heard and saw this week that we, as anthropos have through the ages, can adapt to change, albeit often with pain.

Summary Statement

Peter B. Neubauer, M.D. (U.S.A.)

The theme before us, "Children and Parents in a Changing World," is a most challenging and difficult one. The factors involved are almost too complex, and the approaches to explore them, as we have seen in our conference, can come from almost any direction.

There is the need to assess the changes that occur in the environment, to name a few: overpopulation, migration, mass education, industrialization, the sexual revolution. This assessment in itself would be an exceedingly difficult task, and as has been pointed out, we have insufficiently reliable measurements to do this. Then there are the biological changes. Professor Winik in his paper on social changes and changing psychopathology speaks about the "biological acceleration phenomenon," the change in the rate of change in the maturational timetable. There is the increasing awareness of the nutritional influences; epidemiological studies show disease shifts and many other factors. Surely, we can draw on many professions to give us relevant data. We in the mental health field have a most difficult task. We have to address ourselves to the intervening variable, the psychological experiences and functions that depend on both the biological demand and the environmental condition—we need special instruments to gain access to this inner world of each individual. Even the most detailed information about the biological or environmental factors will not give an understanding of the subjective world of each person who from infancy on creates his own environment. Now we were asked to explore the mental health of the individual when both the biological and environmental conditions undergo significant changes. The introductory or orienting papers referred to the ever-changing conditions of life. It may be useful to differentiate those themes that refer to the average expected biological or environmental change in an average expected environment from those changes that overburden our capacity for adaptation and that make it difficult to maintain our balance of psychic function. The papers and discussions have referred to a variety of changes: the sudden change that meets the individual unprepared and that may disorganize his function and interfere with the synthesizing or integrative function of the ego. There were described the slow changes that put continuous pressure on the individual which may shift his inner balance slowly to deviant behavior or which slowly reaches a breaking point with a loss of ego controls. Then there are the fluctuating changes, when rapid changes are followed by periods of stability, only to be interrupted again. One could continue to outline the various rates of change that may occur and that need to be described.

There were those changes that affect the quality of function; those that render the individual helpless, passive, in which he finds himself to be a victim of events. The psychic consequences will differ sharply when these changes are actively influenced by or controlled by the individual. There are those who left their home voluntarily or because of persecution and who find themselves a new frontier with the hope of creating a new and better life. Much has been written about this frontier modality and values and courage in a transitional period until stability has been achieved.

Are the psychic responses specific when the change occurs under the influence of a powerful ideology that imposes hardships on the individual, which he endures with extraordinary resilience? Israel is a good example of the many conditions of change and various responses to it. When the first settlers came they did it out of their own decision, their choice, and they were acting on conviction and with an aim in mind. Whatever their multiple inner reasons were to leave for Palestine, they became part of actions; they were not victims, nor were they assigned roles, told what to do by the community. Their stamina and endurance were outstanding. The pioneer spirit or the frontier mentality created special patterns of functions. This can be an example of how changes, sometimes rapid changes, can have an activating, organizing effect. The dreamer, the missionary, the builder can have a goal far distant in the future; he will be able to sacrifice or better to subordinate present gratification for future rewards or for rewards for future generations.

In this connection, it was interesting to note that the reactions of widows to the loss of their soldier-husbands was influenced by the conditions of the war, the national response to the war. Those who suffered losses during the Yom Kippur war reacted differently than those who had losses during the previous wars.

It may be advisable to make a preliminary inventory of those psychic conditions that will co-determine the response to change. I suppose our theory of psychic trauma can be of help to us. There are obviously differences as well as similarities between reactions to change and to traumata. When Freud realized that it need not be the external events that create traumata but that fantasies and assumptions about external events can create disruptive influences, a new era in the understanding of psychic life followed. Thus we will have to address ourselves to the fantasies of people under change, the anticipation of a better life or of new disasters and injurious events. There are other aspects of the theory of psychic trauma that may be useful to us: the proposition of psychic economic change; the rapid or slow flooding of ego function by external or internal demands; and the need to understand the pretraumatic condition, the response to the trauma, and the post-traumatic development. Are there ego defenses that are better able to withstand disruption and that allow more adaptive function?

The papers have referred to the relevance of measuring the degree to which psychic autonomy can be achieved or maintained during periods of undue stress, and many have referred to the level of self-esteem as an indicator of internal stability in the face of external assaults on the individual. Others have studied the degree of differentiation that has taken place, and I assume that we can add here as a frame of reference the need to assess the capacity to maintain object constancy and self-constancy. The overendowment of the self with narcissistic involvement may lead to grandiosity that is at times useful against external hardship. At other times it may be a handicap and increase the sense of vulnerability.

We are looking for vantage points, for internal variables that will contribute to our ability to assess the capacity of the individual and to guide us in finding reparative procedures. Another possibility may be the study of defensive maneuvers employed to cope with either internal or external overwhelming stimuli at each stage of development. When we examine, for instance, developmental responses to internal changes during latency we find massive repressive forces to secure ego expansion and coping devices to explore the outer world and accelerate cognitive mastery. During adolescence we can observe ego regression and a need to link earlier modalities of function in order to integrate the past into new dimensions of psychic organization which should lead to maturity and stability. Rapid defensive maneuvers occur and shift from regression to progression, denial and new identification—shifts from gratification to sublimation, fermentations that lead to a secondary individuation and to new ego ideals. These studies could be useful if these defenses against internal rapid changes are seen in reference to changes outside the developmental processes.

Do rapid internal shifts set off responses similar to those we can observe in response to rapid external changes? This reminds me of our study of children in a crisis-intervention program. Here families are placed into a hotel until they find a new residence. Most often they are placed there after a fire has destroyed their house. The family members are in a daze, caught unprepared, and totally dependent on others. The parental passivity and helplessness of a group of people who come from welfare support is transmitted to the children. We organized a day-care program for those children between the ages of 3 and 6 years. Here we could observe their behavior after an acute disruptive event, followed by their placement into a totally new environment. We could outline three steps in their reaction patterns:

1. They seemed to be frozen and physically as well as emotionally repressed. With this there is an alert, visual exploration of the environment, looking, learning about the new, testing the behavior of others before their action takes place.

2. These children, possibly out of their past life experience, turn then to other children as a step of activation in their play or competing for toys or using the swing and the like.
3. After a few more days they may then turn to the adults, either for help or to oppose the routines imposed by the teachers on the group.

I cite these observations because they may give us a clue as to the acute reaction to rapid changes and as to the process of internal adaptability.

First we heard from Mrs. Rabin. I thought it was an important and moving statement, and as Professor Zigler has pointed out, it contained two symbolic statements: Mrs. Rabin's devoted interest in mental health for children in itself is significant, as is her description of the national scene that influences and affects the life of every citizen. She guided us toward a methodology of study when we heard that we came here at a good time—namely, how a single act (the liberation of the hostages at Entebbe) can influence the mood, the self-image of a nation. How can we select and find those actions in the life of a nation or an individual that gain orienting significance and influence motivation? Mrs. Rabin reminds us to study phenomena from the point of view of group psychology, a field we have to bring into our discussions.

Micherlich undertook such investigations into the German society and wrote a book about the fatherless society. He said in a Freud lecture a few months ago that unless we undertake such studies we may not be able to rescue individual children or adults by individual psychotherapy alone, because social dynamic factors may become powerful enough to override individual autonomy and decision making.

The first two papers by Drs. Anthony and Solnit were introduced as orientation presentations. They were more than that. They gave us the platform from which we can view our topic and can integrate the various components.

Dr. Anthony outlined the need for a theory of change—Metabletics—and he reminds us that such a theory has to take into account the continuous struggle between those forces that attempt to maintain continuity and constancy and those that strive for change. Furthermore, any theory of change must address itself to the relationship between change in the individual and change in the environment. But there are difficulties in knowing which of the aspects of the environment gain significance for the individual, or as he states, objective conditions may bear no relation to subjective experiences. Thus we need careful measures of the environment and of the inner world of the individual. Dr. Anthony, therefore, suggests that one should study families exposed to rapid rates of lateration and those who live over a long period of time in a constant and consistent setting. He draws tentative conclusions between environmental change and psychopathology.

1. The environmental effects seem to have their greatest effect before the age of 5.
2. Any change of environment has limits of change for any particular individual in any particular stage of development, since psychic characteristics become increasingly stable with age.
3. There is no such thing as an ideal environment, but what is optimal will vary with the individual child, his stage of development, and his family, society, and culture.

These are significant propositions to be tested by our studies. Such formulations give us the task to investigate the effect of serious environmental changes on early latency or on an adolescent who may barely cope with his own regressive forces.

Dr. Solnit gave us an additional dimension which must be considered in our assessment of reactions to changes. The same environmental change may have different effects dependent on the child's developmental organization. He uses as a measure of the mental health of the child his capacity to proceed with his developmental task. Any interference with development by delaying, deviating, or regressing is, therefore, seen as pathological.

Evaluations of a child that equate social compliance with mental health or social deviance with mental illness ignore the finding that similar behavior may for different children be a reflection of a wide range of different and even opposing psychic factors. Dr. Solnit is quite optimistic about our state of knowledge of child development to justify the establishment of planned opportunities for child health and care facilities.

He formulates the principle that rapid advances are associated with a new phase which is preceded by a period of stability or transient regression.

It is worthwhile to remind us of Dr. Solnit's warning that instead of asking what is wrong with the environment or what is wrong with the child we should instead assess both in their interrelation.

The papers which followed can be divided into five sections:

1. Authors who addressed themselves primarily to the identification of environmental changes, particularly the composition of the family structure, the changing role of parents, their role assignment as to discipline and authority in the Arab and Israeli groups. We heard of a population study in the United States as to family structure, mental disorders, medical technology, and so forth.

2. Papers that correlated *parental changes* and *children's behavior*. These were based on questionnaires and tests, and attempts were made to outline healthy and pathological responses to these changes.

3. The paper that describes intervention services and a most important and burdening emotional experience. Yesterday there was a paper on the airlift of babies and a discussion of the ensuing problems.

4. Dr. Kaplan's paper proposing a method to study families and outlining a *family support system model*. The significance of this paper was stressed; it rests on the opportunity to study families from a new point of view and to provide a systematic guide for planning programs of community mental health. The support systems are defined as attachments among individuals or between individuals and groups or institutions that serve to improve adaptive competence in dealing with short-term crisis and life transitions, as well as long-term challenges, stresses, and privations. As such it has direct relevance to our theme, and it was proposed that it be used and tested by us and our regional study groups so it can be discussed further at our Congress in Australia. Dr. Kaplan surely will be of assistance to those who wish to undertake this.

5. A presentation that discussed the urgency and problems in participating in policy-making decisions on the highest level of government, a function which we too often avoid or give up.

There was obviously an advantage in touching on so many aspects of the theme *problems* of this conference. It allowed us to view the contributions gained from each investigation, and it revealed again the complexity of our topic. The formal discussions as well as the spontaneous response by the participants illustrated the interest and search to coordinate these findings into a fabric of information that will clarify the issues involved into a systematic approach.

The alternating microscopic with macroscopic views profiled the principle of multiple determinants. If we had selected one subtheme for an in-depth exploration we may have gained some focus but lost the perspective. Surely as an additional step one would wish to add focal exploration and, most of all, those data gained from the therapy of children and parents who live under stressful change.

All papers made reference to the family matrix as a primary shield against undue environmental disruptions. As has been stated repeatedly, there should be no polarization between social, biological, and psychological phenomena as we review our themes.

Our general theme, "Children and Parents in a Changing World," can learn much from the many conditions of life in Israel. There are two aspects of the kibbutz that deserve our attention. Collective living was established under a specific ideology that favored a noncompetitive society, a spirit of equality among members, and equal sharing of responsibility as well as benefits. People who originally joined came from a very different society, and it was under the influence of a political-ethical ideology that they searched for a considerable change. Out of this mode of living the kibbutzim established a special educational and child care system. To foster the evolvement of a collective "man" they introduced collective living and education for their children, and thus the newborn were placed into a children's house and into a group. Consideration for others, sharing, interdependency, and an attempt to minimize competition, rivalry, and jealousy are characteristics of this program. The influence of such changes gives us clues as to the effect of new modalities of living on development, psychic function, and the formation of new social structures.

There is another finding which must gain significance for our topic. It has been found that children born into the kibbutz have avoided marrying within the same kibbutz. What is characteristic here is the evolvement of a taboo that was not transmitted by social pressures and was contrary to the preference of the kibbutz society parents that their children stay in the kibbutz in order to provide continuity. This exogamy emerged spontaneously in the generation born there and can be observed in all kibbutzim, independent of the background of the parents. Such findings are in contradiction to the principles outlined by cultural anthropologists who assert that such taboos are transmitted through learning and bylaws that regulate such behavior, or by the sociobiologist who relied on factors of predisposition to explain such taboos. The above finding of exogamy would challenge both assumptions. What is important to us is the exploration of those internal psychological mechanisms that bring about such sudden changes and are responses to changing social conditions.

A rapidly changing world demands theories about processes of change, a new methodology of study, new forms of deliveries of services and treatment modalities. It is my impression that this conference was a step in this direction.

THE AHMEDABAD CONFERENCE*
ON THE EFFECTS OF CHANGE IN A
SLOWLY DEVELOPING COUNTRY

Meeting of the International Study Group on
"Children and Parents in a Changing World"
At the B.M. Institute, Ahmedabad
October 30, 31, November 1–4, 1977

Participants

Chairman: Albert Solnit, M.D.,† President, International Association for Child Psychiatry and Allied Professions

Co-Chairman: E. James Anthony, M.D.†

General Commentator: Reginald Lourie, M.D.

Rapporteur: Peter Neubauer, M.D.

Local Organizers in India: B. K. Ramanujam, M.D., and the Staff of the B.M. Institute, Ahmedabad

Invited Speakers

Alan Roland, M.D.   G. V. Coelho, Ph.D.
G. M. Carstairs, M.D.   C. Chiland, M.D.
C. C. Benninger   Dr. J. Henderson

Official Discussants

Kiyoshi Makita, M.D.   Elisabeth Wann, M.D.
Anna Potamianou, Ph.D.   Joyce Grant, M.S.W.
Winston Rickards, M.D.   C. Chiland, M.D., Ph.D.†
Lionel Hersov, M.D.   S. Lebovici, M.D.
David de Levita, M.D.

* Sponsored by the William T. Grant Foundation.
† Also presented a paper.

Participants from India

B. K. Ramanujam, M.D., and Staff of
the B. M. Institute, Ahmedabad†
E. Hoch, M.D.
M. S. Gore, Ph.D.†

D. M. Bassa, M.D.†
J. S. Neki, M.D.†
Ramlal Parikh, Ph.D.†

Conveners and Resource Persons for Site Visits

Dr. Hansaben Dave
Mr. Bharat Jani
Dr. V. P. Sharma

Mr. Mishra
Mr. M. R. Kulkarni
Mrs. Ilaben Bhatt

Introductory Remarks

Ramlal Parikh, Ph.D. (India)

The International Study Group is considering the impact of change on child development in India at a time when this country is surging ahead in developing its weaker sections, particularly the rural areas. It would be useful for those from abroad to have an overview of the background of Indian conditions so that they can understand the process of change in our society.

First of all, one must recognize that 80 percent of the population is rural and only 20 percent urban. Here in Gujarat, the proportion is 72 percent to 28 percent. The developmental process in India is composite and societal. We are not yet at a stage where we can think of our human beings as units of individual development, as we have such vast numbers still languishing in poverty, illiteracy, and ill health. A decade ago about 44 percent existed below the poverty line; it has now increased to over 60 percent because of our failure to understand the nature of the conditions pertaining to India. The model of industrial society prevailing in the West is not applicable to our circumstances. Our problem, according to Gandhiji, is not mass production but production by the masses.

Secondly, unemployment is widespread. It is hard to find regular jobs for millions of our people, most of whom have barely 4 or 5 months of farm work. Unless we find enough work for them, they cannot achieve the level of development reached by the small, affluent sections, and therefore, the gap between the masses and the handful that make up the elite is widening. The unit of work also cannot be an individual one, since our society is a composite of joint families and closely knit communities. This is an essential ingredient of our development, and any process of change must be observed and understood against this background. The unit of work, therefore, is a family including children, adolescents, youth, and adults working together inseparably as a single unit. They earn together as a unit, and they live together as a unit with an organic unity that must be sustained if any attempt to reduce the gap between rich and poor is to be successful. Change is not feasible if this unity is disrupted into its isolated individual parts.

Thirdly, there is a serious problem of illiteracy in the 230 million people in the age range of 15 to 35. Although the literacy rate is about 30 percent in Gujarat, it is as low as 11 percent in tribal areas, the tribal population constituting about 14 percent of the total population of the state. The literacy rate among tribal women is below 4 percent and less than 11 percent in the slum areas of Ahmedabad, which has a population of 1.8 million and of whom around half a million have no homes of any kind.

The state, however, has a strong tradition of voluntarism, developed by Mahatma Gandhi and other national leaders, so that there is an abundance of voluntary agencies of various kinds serving all ages. Gandhiji advised a system of education that promoted habits of productive work; we cannot afford a professionalization of education on the model of the West because we simply cannot absorb them into professional and white-collar jobs. Although our higher education consists of only 4 percent of the age group, the number of students in all educational institutions from primary to university is about 100 million. This makes for a stupendous task of organization and development and provides a challenge that can only be met with by developing increased work opportunities and more skills. We cannot afford many isolated professional persons. We need many-sided, unspecialized men to deal with the composite society of our poorer communities. The change process in child development is, therefore, inseparable from the change process of total community development.

Theories of Change and Children at High Risk for Change

E. James Anthony, M.D. (U.S.A.)

> *"Change is essential to man, as essential now in our 800th lifetime as it was in our first. Change is life itself. But change rampant, change unguided and unrestrained, accelerated change overwhelming not only man's physical defenses but his decisional processes—such change is the evening of life."*
>
> (*A. Toffler*, Future Shock
> *New York, Random House, 1970*)

All of us, whether we recognize it or not, are living in an increasingly extraordinary world, extraordinary by the very nature of the rapid changes—social, political, and technological—taking place in our time. The accelerations of change seem liable in every new decade to overwhelm us, and our adaptabilities are strained at times to breaking point. What aggravates the problem is that the changes outside are paralleled by the changes that take place within us, and the two intensities are closely correlated. From being essential to man and part of his human characteristics, change, when rampant, can become inimical and a hazard to mental and physical health. Yet, under ordinary circumstances or within the range of adaptation change is a stimulus and a pleasure, and man is unique among the animal species in being able to cope with both the internal and external changes that confront him like "the great and true amphibium, whose nature is disposed to live, not only like other creatures, in diverse elements, but in divided and distinguished worlds." This is the way in which Sir Thomas Browne described him centuries ago, and it is only today that research has enabled us to understand something of this psychological amphibian state.

From the moment of birth, the infant, as described by Piaget, reaches out to the world through his senses and gradually constructs within himself a conception, at first rudimentary and incomplete, of how the world is and of how it works. This internal representation or model that he gradually assimilates helps him to differentiate the familiar from the unfamiliar, the regular from the irregular, and the animate from the inanimate, but it has the additional advantage of being fed from both reality and fantasy sources. This world model the child creates has, therefore, an extensive range of all "possible" worlds at any particular stage of development, and they serve him differently at different times according to his needs.

It is, however, his attempt at realistic constructions that prepare him for the problems of living, and it is these so-called "assumptive" models that permit him to make provisional predictions about what actually exists and about what actually has to be faced. These assumptive worlds are valuable as rehearsal grounds for possible strategies of behavior, and the child's curiosity and exploratory zeal constantly refurbish and update his working models which may be at times, to greater or lesser degrees, contaminated with wishful expectations.

We next try to consider what takes place when change impinges on the individual; we must consider in turn the situation involved, the different levels affected by the impact, and the modifications required in both the assumptive and fantasied worlds. If the change has been approximately anticipated in terms of its nature, its amount, and its rate, accommodation (in Piaget's terms) can be easily made with only minor adjustments to the inner conceptual framework. The child can thus deal with the novel aspects of his life space by this process of familiarization based on structural alterations. Adaptation to change that is not catastrophic consists essentially in rendering the unfamiliar familiar.

The Meaning of Change

Change is not only an essential part of life: it *is* life, and it is knowledge since only through change can we learn to know the dimensions of existence and environment. Yet, like any natural phenomenon, it contains a potential for pathology depending on whether an individual or group of individuals can cope with its excesses.

On an empirical basis we can summarize some of the meanings that change may have for us from a nonclinical and clinical viewpoint:

1. The child constructs conceptual models of the universe in order to be able to anticipate and familiarize himself with his living environment.

2. These constructs or world models reflect the level of sophistication at different stages of development and also reflect the wishful and realistic components that feed into all mental life.

3. Experience with change leads to gradual alterations in the various conceptual models erected within the individual, and in the "average expectable universe," the construction requires relatively little adjustment to enable it to fulfill its familiarizing and predicting role.

4. Under abnormal conditions of change, the discrepancy between the external circumstance and the internal construction becomes too great for the individual to handle comfortably, and various clinical states ensue, accompanied by their own system of senses (denial, withdrawal, confusion, etc.) and their own system of affects (anxiety, apprehensiveness, fearfulness, shame, etc.). Whereas nonclinical changes tend to provoke pleasantly toned feelings, clinical changes can create disturbing feelings of unpleasure.

5. Every change can, therefore, possibly have two meanings: that our internal model is adequate to deal with it with perhaps only minor modifications or that our internal model is inadequate, incorrect, or redundant and that the construction lacks explanatory power and consequently leaves us ill-equipped to deal with the alteration. In the first instance the change is experienced positively as a gain, something adding to our wealth of knowledge, pleasure and competence, but in the other change is experienced as a loss with all the meaning that loss signifies to the individual at any stage of his development. In this matter of gain or loss there is no need for an internal accounting system, since our affects of pleasure or unpleasure are a sure guide to the direction of the change.

6. Changes may be either the outcome or the cause of pathology, both physical and mental. With somatic illness our bodies

change and the environment around us changes in accordance with our needs and sufferings. On the other hand, when adaptation to change fails, then somatic, psychosomatic, and psychiatric illnesses may supervene. It has been more than amply demonstrated by various investigators that life changes are associated statistically with an increased risk to physical and mental health. The changes, according to Rahe, set up "clusters of illness," and within any given population certain susceptible individuals appear to be more prone in such clustering.

7. Change is confronted differently by different individuals, depending on certain immunities that are inherent or learned. This aspect of change brings it into the category of risk and vulnerability where change is regarded as a stress, a risk to well-being, a threat to physical or psychological survival, and a liability with respect to breakdown. Certain individuals are more vulnerable to the effects of change than others.

Vulnerability to Change

Somewhat paradoxically, children are both more adaptable to change and yet more likely to suffer lasting damages if faced with major specific changes, especially those involving loss of significant figures. In addition to bereavements, children also suffer from changes brought about by divorce and separation, residential relocations, emigrations, and disasters, but as Freud and Burlingham first pointed out in their London studies, change can be tolerated by the child when the support system of family and familiars act as a buttress.

In summarizing the vulnerability to the risk of change, we can point to certain constitutional and learned factors that affect the immunity process:

1. Age is an important factor in vulnerability. As already mentioned, the younger the child, the greater the upheaval and the more deficient the support, the more catastrophic is the reaction to change. At the other end of life, the same becomes true again, as the resistance to change increases with aging and the rigidity of the personality.

2. Early experience of massive or recurrent changes may predispose to chronic insecurity and the absence of any feeling of

safety. Such individuals are later highly resistant to change in any form and unduly apprehensive when confronted with it. Such sequences are not always the case; in some, frequent changes during the formative years may habituate the individual to the experience or, to put it colloquially, "toughen him up." It is a common clinical experience that children who have been exposed to multiple placements in different foster settings become curiously detached and dispassionate in their reactions to change.

3. Heider, Thomas and Chess, Wolff, and others working in the constitutional field, have pointed to a class of vulnerable children who seem from the beginning of life to be unduly sensitive to sensory impingements, changes in routine, unfamiliar environments, and strangers, becoming both hyperactive and hyperreactive. They exhibit an unduly low threshold to all stimulations and insist on conservative modes of behavior: everything must be "just so" and every aspect of the environment must be kept "exactly the same." In their more extreme forms, they are seen later by the clinician as autistic or obsessional children.

4. Parental attitudes and behavior may also predispose the child to become change resistant. Oversolicitous parents, lacking in self-confidence, insecure and unsure in themselves and living constricted lives, may so imbue their offspring with visions of a potentially dangerous world that every novelty becomes a threat.

5. It used to be thought that exposure to disaster was a transient effect, but recent work in the follow-up of cases suggests that such individuals remain more or less permanently prone to vulnerability with any risk of change. This means that situational disorders can bring about internal structural modifications, at least in some individuals.

6. The sex of the individual may sometimes ensure overprotection from a changing environment. In some traditional settings female children tend to have their lives reduced to routine, so that in later years they become unduly susceptible to even minimal changes and may retreat once again to routine activity to escape the disturbances of change. The procreative aspects of their lives may also render them vulnerable to change, such as failure to accept the menstrual cycle and the changes introduced by it; failure to accept the maternal role and the vast changes

introduced by pregnancy, parturition, and parenthood; and finally failure to accept the narcissistic hurt of aging as is signified in the menopause.

The Situation of Change

With the increasing acceleration of change affecting all aspects of modern living, the amount of pathology that can be attributable to this appears to be on the increase. The accelerative thrust invades all aspects of a situation, and the increased acceleration outside, as the pace of life quickens with advancing technology, the internal milieu may become equally infected with a state of unrest.

In analyzing the situation of change, a number of separate factors must be considered:

1. The total setting of the change event—social, historical, cultural, and developmental must be taken into account. Each of these factors adds its own particular component to the change, and without an understanding of their influence, the effects of change may seem more mystifying.
2. The place in which the change occurs may actually undergo change itself or be perceived as changed by the individual in the process.
3. The things, both natural or man made, that furnish the place may become defamiliarized by change, and in some cases socalled "transitional objects" are needed to tide the individual through such a predicament of change.
4. The people in the situation represent its most important feature, since the security and safety of the individual are closely bound up with the stability and continuity of the human inhabitants and caretakers.
5. The ideas and information that pervade the living space of the situation may also undergo revolutionary changes and leave the individuals disoriented and confused.
6. The duration of change within the situation is a crucial factor, since short-term changes are often more able to be dealt with than long-term ones, although in the latter case habituation may gradually make the task easier.

The general adaptability to change, therefore, is dependent not only on the inherent and learned change sensitivity of the individual but also on the vicissitudes of the various situations to which he is recurrently exposed. An overall factor which is hard to conceptualize or assess is the time sense that develops and is related, among other things, to biological rhythms, to psychosocial management, to the experiences of growing up, to parental attitudes and behavior, and to the establishment of enduring relationships. The time sense in some may remain predominantly subjective and may add an additional quota of confusion to that brought about by change.

The Assessment of Change

Experience has taught us that the capacity for adaptability to change is limited in the biosystem we call man. The human tolerance for stimulation (or to put it in other terms, for change and novelty) has an adaptive range below which the individual suffers from sensory deprivation, disorientation, and hallucinosis, and above which becomes overstimulated, disorganized, chaotically functioning, and numb. Too much change as well as too little change predisposes to morbidity.

The pathology engendered can be looked at from three different points of study:

1. Sensory input is assimilated and the input is transformed into structure-determining further behavior. There is a gradual development of a selection process that excludes the major part of the sensory bombardment and allows the individual to attend and concentrate on his environment sufficiently to make sense of it.

2. The information processing, storage, and retrieval that grows out of the stream of change from "bits" are abstracted. Here, too, the channel capacity is limited, and "glutting" is liable to occur.

3. Within the same theoretical system, the individual who is exposed to change is frequently required to make some decision. This may require no more than the application of old routines and habits (programmed decisions), or it may demand innovative activity, problem solving, and the making of choice. If this is overloaded by change, the individual rapidly becomes exhausted and disorganized; if underloaded, he becomes bored, apathetic, and disinterested.

The recent research on change has tended to focus on measures of adaptability, vulnerability, and change tolerance, together with somatic and psychological concomitants. Changes in the external environment are correlated with changes in the internal environment. These correlational sets can be summarized under the following headings:

1. Various brain changes have been found in response to environmental changes. The first account of such brain changes is to be found in the work of the Italian anatomist Malcarne in the 1780s. He worked with two dogs from the same litter and two parrots, two goldfinches, and two blackbirds from the same respective clutches of eggs. He then trained one member of each pair for a long period and left the other untrained. The animals were subsequently killed and their brains examined. Malcarne reported that there were more folds in the cerebellum of the trained than of the untrained animals. A hundred years later Broca found that medical students had larger head circumferences than nurses and attributed this to differences in the amount of medical training. Modern work is more decisive. Rats exposed to a rapidly changing environment were compared to rats who were left in an unchanging isolate. The first group had heavier brains that showed more enzymatic activity, a greater number of glial cells, larger neurons, and a significant increase in the RNA/DNA ratio. There was also an increase in the weight of the adrenal glands. In this, still somewhat tentative work, there are the makings of a neurobiology of change that would eventually link brain changes, psychological changes, and changes in the environment.

2. Psychophysiological changes in response to environmental changes can be categorized under two headings: the orientation response (OR) and the adaptation response (AR). The first is an immediate initial response that Sokolov has explained ingeniously in terms of the establishment of cortical neural models that process the intensity, duration, quality, and sequence of incoming stimuli. If the stimuli are familiar and matching reveals their similarity to previously stored models, the OR is inhibited for minimal and transient, but if the stimuli are novel and unmatchable, the OR takes place and can be observed as well as recorded electrophysiologically. The OR

triggers a release of stored energy in muscles, sweat glands, and so on. Therefore, OR is an index of change. The adaptation response (AR) follows on the OR, and the two processes are so intertwined that the OR can be regarded as the initial phase of the larger and more encompassing AR. The former is mainly a neural response, whereas the latter involves the neuroendocrine system. When individuals are forced to make repeated adaptations to change and novelty or are compelled to adapt to certain situations involving conflict and uncertainty, a hormonal sequence results in which ACTH of the pituitary goes to the adrenals which in turn release corticosteroids that raise the blood pressure, increase the amount of anti-inflammatory substances, and begin to turn fat and protein into dispersible energy. Even quite small changes in emotional climate or interpersonal relationships can increase the amount of corticosteroids and catecholamines found in the blood and urine. The AR, therefore, provides a much more potent and sustained output of energy than the OR.

3. These chains of biological events touched off by efforts to adapt to change and novelty are linked to psychological responses that can be measured in so-called "Life-Change" Units Scales, "Life-Change" Questionnaires, and retrospective assessments of any alterations in life style that require adjustments and coping. This brought "human ecology" into the field of medicine and psychiatry and required a new evaluation of environmental factors. It was Holmes who first came up with the critical idea that change itself, its amount and rate, rather than any specific change was the major factor in stress. The Life-Change Units Scale (invented by Holmes and Rahe) was a device for measuring how much change an individual has experienced in a given span of time and, in a relatively crude way, has provided us with our first index of change. Not only did it link psychiatric illness with change, but it also allowed for the prediction of illness following change and established a connection between the body's defenses and the demands for change that society imposes. Since all change was stressful and since some changes like the loss of a spouse were more stressful than other changes such as going on a vacation, the changes were not categorized as "good" or "bad." One shortcoming in the scale is its failure to differentiate between subjective and objective assessments, and what we find in clinical work is that the fantasied world models

swamp the assumptive models so that what is pleasure to one is poison to another.

Some Failures in the Adaptability to Change

Change can be evaluated objectively in terms of the somatic and psychological responses or subjectively by the impressions of impactfulness, changefulness, unexpectedness, unpreparedness, suddenness, meaningfulness, or meaninglessness as experienced by the individual. One can describe a number of syndromes of psychopathology under the heading of change syndromes. As mentioned earlier, the nature of the change has less significance than the amount and rate of change in determining the extent of the psychopathology induced.

The bereavement syndrome relating to the loss of a significant person has been described by Bowlby [1] and Parkes [4] among others. Bowlby described the response to changes brought about by separation as involving a phase of protest, a phase of resignation and finally a phase of detachment. Parkes has a somewhat less categorical evolution. If the change is sudden or unexpected, the individual is likely to respond immediately by shock or disbelief and may speak of his feelings as being numb or blunted. This is followed by a gradual process of realization in which, little by little, reality is confronted. There is still a tendency to resist the actuality of change and to continue to pine for the world that is no longer there, and at this time feelings of anxiety, anger, and frustration are very common. The intensity of these unrealistic strivings diminish with time, but there is a new element of defeat, apathy, and despair, frequently associated with depression, as the individual increasingly realizes the discrepancy between the world that is and the world that once was. The person feels as he had been forced away from a relatively safe and familiar world into one in which he has lost his bearings and the "structure of meaning" that has been carefully built up over the years. As Parkes states, the sequence of denial, struggle, acceptance, and reorganization is never clear-cut, and most individuals oscillate back and forth in their feelings.

Cultural shock syndrome has been described by Lundstedt as a form of personality maladjustment in relation to new surroundings and people. The individual is forced to grapple with unfamiliar and unpredictable events, relationships, and objects, and he is left feeling fatigued, uncertain, isolated, and lonely. His sense of reality is undermined, and he can no longer predict even the immediate future. For a time he may wander around anxiously, confused, apathetic, and emotionally and intellectually withdrawn. There is an overwhelming sense of loss.

The immigrant syndrome has been classified by Tyhurst into three phases. In the first the individual is mainly concerned with survival and the necessity of obtaining a job and a home and a sufficiency of food. At this stage he is restless and unhappy and feels alienated from the environment. In the second stage there are symptomatic developments with anxiety and depression, somatic preoccupation, feelings of being different from others, concerned only with his own problems, and lapsing into withdrawal and helplessness. In the third stage a relative adjustment may take place, or serious psychiatric disorder may result even to the point of psychosis.

The relocation syndrome occurs when an employee is compelled to seek a job in a new location, and the essentials of the syndrome have been carefully described by Fried. It involves expressions of grief; feelings of painful loss; continued longing for the past; a generally depressed affect; psychological, social, and physical disturbances; a sense of helplessness; a lot of undischarged anger; and idealization of the lost location. In many ways, Fried emphasizes that there is a striking resemblance to the mourning for a lost person, as if the loss of a person and the loss of a place were treated symptomatically in the same way.

The syndrome of "future shock" was described by Toffler as a "new psychological disease," somewhat comparable to culture shock in which unprepared individuals are immersed in strange environments where everything seems to be turned upside down or roundabout. In this situation, the individual experiences bewilderment, frustration, and disorientation, a misreading of reality, an inability to cope, and a breakdown in communication. According to him "future shock" is a malady brought on by "the premature arrival of the future into a present that is largely unprepared for it," and he sees this as the most important disease entity of tomorrow. Like others, he blames the new technologies that have precipitated a second industrial revolution. It was not merely that the scope and scale of change had been extended but that its space had been radically altered. The pathology that stems from it is an increasing inability to deal rationally with the environment or competently with its problems associated with a tendency to resort to violence as a way of solution or else mass neurosis. To quote him: "We have in our time released a totally new social force—a stream of change so accelerated that it influences our sense of time, revolutionizes the tempo of daily life, and affects the very way we 'feel' the world around us. We no longer 'feel' life as men did in the past."

Combat syndrome reduces the soldier who suffers from it into a state of being "incapable of doing the simplest thing for himself" and of seeming "to have the mind of a child." The stages are once again familiar to us. It often begins with fatigue, followed by confusion and irritability. There is hypersensitivity to the slightest stimulus around and a tendency to leap for cover at the least provocation. Bewilderment makes it difficult to distinguish enemy fire from less-threatening sounds, and all sounds make him tense, anxious, irascible, and likely to flail out in anger and violence. Finally, a state of emotional exhaustion sets in in which the soldier appears to lose the very will to live, appearing dull, listless, mentally and physically retarded and totally withdrawn.

The disaster syndrome has been well delineated by Lifton in the context of Hiroshima and Erikson [2] with regard to the destruction of a coal mining community by a flood. Once again we have the same immediate responses, the same psychic numbness, the same acute blow to the psyche that breaks through defenses, reduces efficiency, and alters the personality. The stage of shock is followed by feelings of guilt and shame on the part of the survivors, of death anxiety as predominantly expressed in terms of abandonment, helplessness, and desensitization that seems to drain off all compassion, and then a stage following the disaster where there is a utopian response in which everyone helps and feelings of pity are once more evoked in the face of the "ultimate horror." The disaster syndrome carries people to the very roots of existence, and at such times their emotions are profoundly simplified. Survivors often conclude that they have lived because others have died, and this may be one of the most fundamental expressions of human existence. The loss of the sense of invulnerability is movingly expressed by Erikson [2]: "Among the symptoms of external trauma is a sense of vulnerability, a feeling that one has lost a certain natural immunity to misfortune, a growing conviction, even, that the world is no longer a safe place to be, and the feeling often grows into a prediction that something terrible is bound to happen." It is sudden, unexpected change that brings about the sense of vulnerability and insecurity.

Preventive Measures in the Clinical Crises of Change

The clinical aspects of change are related to an excessive rate of change, an increased amount of change, and an intensive experience of change. The preventive measures to counteract these effects follow logically from what has preceded this section.

1. As with all conditions of high risk, one needs to identify the vulnerable subject from his past history of overreaction to minor and expectable developmental changes.
2. Having identified the vulnerable subject, one must monitor and guide his progress carefully through periods of change. Many subjects require permission to experience feelings at such times of crisis and to abreact their affects.
3. The world models of the children, both real and fantasied, must be greatly explored and the discrepancies induced by change brought into the open and discussed.
4. When undue change is anticipated, stressful by reason of rate and amount, preparation for change must be an integral part of the total prophylactic program. (It has been found that the preparation of children for surgery can reduce the time spent in hospital, the amount of postoperative medication administered, the risk from complications, and the development of lasting psychiatric disturbances.) Preparation requires detailed explanation and demonstration.
5. An effective preventive program, like an effective therapeutic program, must be based on a sound and trustful alliance between subject and clinician. Sometimes anticipatory guidance is best accomplished by the use of a preventive team so that somatic, psychological, social, and psychiatric aspects of change are all considered.
6. In the case of females the period of the menstruum is especially vulnerable to the impact of change, as work with immigrant

adolescents in Israel has shown. The clinician should be ready to succour at such times.

7. When the anxiety and tension titer is especially high, the judicious use of tranquillizers and preventive medication over the period of change may be considered with certain individuals who are psychologically hard to reach.

8. With change-sensitive individuals about to be exposed to significant change, as many support systems as possible within the family and outside the family must be mobilized on behalf of the vulnerable ones.

9. The empathic management of expected change can help to mitigate some of the unpleasant side effects and reduce the casualty rate.

In general, a care-oriented and family-centered approach to the crisis of change coupled with an extended support system in the community will do much to prevent the psychopathology ensuing from change.

Conclusion

Change is often confused with progress and with the optimism and utopianism generally associated with this term. It is often conjoined with progress and considered conducive to it. Let us look first at the notion of change. We hear that the world hates change and yet that is the only thing that brings progress; that change is inevitable, ubiquitous, and constant; that change is permanent and that nothing endures but change; that everything takes place through change and that not only do we live by the great laws of change but that the universe itself loves nothing better than to change; and that whosoever would seek to change men must first change the conditions of their lives. Next, we turn to progress, and what we hear is that it, too, is the law of life, the way of the universe, the integral part of nature; that without it "life is a corrupting marsh"; that, in the course of its development, it follows not a straight ascending line but a spiral with rhythms of progression and retrogression, of evolution and dissolution. Now let me mention the illustrious names of all those who made these confident statements about the nature of change and progress: they include Kettering, Burke, Disraeli, Heraclitus, Hertzl,

Marcus Aurelius, Browning, Goethe, Spencer, and H. G. Wells, so often described as the prophet of change. It was left to Bertrand Russell to try and differentiate these two terms that appear to have so much overlapping meaning. According to him, "change is one thing, progress is another, change is scientific, progress is ethical, change is indubitable, whereas progress is a matter of controversy." In this presentation we have attempted to deal not with progress with all its built-in value judgments but with the scientific nature of change regarded both as an existential phenomenon and as an observable and even measurable reality.

In India, with its age-old reputation for changelessness in the midst of change, the spirit of change is now very much in the air. As early as 1958 Nehru remarked that "the basic fact of today is the tremendous pace of change in human life," which implied that the country was in the process of being confronted with some very conflicting choices: were the old traditions to be maintained, consolidated, and sanctified? Were the people to continue to do the things in the way they had always been done? Or were they to open themselves to the seductive winds of change from the West? Could West and East affect the workable synthesis that allowed for both tradition and change to precede amicably, hand-in-hand?

Rabindranath Tagore was well aware of this dilemma and reacted to it characteristically in his own fashion:

We were, at one time, (he said), overwhelmed by the splendor of Europe and accepted its gifts without discrimination, like beggars. That was not the way to make any real gain. Whether it is knowledge or a political right, it must be earned; that is, it can be real for us only if we win it by struggle with obstructing forces. If someone places it in our hands, by way of alms, we shall not be able to keep it in our possession. We insult ourselves by accepting a thing like that and it does more harm than good. This revulsion has been necessary for the purposes of the history which time is evolving in this land of India. The things we have been accepting from the West without question, in sheer poverty of spirit, could never become our own, since we failed to assess their value and used them only as objects for show. As we realized this, *it was only natural that we should ask for a change.*

We can add to this a powerful voice from the West that says, in the words of Goethe, "what you have inherited from your fathers, earn over again for yourself or it will not be yours." If we now put these two admonitions together, we must learn that in order to construct our own dynamic way of life, suitable for our own changing needs and applicable to the changes that we wish to bring about, we have to earn the knowledge that we borrow from others, and we have to earn the knowledge transmitted to us from our own past. Only then can change be truly assimilated and made our own.

References

1. Bowlby, J. *Attachment and Loss,* Vol. 1, 2, 3. Hogarth, London, 1969, 1973, 1977.
2. Erikson, K. *Everything in Its Path.* Simon and Schuster, New York, 1976.
3. Morris, P. *Loss and Change.* Routledge, Kegan and Paul, London, 1974.
4. Parkes, C. M. What becomes of my redundant world models: a contribution to the study of change. *Brit. J. Med. Psychol.* 48 (1975), 131.
5. Rahe, R. H. In *Life Crises and Health Change in Psychotropic Drug Response Advances in Prediction,* P. May and J. Wittenhorn, Eds. Charles Thomas, Springfield, Ill., 1969.

The Meaning of Change in Child Development

Albert J. Solnit, M.D. (U.S.A.)

Although cultural expectations and guidance invariably make unique demands from society to society and within the differing subcultures of each society, our aim is to search for the change dimensions of human development that are found in children and their parents in every culture and society. We are bound to some extent by the characteristics of a particular historical epoch and the options that epoch provides for the alternative ways in which men can develop. These alternative patterns of development represent, as always, man's unfolding genetic potential interacting with the shaping experiences of his social and physical world. In regard to the latter, human development has been sharply influenced in the past by the pandemic pestilential diseases that have shaped civilization as well as individual development. Such catastrophes influence the psychological meaning of life—the value of the individual person and his life expectations.

Endemic infections and parasitic infestations such as malaria, trypanosomiasis, and schistosomiasis currently shape human development through the high incidence of physical impairment and life curtailment that such diseases bring in their wake. The same can be said about starvation conditions associated with a drastic deficit of food.

In this Chapter questions are raised and windows provided through which we can look at issues and questions about the powerful forces within man, the internal changes, as they express themselves in attitudes and behavior (i.e., in the personality) of children and parents (i.e., children in families). The psychology of change is an elusive one, often tending to evoke a predominantly sociological, anthropological view of change.

The macroscopic view offered by the social sciences, as crucial as it is, is a secondary one. It can be more useful heuristically to presume that man shapes his environment more than he is changed by it. At least such a presumption requires a more detailed and painful awareness of what we tend to overlook, though that is not to say that we are dealing with an either/or proposition. Man shapes his environment, which in turn shapes man. The way in which nature and nurture are always present in a dynamic resonance can be spoken of as a complemental series. The resonating influences of personality and environment can be consonant with healthy development, or they can set up a dissonance of stunted or distorted development.

Our clinical method is like a microscope as compared to the macroscope of sociological magnifications. In using the clinical magnification, we evaluate individuals and can use our understanding of individual differences to assess health and illness, weaknesses and strengths in that person. This account of the individual's resources is most useful and best inferred as a dynamic, not a static, inventory during conditions of internal and external change.

The unfolding changes of the human personality that proceed from the genetic template, tempered by the intrauterine experiences and by the impact of the labor and birth process at the end of pregnancy, constitute maturation. Development consists of the patterned changes that take place as the child's maturational forces are influenced by the stimulation, demand, and challenge of the psychosocial environment, especially as mediated in the early years by adults, the parents. Thus the shaping of human personality, referred to as human development, can be viewed along several continua:

1. The strengths of the maturing child as supported by the care provided for that child or the strengths of the maturing child as dampened, diluted or distorted by the care provided.
2. The weaknesses of the maturing child as exaggerated by the

care provided for that child or the weaknesses of the maturing child as mitigated, minimized, and gradually transformed into adequacies by the care provided.

3. The degree to which parents and others who provide care for the children adapt to the "needs" of children and the degree to which parents and others demand or expect the child to adapt to the family and society in which they live as not only a variable of the child's age and developmental capabilities and tolerances, but also often as the patterned expression of a given culture or subculture. These evolving patterns reflect what that society expects of a developing child in regard to care of the bodily, social, and cognitive skills and work and play activities.

In this continuum there are changing expectations according to the child's age, sex, and ordinal position in the family. These expectations, culturally shaped and individually mediated and modified, have a powerful influence on the individual personality and on the transmission from one generation to the next of cultural and idiosyncratic characteristics. Such expectations, socially institutionalized and individually transmitted, can be viewed as a definition (or even a prediction) of what kind of adult the child should become, that is, how the child will change into the adult who becomes an essential part of the continuity of his family and culture.

In the individual child, internal changes (e.g., moods and attitudes) and external changes (e.g., physical growth or environmental changes), which proceed gradually and along the lines of what the dominant adults expect, usually are quiet, subtle, and harmonious. Conversely, in the individual child changes that are sudden and unexpected in form and intensity and that approach or exceed the child's tolerances often constitute crises, albeit many of these crises are normative, markers of rapid advances in development (e.g., puberty). During such crises, the intensity and rapidity of the changes often also illuminate the individual's past difficulties and accomplishments in terms of adequate and inadequate mastery of past developmental tasks. Normal developmental crises include separation anxiety in many children toward the end of the first year of life and the transient regressions of puberty.

Developmental changes often cannot be detected by observing manifest behavior alone, nor do changes in overt behavior always reflect developmental changes. More generally, behavioral changes in man are not reliable indicators of mental changes, and what appears as behavioral change may not be accompanied by predictable psychological or emotional changes. Conversely, as in many adolescents, smooth, gradual behavioral changes may be accompanied by erratic and powerful mental changes in terms of underlying attitudes, phantasies, cognitive operations, and emotional states that are far-reaching. This discrepancy between manifest behavior and internal mental states fosters the need for theories and theoretical systems that explain and predict what happens in the mind. Mental activity can be inferred from the evidence that the human being remembers, symbolizes, and communicates symbolically in order to cope with past and anticipated tensional experiences and conflicts and in order to transmit memories to others. Man's mental activity is also demonstrable through noting his self-observing and self-critical capabilities.

There are also changes in the level of abstract thinking that accompany and are a reflection of maturational and developmental advances. This is also acknowledged in Dr. Anthony's chapter when he referred to how children develop the mental capacity to form internal constructions or representations, an average expectable universe or world model, as a coping capacity in preparing for change.

As psychoanalysis has made clear, mental activities cannot be adequately explained by what we are conscious or aware of. Thus mental activities can be characterized as:

1. Not directly observable.
2. Not adequately explained by what is noted as conscious.
3. Having a motivational quality that is both conscious and unconscious.
4. Having the capacity for self-observing and self-critical functions that are conscious and unconscious.
5. Having the capacity to be influenced by past experiences (memory) and to cope with present and anticipated problems (changes) by using thought as a trial action.

Mental changes also reflect several bodily and mental rhythms, those of hour-to-hour changes (e.g., hunger and arousal), daily changes (e.g., sleeping and dreaming), and changes that may be monthly, seasonal, and in terms of years or decades. The changes may be within the individual and between individuals, (i.e., interpersonal). Thus rhythm, regularity, and predictability or unpredictability of rate and direction of change are significant components of inner as well as of outer changes.

Just as external changes may exceed the individual's tolerances (e.g., oxygen deficit in a rapid ascent), internal changes (e.g., sexual maturation) at times may exceed the individual's tolerances. For example, the advent of the sexual drives during puberty may come about more rapidly and with more intensity at a given point in time than that individual's emotional, regulatory, and defensive resources can bear without slipping into neurotic or regressive holding patterns to cope with the demands of these sexual drives and needs. Usually such an unbalance of change rates and intensities is transient. When they persist, it may be evidence of developmental disturbance or psychopathology. More generally, in puberty the rapid biological changes, initiated by a ripening of endocrine organs and by a change in the hormonal spectrum, are accompanied by rapid physical growth and by rapid changes in the emotional and cognitive resources of the individual child. Since these changes are usually not balanced (i.e., orchestrated in a harmonious way), one or more of the capabilities or tolerances (e.g., emotional intensity, sexual longings, intellectual insights, physical strength and durability) usually lag behind the others. The individual child may be able to tolerate the physical growth but at that time have less tolerance of sexual appetite arousal.[1] This may be reflected in overt behavior but more commonly also requires access to that individual's mental activities—phantasies, moods, longings, and efforts to hold back or to modify through mental mechanisms. In psychoanalytic theory the latter is conceptualized as defensive functions of the ego.

As adolescence proceeds, the individual's developmental tolerances and their expression are not in a steady state but are like a horse race, with physical, emotional, and intellectual resources moving at differing bursts of speed, first one then the other moving ahead or lagging. In a manner of speaking, adolescent development culminates as healthy adulthood when the repertoire of drives, regulatory, and self-observing capabilities and preferences for work and loving rela-

---

[1] In psychoanalytic terms, this would be referred to as the sexual instinctual drive.

tionships are in balance, a unique one for that particular adult. The healthy adult then can be characterized as relatively dependable, with a more permanent identity and as developing (changing) more gradually with relatively stable tolerances, as he lives his life and does not feel lived out by the change forces within himself.

Developmental tolerances [6, 7, 8, 20] are further elucidated by examining the concepts of vulnerability and at-risk environment in early childhood. Vulnerability refers to those characteristics of the individual that are weaknesses or deficits of the individual's equipment. These can also be described in terms of tolerances and intolerances. However, the person's resources can never be understood without relating them to the social environment in which he or she functions and develops. An at-risk environment refers to the deprivations, traumas, and disruptions (i.e., changes) that characterize that environment. Thus the individual's resources must be assessed and understood in relationship to the changes, demands, deficits, dangers, and nurture provided by the environment as well as the changing instinctual demands and ego vulnerabilities that characterize the inner resources of and demands on the individual.

Mythology and religious custom reflect the ubiquity of our sense of vulnerability and at-risk environments in early childhood. For example, if a young child has a serious or fatal illness, it has been the custom of orthodox Jews to attempt to change a tragic fate by deceiving its messenger, the Angel of Death. The sick or vulnerable child, under the shadow of a fatal outcome, is given an additional name to deceive the Angel of Death. When the Angel of Death appears, he will not recognize the sick or vulnerable child "changed" by the "new" name. The additional name also may convey a wish or "immunizing" effect by its content which can refer to the wish that the child should have a long life or be healthy and strong.

In a recent paper [26] we formulated a subtitle that emphasizes the goal and power of change and continuity, "Care for your children as you wish them to care for your grandchildren." This goal implies that there is some consensus about what we wish our children to become, further suggesting that we can have substantial agreement about the change patterns implied by our concepts of health, vulnerability, resilience, and at-risk conditions in childhood. These agreements are based on the following: Health is characterized by a progression of maturation and development, that is, changes in the mental and emotional spheres as well as in the physical sphere. When there is a failure of developmental progress (healthy change) that is more than transient, ideally the expert observer would detect it before the deviation has created its own complications. Of course, if the child and parents start off with the child poorly or incompletely equipped or with the parents unable to respond with competence and affection to a healthy child, the vulnerability of the child or the at-risk environment created by the parents may set up a deviant or impaired development that has its own momentum and pattern.

Thus vulnerability refers particularly to the weaknesses, deficits, or defects of the child, whereas risks refer to the interaction of the environment and the child. For example, a premature infant is vulnerable, and usually the environment is a risky one because most hospitals have no program for keeping mother and premature child close together. Here the emphasis is on the need for change with continuity of relationships. As the work of Klaus and Kennell [17] has demonstrated, a mother who is deprived of contacting and caring for her child in the newborn period is a vulnerable mother. The premature child of low birth weight is also vulnerable, or if the child is well and the mother is not able to begin the bonding immediately after birth, the mother's vulnerability becomes the child's at-risk environment.

As Lois Barclay Murphy has put it in her recent publication [18], "Few are so robust as to be free from some zone of vulnerability. . . . Most children have a checkerboard of strengths and weaknesses, or an 'Achilles heel' or a cluster of tendencies that interact in such a way as to produce one or another pattern of vulnerability as well as strength."

Healthy development or change is not a straight-line affair but is characterized by advances, plateaus, and temporary regressions. For example, rapid advances are often associated with the advent of a new phase of development (latency, adolescence) which is usually preceded by transient regression. It is as though the developmental push forward (i.e., the maturational change) is prepared for and aided by a regressive "resting" behavior from which emerges the mobilization of developmental energies and capacities.

In the first months of life the child's psychic functioning is not sufficiently differentiated to separate it from his physiologic functioning. Born helpless, an infant develops and grows in a social setting that, in order for him to survive, requires that an adult provide nurture, regulatory, and filtering functions and expectations that are the basis for socializing (i.e., helping the changing child become fit for a particular human community). Of course, the community also changes, but usually more gradually.

Thus the infant's helplessness becomes a powerful stimulus that evokes the nurturing care and protection of the adult, a person who also changes, develops, and becomes a parent [27]. As the child matures and as earlier care is associated with the child's developmental progress, the parents find satisfaction and fulfillment that evoke the continuity of affectionate care of the child by the ordinary devoted parents [28] who gradually and intuitively enable the child to become more active in mastering daily and developmental tasks. The child's competence emerges from this mutuality of parent-child relationship [2]. How successfully he develops this confidence is largely based on the care provided him by parental adults and older siblings, themselves a family unit, who to one degree or another are representatives of that community.

We further assume that, under the crucial impact of these early environmental influences and demands, biological and social factors are uniquely combined in and mediated for change by the individual child as he forms his own unique personality. This mediating capacity is itself a product of the child's biological makeup and environmental experiences. The hypothetical agency which is responsible for mediating and integrating social change experiences is the ego. The parent is the auxiliary ego until the child's ego capabilities are able to take over these mediating, regulating, tolerating functions. With the ongoing development of the ego, the child changes through perceiving, registering, storing, and reacting to the pattern of his experiences and needs, especially through his identifications with his parents and siblings. Normatively these changes enable him to develop a useful memory, to differentiate his social environment from his internal or mental representations and experiences and through his past identifications with those who care for him to become like them but a unique person in his own right.

The capacity for differentiating an inner-changing psychic life from his changing social experience enables the child to develop other capacities that are essential for mental and social development. Included in these later developments—starting in infancy but becoming crystallized in later life—are the maturing capacities for thinking logically, remembering selectively, and finding those alternate pathways that lead to gratification, problem solving, and adaptation. These are discernable consequences of the child's gradually dawning capacities, after infancy, to harness his instinctual energies for learning, for expressing his ideas, and for developing his repertoire of affects—including humor, sadness, joy, and concern (empathy). The child develops the ability to anticipate change by constructing a world model or an expectation of what will happen next that prepares him to deal with similarities, differences, and discrepancies (Anthony, this volume).

The concept of risks requires further considerations. If the environment changes too slowly, is relatively monotonous, the child is at risk of not having sufficient stimulation to foster a healthy development. Conversely, if the changes are too intense, rapid, chaotic, or erratic, exceeding the child's developmental tolerances, the environment is experienced as overstimulating, disorganized, or lacking in nurture and support, and the risk of retarded or deviant development will be high. For example, children born out of wedlock or born into families disorganized by poverty or psychopathology are more likely to become deviant. When it is recognized that the environment is likely to cause deviant or stunted development, anticipatory interventions, i.e., change agents, should be mobilized to supplement or correct the child's experiential deficits and distortions.

On the other hand, if the child is born into an average expectable environment (one in which change is predictable), but is vulnerable because of a biological or constitutional disadvantage, then special guidance with educational and rehabilitative assistance may be necessary. For example, a child who is very premature and has a congenital defect or suffers from an inherited metabolic disorder will be vulnerable, the susceptibility stemming from his biological equipment rather than from the environment. Our assumption is that healthy development will be threatened if either the child's environment or his equipment is disadvantageous. In either case change is more challenging and more threatening for such a child.

In outlining the criteria for healthy psychological development, we view social development as a composite of psychological, emotional, and intellectual capabilities. Perceptual, motoric, emotional, and intellectual functioning are assessed in a social context. Change is one of the basic characteristics of such a context.

Interactional experiences and change patterns between babies and their parents can be viewed in terms of developmental processes in the child and in the adult. Following the traditional medical pathological model we have learned a great deal about vulnerability and the concept of "at risk" by observing and intervening as best we can when the conditions are severely deviant, as in the battered-child syndrome or where a child has a significant physical handicap such as in very young deaf infants. All the same, one cannot think of young children without thinking about their parents, mother and father (i.e., vulnerability and at-risk environments are parts of the whole; you cannot estimate vulnerability without knowing the risks).

The weaknesses and intolerances of the infant often serve as a magnet and magnifier for environmental actions and reactions, for parental perceptions of and responses to the baby. In this sense, the infant plays an evocative role as a change agent [27]. Included in this focus are vital past experiences that influence parental behavior and that tend to utilize the newborn and young infant as a screen on which past feelings and attitudes, ofttimes inappropriate ones, are projected onto the baby and distort the current reality of infant and parent. Such adult behavior is not only an inappropriate reaction (change) to the child, but tends to promote the repetition and continuation of the adult's deviant behavior.

What starts out for the child as a weakness or vulnerability may be magnified and elaborated by the parents' responses either because the parents lack resources or because the parents transfer inappropriate past attitudes or expectations onto the child. For example, the child may be experienced unconsciously as a rivalrous sibling or as a tyrannical parent, despite the reality of the infant's needs and behavior. Conversely, in many of these instances, the child's vulnerabilities activate potential resources within the parents. The child's deficit becomes a challenge to which such parents respond (i.e., change appropriately) by helping the child to gradually overcome a congenital deficit or vulnerability, enabling the child, often with the help of special services in the community, to optimize his or her development. These assets of the parents, or what could be termed their autonomous ego functions, serve as a counterbalance to the vulnerable tendencies in the same child.

Thus the child who is weak, handicapped, or deficient in strength and balance of capacities and equipment may evoke the sensitive, extra attention of a competent parent in which the disadvantageous start becomes a challenge that is well met. In these instances the challenge leads to mastery. What begins as a potential defeat in early functioning with the care of successful parents can lead to an exuberant development. Usually these are the quiet cases that we do not see or hear about.

A vulnerable child encounters common tendencies or patterned responses by parents, especially the mother, when the infant's weakness or deficiency appears at birth. Parental expectations that are not fulfilled by the infant become challenging and threatening changes. In such circumstances parents frequently respond with changes (i.e., depressive reactions), defensively and with resentment. They often feel defective, helpless, and hopeless.

Parents are often vulnerable when a child is being born because their preparation for the labor and delivery is associated with an intense review of their past and with the effort to anticipate what lies ahead. The birth of the baby and the parents' contact with their child completes the preparation for parenthood and establishes the parent-child relationship. This psychological process of becoming a parent, what I have termed preparation for parenthood, is most intense for the first child, but also is significantly unique and essential for each subsequent child. The process or preparation is completed or has its last phase after the child is born and there have been the first interactions between parent and child. This preparation, in its final phase, also should be the basis for working through the discrepancies between the phantasies about each child and the realities of that child. The phantasies, a preparation for expected change, are both positive and negative, touching on both the idealized child (preferred sex, complexion, height, temperament, etc.) and the feared child (tyrannical, weak, passive, defective, retarded, grotesque, etc.). Theoretically, the greater the discrepancy between the expected child and the child that is actually born, the more difficult it is for the parents to establish a sound psychological parent-child relationship.

These discrepancies are also heightened or minimized by the parents' emotional resources and state of health. For example, a mother suffering from a depressive reaction in the postpartum period or concerned with marital conflicts may not provide appropriate stimulation and nurturance to a passive child, and a pattern of pseudoretardation may unfold. In a sense, the vulnerable mother is at risk, and if she feels rejected by her child's passivity or by an actual deficiency, a vicious resonance is set into motion—the mother feels rejected and is unable to work patiently and hopefully with her child. Conversely, a more active child, demanding more attention, can provide such a mother with more opportunities to demonstrate her competence and can keep her busy enough to ward off transient depressive reactions.

The child with a vulnerability has a narrower range of resources available to extract adequate development-promoting experiences from the environment (i.e., such a child has fewer resources to cope with change); whereas a relatively invulnerable child can make do with a wide range of responses, stimuli, expectations, and satisfaction-frustration options. Thus vulnerability in childhood can be defined by the child's need for more specific growth-promoting experiences, for example, environmental changes should be more modulated, prepared for, and less complex to enable a vulnerable child to utilize external change in the service of development, that is, internal progressive changes. The vulnerable child is not as resilient or resourceful an extractor of development-promoting experiences, lacking the degree of autonomous ego functions [14] and the range of adaptive responses that the less vulnerable child brings to life experiences. In fact, we can conceptualize the child's healthy equipment and functioning by how he or she can respond well to a limited parental repertoire of stimulation, affection, protection, and nurturant care. Thus when a child thrives, even though the mother is mildly depressed and feels exhausted, in a situation where father, grandparents, and others fill in for the mother, we assume that the child was able to extract what it needed to activate a healthy development. Similarly, when the child is vulnerable, he needs a human environment that can elicit healthy development from the nonvulnerable elements of his makeup, while gradually compensating for and transforming the weakness into adequate functioning. In this way change energies can be harnessed, and vulnerability can be compensated for or mastered in a low-risk, resourceful, mothering environment.

Freud's concepts of trauma [9, 10, 11, 12] and of traumatic neurosis have been durable and are useful as another approach to the psychology of change and as an extension of our concern with developmental tolerances. These concepts are derived from psychoanalytic treatment, a "microscopic" view of inner change, especially reconstructive data, from empirical observational data. These observations are recorded in the psychoanalytic treatment through the analysand's account of ordinary, day-to-day living situations (e.g., rivalry, ambition, disappointments, observations of or phantasies about primal scenes and birth, illness, injury, or death in a family). "Macroscopic" observations of individual reactions to extraordinary conditions (e.g., war, earthquakes, floods, medical emergencies, and medical treatment as in intensive-care units) are also very useful. In addition to their durability, these psychoanalytic concepts of trauma derived from the study of changes in individuals have also been useful as formulations that lead logically to an elaboration of our psychoanalytic theories of mental functions, such as psychic energy, defense, stimulus barrier, and developmental tolerances. Further support has been derived from the utility of applying trauma theory to issues of child rearing, the limits of adult tolerances, and the use of education to enable children and adults to prevent or resist trauma. The psychiatric treatments of posttraumatic neuroses have also illuminated and refined trauma theory.

According to the psychoanalytic theory of trauma, the individual can be overwhelmed by the amount of emotional stimuli that impinges on him either suddenly or cumulatively. The stimuli may be initiated by a demand from another person or persons (e.g., sexual seduction, battle fatigue) or by the demand the individual experiences from his own feelings in a neutral environment (e.g., sensory deprivation). These demands, inner and outer, are filtered by a capacity that Freud [11] referred to as the stimulus barrier. Freud's assumption of a stimulus barrier in "Beyond the Pleasure Principle" called attention to observations that each person has a barrier or filter that selects and excludes stimuli that can be registered psychically at any given point in time. This barrier also functions in terms of the tolerances each individual has for demands or challenges, beyond which he is overwhelmed by the intensity, the magnitude, and the cumulative or sudden total impact of such challenges. Clinically, the overwhelming or traumatic impact can be recognized by the marked change in functioning of the individual. These changes include: disorganized, regressive, and constricted or inhibited behavior; recurrent nightmares; anxiety states; and many other equivalent changes in which the continuing impact of the overwhelming past experiences dominates the individual's current functioning.

The concept of developmental tolerances has been given added usefulness by Hartmann's interest in the stimulus barrier [14]. Hartmann's assumption that neutralized aggressive drive energy is the basis for the defensive and adaptive functions of the ego suggests that the stimulus barrier, as one of the ego's regulatory functions, wards off or accepts certain internal or external challenges according to the availability of its neutralized aggressive energy barrier.

As Hartmann pointed out, the infant's blinking of the eye is a prototype of later regulatory or defensive maneuvers under the ego's control. Thus the demands of perceptual stimuli, the instinctual drives, and life-threatening dangers are on a continuum of challenges to the individual who has varying ego capacities according to his developmental tolerances and resources, his neurophysiological and psychological endowment, and the impact of his life experiences.

For example, the person exposed to a severe and sustained sensory deprivation may be traumatized by the instinctual drive demands and by being flooded with primary process thinking. Under such circumstances the stimulus barrier, relatively speaking, is lowered and overwhelmed as the supportive environmental "shield" is removed (sensory deprivation) and the resources of neutralized aggressive energies (the stimulus barrier included) are exceeded by the internal demands. Under these circumstances the internal pressures have been strengthened relative to the monotony and lack of demand by the external environment.

When the neutralized aggression that provides the energy for the stimulus barrier is deneutralized or its protective capability is exceeded, as in states of exhaustion or regression, we can speak of an uneven match between the weakened ego's capacity and the challenging demands made on the ego to select, channel, or ward off such demands with its limited resources.

In psychoanalytic theory we speak of those traumatic experiences that involve gratification of instinctual wishes (e.g., seduction) and of those traumatic experiences that are imposed from without and which do not involve the gratification of unacceptable instinctual wishes (e.g., automobile accident). In the latter we can more clearly see the heuristic value of assuming that the repetition in dream, phantasy, and partial or symbolic ways of recreating the trauma is an effort to heal the founded, penetrated ego defenses by practicing how to cope in order to achieve mastery of the trauma. In this process passivity is turned into activity, and the impact of the residual trauma is reduced by strengthening the ego either in treatment or spontaneously by practicing until mastery is achieved.

In this hypothesis it is not that mastery is an instinctual drive, but that repetition (the repetition compulsion) becomes practice that can achieve mastery. In this way the stimulus barrier is "healed," and the person's ego or regulatory functions are restored.

The psychoanalytic theory of trauma also has been useful to others concerned with social planning and with the critical analyses of social policies. This application is currently seen in planning and evaluating programs for day care for young children, the hospitalization of children and the elderly persons, and a community's planning for and response to natural or man-made catastrophes. Thus the study of mental changes in individuals has social as well as clinical applications.

For example, the following, clearly influenced by the psychoanalytic theory of trauma, was formulated by Kai Erikson, a prominent sociologist, who reported on the aftermath of a disastrous flood in 1972, known in the United States as the Buffalo Creek Disaster, that, without warning, wiped out a community and 125 lives:

We live in a precarious world, and those people who must make their way through it without the capacity to forget those perils from time to time are doomed to a good deal of anxiety. And this feeling is what the flood seems to have brought on Buffalo Creek. It stripped people of their communal supports and, in so doing, it stripped them of the illusion that they could be safe [3].

The people of Buffalo Creek come from a land where dreams are thought to have a special portent, so they may have been prepared for the fact that the black water would come back to haunt them at night. Most of these dreams are hazy reenactments of scenes witnessed on the day of the disaster or general dramatizations of the horror they provoked. As one might expect, children both known and unknown, play a prominent part in those dreams.

One theme that appears again and again in those dreams is the feeling that one is dead and is being buried by people who were once quite close. It is as if one's alienation from others is a form of death—a grim rehearsal for that final act of separation.

The dreams of the night, then relive the terrors of the day; but they also serve to remind people that the fears and uncertainties derived from the events of February 26, 1972 are still a part of their lives now. In dreams the disaster becomes a kind of vortex into which other problems are drawn, a repetitive drama in which unsettled anxieties of the past and the newer anxieties of the present fuse together in a chronology that knows no time [4].

Thus the psychoanalytic theory of trauma focuses on the inner changes of the individual person, in the social and behavioral sciences, in the daily work of the clinician, and in the work of the psychobiologist who is concerned with the mediating mechanisms through which the process of trauma operates.

A bridge between two major avenues for the application of trauma theory to the understanding of change was suggested in 1969 by Professor Irving Janis [16] in his use of psychoanalytic theory to understand reactions of patients to the changes associated with surgical procedures. Through his study of a number of individuals he was able to demonstrate the role of preparation, including what he termed "the work of worrying," in the prevention of trauma and in understanding the psychological meaning of surgery for adult patients. In regard to the concept of chronic traumatic neurosis he stated, (it is) ". . . a generalized form of apprehensiveness and timidity that seems to extend to the whole social and physical environment, indicating that the traumatized person now regards his entire world as an unsafe place." Preparation for change, an intrinsic capacity, can be mobilized or impaired by the ways in which physicians, nurses, and hospital administrators are sensitive or insensitive to the "work of worrying." Educational and psychological preparation for surgery obviously helps the patient use his "worrying work" to prepare for the "changes" of hospitalization, anaesthesia, surgery and postoperative care, and in this way to avoid being traumatized. For the child, vulnerable to such trauma, preparation for hospitalization and surgery has been demonstrated to be crucial if psychological trauma is to be prevented [5, 19, 22, 23, 13, 24, 25].

Conclusions and Summary

The meaning of change in child development can be enriched and refined by our understanding of developmental tolerances, vulnerability, at-risk environments, and the applications of the psychoanalytic theory of trauma. In turn, this understanding should enable us to advance our knowledge about resilience, deprivation, and developmental phase specificity, the criteria for healthy adaptation and maladaption of children and their parents in differing social and cultural environments.

Our studies have reaffirmed the utility of the following assumptions:

1. At-risk environments tend to accentuate a child and family's weaknesses and interfere with the emergence and effectiveness of their coping capacities through presenting sudden or overwhelming changes, traumatic or/and deprivations.
2. Vulnerability in the newborn tends to create unusual stresses for parents in their nurturing activities and to require that parents adapt the environment more and for a longer time than in a nonvulnerable child, in order to support changes leading to compensation and mastery through rehabilitative measures and the practiced use of by the child of his intact resources. Many parents, though not all, respond in ways that bring out the risk factors in the social environment more than the supporting resources of that environment.
3. Clinical interventions adapted to the vulnerabilities of children and the at-risk environment as opportunities for parents to be active in helping their children can lessen the vulnerabilities and transform the risk of a social environment into experiences which promote rather than impede development.

The psychology of change, especially when one tries to give balanced attention to maturational and developmental changes in apposition to the changes in the social environment, can be usefully approached through an understanding of the interaction between the characteristics of the child and the environment along the continuum of vulnerability-invulnerability and high-risk to low-risk environments.

References

1. Anthony, E. J. A risk-vulnerability intervention model for children of psychotic parents. In *The Child in His Family: Children at Psychiatric Risk*, Vol. III, Yearbook of the International Association for Child Psychiatry and Allied Professions, E. J. Anthony and C. Koupernik, Eds. Wiley, New York, 1974, p. 100.
2. Erikson, E. *Insight and Responsibility*. Norton, New York, 1964, p. 113.
3. Erikson, K. T. Trauma at Buffalo Creek, *Society*, Sept./Oct. (1976), 58–65.
4. Erikson, K. T. *Everything in Its Path: Destruction of a Community in the Buffalo Creek Flood*. Simon and Schuster, New York, 1976.
5. Freud, A. The role of bodily illness in the mental life of children, *Psychoanal. Study Child*, 7 (1952), 69–81.
6. Freud, A. Assessment of childhood disturbances, *Psychoanal. Study Child*, 17 (1962), 149–158.
7. Freud, A. The concept of developmental lines, *Psychoanal. Study Child*, 18 (1963), 245–265.
8. Freud, A. *Normality and Pathology in Childhood*. International Universities Press, New York, 1965.
9. Freud, S. Introductory lectures, *S.E.* 16. Hogarth Press, London, 1916–1917, pp. 284–285.
10. Freud, S. Introduction to the psychoanalysis of war neuroses, *S.E.* 17. Hogarth Press, London, 1918, p. 202.
11. Freud, S. Beyond the pleasure principle, *S.E.* 18. Hogarth Press, London, 1920.
12. Freud, S. Outline of psychoanalysis, *S.E.* 23. Hogarth Press, London, 1940.
13. Green, M. and Solnit, A. J. Reactions to the threatened loss of a child: A vulnerable child syndrome, pediatric management of the dying child, Part III, *Pediatrics*, 34 (1964), July, 58–66.
14. Hartmann, H. Contribution to the metapsychology of schizophrenia. In *The Psychoanalytic Study of the Child*, Vol. 8, 1953.
15. Hartmann, H. *Ego Psychology and the Problem of Adaptation*. International Universities Press, New York, 1958.
16. Janis, I., *Stress and Frustration*. Harcourt, Brace Jovanovich, New York, 1969.
17. Klaus, M. H. and Kennell, J. H. *Maternal-Infant Bonding*. Mosby, St. Louis, 1976.

18. Murphy, L. B. *Vulnerability, Coping and Growth from Infancy to Adolescence.* Yale University Press, New Haven, 1976.
19. Oremland, E. K. and Oremland, J. D., Eds. *The Effects of Hospitalization on Children—Models for Their Care.* Charles C. Thomas, Springfield, Ill., 1973.
20. Provence, S. and Lipton, R. C. *Infants in Institutions—A Comparison of Their Development with Family-Reared Infants During the First Year of Life.* International Universities Press, New York, 1962.
21. Prugh, D. G. et al. A study of the emotional reactions of children and families to hospitalization and illness, *Amer. J. Orthopsychiat.,* 23 (1953), 70–106.
22. Richmond, J. B. and Waisman, H. A. Psychologic aspects of management of children with malignant diseases, *A.M.A. J. Dis. Children,* 89 (1955), 42–47.
23. Robertson, J. *A 2-Year-Old Goes to Hospital,* 16 mm film, sound, 45 minutes, English or French. New York University Film Library, New York, 1953.
24. Senn, M. J. E. and Green, M. Teaching of comprehensive pediatrics on an inpatient hospital service, *Pediatrics,* 21 (1958), 476–490.
25. Solnit, A. J. Hospitalization—An aid to physical and psychological health in childhood, *A.M.A. J. Dis. Children,* 99 (1960), 155–163.
26. Solnit, A. J. A summing up of the Dakar conference. In *The Child in His Family: Children at Psychiatric Risk,* Vol. III, Yearbook of the International Association of Child Psychiatry and Allied Professions, E. J. Anthony and C. Koupernik, Eds. Wiley, New York, p. 405.
27. Solnit, A. J. and Provence, S. Vulnerability and risk in early childhood. In *The Handbook of Infant Development,* J. D. Osofsky, Ed. Wiley-Interscience, New York, in press.
28. Winnicott, D. W. *Mother and Child.* Basic Books, New York, 1957, pp. vii, 3–115.

Images of the Life Cycle and Adulthood in Hindu India

Sudhir Kakar, Ph.D. (India)

The increasing interest in a holistic approach to the human life cycle, notably in the work of Erik H. Erikson, has important consequences for the practice of psychoanalytic therapy in non-Western cultures, for example, in India. As long as we non-Western psychotherapists could exclusively concentrate on the early stages of childhood, on man's "pre-history" as it were, the practice of psychoanalysis could be more or less acultural without involving any substantial loss in understanding the dynamics of human development or in the effectiveness of the therapy. In our clinical work we could recognize what we had been trained to see, that the preoccupation of Indian children with birth, bodily functions (and the pleasure or guilt associated with them), sexual organs and sexual feelings, and relationships within the family were preoccupations of all children everywhere. We could see that the fundamental intrapsychic processes, defense mechanisms, and conflicts in development were universal, although there were observable cultural differences in the *Ablauf* of these processes, in the relative importance of the various defense mechanisms as well as in the intensity and form of different conflicts [1].

In the holistic approach, however, which emphasizes the importance of *each* stage of life for the life cycle as a whole, which looks at the *mutual* relationships between the stages as well as the relationships of these stages to the structure of society, we can no longer ignore the cultural context of human development and of psychoanalytic therapy. For in many ancient non-Western societies there exist traditional world images that define personal identity and the goals of adulthood, the ways to reach these goals, the errors to be avoided, and the obstacles to be expected—a world image that is dramatically conveyed to children, and to their adult caretakers, as inescapable truths of human existence. I am not talking here (in the case of India) of Hindu philosophy in the sense of abstract, intellectualized concepts accessible only to an elite priesthood of interpreters, but of the prescriptive configuration of ideal purposes, values and beliefs on the life cycle that percolates down into everyday life of the ordinary people and gives it form and meaning.

As practicing psychotherapists we could no longer avoid an inquiry into the contents of these traditional images of the life cycle and also their comparison with the psychoanalytic image in which we had been trained. We became increasingly sensitive to the residual power of such traditional images on the behavior of even Westernized Hindus and on the relationships between the generations in Hindu India. Thus, to take one example, in the Hindu image of the life cycle the newborn infant is not considered as a *tabula rasa* but comes equipped, as it were, with innate psychological predispositions (*samskaras*) as a result of previous lives. Thus Hindus do not view infant nature as universal or infinitely malleable. With the cultural acceptance of the notion of *samskaras*, there is little social pressure to foster the belief that if only the caretakers were "good enough" and constantly on their toes, the child's potentialities would be boundlessly fulfilled. With the Hindu emphasis on man's inner limits, there is not that sense of urgency and struggle against the outside world—with prospects of sudden metamorphoses and great achievements just around the corner—which often seem to propel the relationships of Western adults to their children.

In our inquiries we also became more aware that culturally different images of the life cycle shape human development in different ways—a culture "choosing" whether childhood, youth, or adulthood is to be a period of maximum or minimum stress. In India, for instance, in contrast with Germany or France, it is early childhood rather than adulthood which is the "golden age" of individual life history. Such preferential imagery influences a cultures' perspective on the different stages of the human life cycle—whether the emphasis is on the child in the adult or on the adult in the child—and on the intensity of individual nostalgia for the "lost paradise" of childhood in a particular culture. My purpose here, however, is not to list out all the questions facing a non-Western psychotherapist practicing in a non-Western culture but to provide a brief account of the Hindu image of the life cycle, especially of the stage of adulthood, and to examine its convergences and divergences with its counterpart in the psychoanalytic tradition.

The Traditional Hindu Image of the Life Cycle

The traditional Hindu scheme of the life cycle (*ashramadharma*) conceptualizes human development in a succession of four stages. It holds that development proceeds not at a steady pace in a smooth continuum but in discontinuous steps, with marked changes as the individual moves into each new phase of life. Essentially, *ashrama-dharma* is the Hindu counterpart of the epigenetic principle applied to man's development in relation to his society and, as I have shown in detail elsewhere, it is very similar to Erikson's theory of psychoso-cial stages of growth [2]. Contrasting with Erikson's model, which is clinical and developmental, the Hindu view proposes "ideal" images in the Platonic sense. In outlining the stages of life and the specific tasks of each stage, the Hindu model does not chart the implications for mental health if the tasks remain unfulfilled, but emphasizes the importance of the scrupulous progression from task to task and from stage to stage in the ultimate realization of *moksha* ("liberation," "self-transcendence), the goal of the Hindu life cycle. Or, in the pop-ular saying—"It is only he who has built a house, planted a tree and brought up a son, who is ready for the final effort" (toward *moksha*). Since I have compared the Hindu scriptural model with Erikson's theory in detail elsewhere, here I would content myself with repro-ducing a schematic comparison that shows their basic convergence. In itself this convergence should not seem remarkable since both the religious endeavour to give meaning to the stages of life and the clini-

Erikson's Scheme		Hindu Scheme	
Stage	Specific Task and "Virtue"	Stage	Specific Task and "Virtue"
1. Infancy	Basic trust versus mistrust: hope	Individual's "prehistory" not explicitly considered	Preparation of the capacity to comprehend *dharma*
2. Early childhood	Autonomy versus shame, doubt: will-power		
3. Play age	Initiative versus guilt: purpose		
4. School age	Industry versus inferiority: competence	1. Apprenticeship (brahma-chārya)	Knowledge of *dharma:* competence and fidelity
5. Adolescence	Identity versus identity diffusion: fidelity		
6. Young adulthood	Intimacy versus isolation: love	2. Householder (gārhasthya)	Practice of *dharma:* love and care
7. Adulthood	Generativity versus stagnation: care	3. Withdrawal (vānaprastha)	Teaching of *dharma:* extended care
8. Old age	Integrity versus despair: wisdom	4. Renunciation (Samnyasa)	Realization of *dharma:* wisdom

Figure 1.

cian's attempt to connect and correlate the attributes of these stages must be based on what evolution has created: human growth and development.

The image of the course of an ideal life cycle, as described in the stages of *ashramadharma,* is deeply etched on the Hindu psyche. The strength and persistence of this tradition was brought home vividly to me in a series of interviews with four brothers running a large business in Calcutta. The eldest brother, in his early 60s, was increasingly turning away from family and business affairs to concentrate on matters of spiritual development. He did not talk of *retiring* from his work and his role as head of the extended family, which had involved him profoundly during the major part of his adulthood, but of an *active* renunciation of his previous concerns. The transition certainly contained elements of grief and discontent; yet the eldest brother's subjective experience of the step he was taking had an overall quality of hopeful renewal rather than a regretted end. The second eldest brother, in his 50s, who had taken over the responsibilities of chief executive of the family firm a couple of years before, was beginning to see his major task more and more as encouraging and nurturing the growth and development of his younger brothers and others of the next generation coming into business, rather than gathering personal laurels through a spectacular increase in the company's profits or other financial feats. The two younger brothers, in their late 30s, were immersed in their work and their families, while fully enjoying a hectic social life and all the sensual pleasures that great wealth can provide in India. These four modern, highly Westernized brothers were living out their respective *dharma* ("moral duty," "conformity with the truth of things") as businessmen, thereby unconsciously realizing—with feelings of inner well being—the ancient tradition of *ashramadharma*. Nor is this an isolated incident. The traditional image of the human life cycle is so much in a Hindu's bones, whether or not he is conscious of it, that one often finds in clinical work that the failure to renounce the life—concerns of an outlived life stage, as well as a premature commitment to tasks that are appropriate only for a later stage of life, as defined by *ashramadharma*—contribute to the "dis-ease" in the individual.

Psychoanalytic and Hindu Views of Adulthood

Although psychoanalysts often stress goallessness as the hallmark of the psychoanalytic technique, psychoanalysis as a body of knowledge on the development and structure of the human psyche has a well-defined conception of the goals of psychological maturity, even when it concedes that these goals are more to be striven for rather than achieved in any absolute fashion. Depending on the metapsychological leanings of the individual psychoanalyst, emphasis may be placed on adulthood within the individual life cycle—the goals of the individual psyche—or on adulthood within a social matrix, that is, on the adult's functioning within his social environment. Both these sets of goals develop together; they are, in fact, intimately interwoven, and any separation between the two, such as the one I make here, is only for the purposes of analysis and description. What is, however, rarely articulated in psychoanalytic writings is the fact that both sets of goals are themselves embedded in what Roy Schaeffer calls a "vision of reality" [3], a shared image on the nature of man and the world he lives in. Such a vision of reality—a composite of certain verifiable facts, acts of speculation, and articles of faith—unite group of human beings in specific cultural consolidations. They necessarily involve looking at inner and outer reality from certain angles while ignoring others, and appeals to the "evidence" by adherents of the one or the other vision rarely lead to a more inclusive, universal vision but only succeed in emphasizing their essential relativity. I shall come back to this later.

In their individual aspect, the psychoanalytic goals of adulthood and psychological maturity are encapsulated in Freud's well-known dictum "where id was, there shall ego be" or "to make the unconscious, conscious." Other writers have elaborated on these terse formulations. The "healthy" adult (and I equate "healthy" with the "moral" and the "ideal") has the ability to tolerate anxiety without being crippled. He has the capacity to experience pleasure without guilt and can adequately distinguish between his fantasies and the objective reality, irrespective of the reality's painfulness and the intensity of his own needs. He has insight into his conflicts and an acceptance of his strengths and weaknesses, and he can use his aggressive energies for achievement, competition, and the protection of his rights [4].

On this broad canvas of healthy adulthood, individual writers have emphasized one or the other detail they consider central to the picture of adulthood and a sine qua non for psychological maturity. Thus Michael Balint speaks of the development of a reliable reality testing that enables the individual to maintain an uninterrupted contact with reality, even under strain [5]; Ernst Kris stresses the achievement of an irreversible insight into one's conflicts [6]; Annie Reich emphasizes the acceptance of one's limitations as the hallmark of an adult [7]; while from her particular metapsychological perspective, Melanie Klein talks of a reduction in the two basic (depressive and persecutory) anxieties and the development of a capacity to mourn [8]. I must emphasize that I have confined myself here to the goals of psychological maturity in the classical tradition and have ignored some of the newer departures such as those of Bion and Kohut.

In their *social* aspect, the psychoanalytic ideals of adulthood are condensed in another one of Freud's maxims—to be able to love and work. Elaborated, this would imply that the healthy adult has the capacity for loyal and enduring relationships; can use his or her talents, free from paralyzing inhibitions, in productive work; and is capable of heterosexual pleasure and potency. Once again, individual analysts may stress one or the other aspect of the adult's functioning in his social environment. Thus Wilhelm Reich subsumes all social aspects of ideal maturity under an overarching concept of "orgiastic potency"—the ability to have frequent, "good and satisfactory" orgasms with a loving and beloved partner. As Reich baldly puts it: "A healthy individual who has enough to eat does not steal. An individual who is sexually happy does not need an inhibiting "morality" or a supernatural religious experience. Basically, life is as simple as that" [9]. More comprehensively, Erikson writes of a development of the capacity for *intimacy,* "a mutuality of orgasm with a loved partner of the other sex, with whom one is able and willing to share a mutual trust and with whom one is able and willing to regulate the cycles of work, procreation and recreation so as to secure to the offspring too, all the stages of satisfactory development" [10].

Thus in their interpersonal aspect the psychoanalytic goals of adulthood shift their focus from the individual adult to an intermeshing of adult lives. With this concept of care, arising out of the crisis of generativity versus stagnation in late adulthood, Erikson goes beyond the intermeshing of adults to give meaning to adulthood within the cycle of generations as he proceeds to describe the ideals of adulthood in relation to those who are not yet adult and in relation to society's institutions. Care, as described by Erikson, is the unfolding capacity of the adult to "bring up," guard, preserve (and eventually transcend) all that he has generated, produced, or helped to produce in the past [11]. This care extends to the adult's work, his ideas, but above all to the younger generation; it is the essential provision of the support for developing egos.

In reviewing the psychoanalytic notions of adulthood, both in their individual and social aspects, one is struck by the pervasiveness of the humanistic ideals of moderation, control, and responsibility—by the preponderance of the Appollonian "golden mean." For instance, instinctual activity and passions—except perhaps those of the mind—are certainly not denied but controlled, channelled, postponed, or sublimated. As Erikson in writing of adulthood says, "A human being should be potentially able to accomplish a mutuality of genital orgasm, but he should also be so constituted as to bear a certain amount of frustration in the matter without undue regression wherever emotional preference or considerations of duty and loyalty call for it" [12]. The guiding principle of adulthood in psychoanalysis is perhaps best expressed by the Latin hexameter, *Quidquid agis prudenter agas et respice finem* (Whatever you do, do it with prudence and consider the consequences). Even one of the most radical of psychoanalysts and a cult figure for many new forms of psychotherapy, Wilhelm Reich, whose emphasis on the orgasm has become an article of faith with many, does not advocate any wild indiscriminate Dionysian sexuality—tho glorification of the instinct without regards for its objects—but looks at promiscuity, homosexuality, perversions, and the like as neurotic and, at most, accords his approval to a kind of serial monogamy.

The prudent adult of psychoanalysis would be a welcome and compatible guest in the Hindu scriptural tradition. In their preparatory stages, all the Yoga schools of "liberation," irrespective of whether they focus on the way of knowledge and discrimination (Jnana Yoga), detached work and activity (Karma Yoga), devotion (Bhakti Yoga), or meditation (Raja Yoga) emphasize the development of certain common adult virtues that do not markedly differ from those possessed by a healthy adult in the psychoanalytic tradition. Thus Jnana Yoga stresses and expects the development of discrimination (*viveka*), dispassion (*variagya*), tranquility (*sama*), restraint (*dama*), and so on. Bhakti Yoga talks of discrimination, freedom from passions (*vimukha*), cheerful acceptance (*anavasada*), and absence of manic exuberance (*anuddharsha*). Karma Yoga, too, stresses a similar constellation of adult virtues in which psychic balance, restraint, and freedom from anxiety and passions are the core for the seeker (*sadhak*) of liberation. Similarly, in its first two steps of *yama* and *niyama,* Raja Yoga demands the development of the ethical (as distinct from the moralistic) adult.

Although the principal Yoga schools (excepting perhaps Karma Yoga) are relatively more concerned with the development of the individual, the social goals of adulthood have been highlighted in the duties prescribed for the householder (*grahstha*) in the Dharmasastras. Again, both sets of goals—individual and social—must be seen as being complementary and evolving together. In a certain sense, whereas the Yogas are the "psychology" of man in the Hindu world view, the Dharmasastras constitute the normative "sociology," an ideal model of social relations based on a common vision of the nature of man and the world he lives in.

The adult of the Dharmasastras, consistent with the social focus of these texts, is not an isolated being but an individual embedded in a multiplicity of relationships. He is a partner (to the spouse), a parent to his children (and a child to his parents), and a link in the chain of generations and in the history of the race. The personal requirements for adulthood, implicit in the prescribed duties and symbolized in the rituals specific to this stage, are "loving" and "caring." Loving and caring are, of course, omnibus words with certain specific meanings in the Western tradition. We need to look at their contents and connotations in the Hindu view more closely, lest we succumb to the illusion of understanding that the use of familiar concepts in a different context is often apt to give us.

The characteristics of a loving relationship, as reflected in the various marriage rituals, are manifold. First of all, the adult is expected to transcend childhood (and childish) attachments and to enter an intimacy in which he is both a separate person and part of a new configuration. As a scholar of Hindu rituals somewhat lyrically expresses, "They (the man and the woman) are united like two young plants, which are uprooted from two different pots and are transplanted into a new one" [13]. The theme of separate yet fused identities comes out clearly in the verses that the couple repeats in the marriage ceremonies of *samanjana* (anointment), *panigrahana* (grasping the bride's hand), and *hrdyasparsa* (touching the heart): "This I am, that art thou, that art thou, this am I. The *saman* am I, the *rk* thou; the heaven I, the earth thou. Come let us unite" [14];

"I add my breath to thy breath, bones to thy bones, flesh to thy flesh, skin to thy skin" [15] and "Into my will I take thy heart, thy mind shall dwell in my mind. May Prajapati join thee to me" [16]; and so on. In addition, the *vivaha* rituals also emphasize stability, procreation, efforts toward worldly prosperity, and the ability to bear sexual frustration as the requirements of married intimacy.

Caring for the children, parents, ancestors, gods, and all those who need care is, of course, the chief quality of the householder. As the etmylogy of the world *vivaha* (to support, to sustain) suggests, even the intimacy of marriage is not a goal in itself but a necessary step toward the development of adult care and generativity. Caring gives the householder the central position in the Hindu scheme of the life cycle. "And in accordance with the precepts of the Vedas, the householder is declared to be superior to all of them; for he supports the other three. As all rivers, both great and small, find a resting place in the ocean, even so men of all orders find protection with the householders" [17] say the *Laws of Manu,* while Vivekananda writes, "The householder is the basis, the prop, of whole society. The poor, the weak, and the women and children, who do not work—all live upon the householder. . . . The householder is the centre of life and society. It is a kind of worship for him to acquire and spend wealth nobly; for the householder who struggles to become rich by good means and for good purposes is doing practically the same thing for attainment of salvation as the anchorite does in his cell when he prays" [18].

In summary, the ideals of the first stage of Hindu adulthood—psychic balance, instinctual restraint, freedom from anxiety, development of the capacities for loving and caring—show a marked convergence with what psychoanalysis has come to regard as the qualities of the healthy adult. Yet in the Hindu view the healthy adult is only a prelude to the "liberated" adult. Ideally, adulthood does not stop at prudence but must lead toward liberation. It is in elaboration of the goals of the liberated adult that the Hindu scriptures sharply diverge from psychoanalytic and psychoanalytically influenced forms of Western psychotherapy.

The concerns of the individual in the second stage of Hindu adulthood are radically different from those of the preceding one. This change, as I have shown elsewhere [19], is dictated by the looming realization of the fact of man's mortality and the approaching end of the life cycle. The essence of this change is an unambivalent emotional (and sometimes even physical) withdrawal from the outside world and a concentration of mental interest on the discovery of the "real" relationship between the self and the world. As Vivekananda puts it, "When the human soul draws back from the things of the world and tries to go into deeper things; when man, the spirit, which has somehow become concretized and materialized, understands that he is going to be destroyed and reduced almost to mere matter, and turns his face away from mere matter—then begins renunciation, then begins real spiritual growth" [20].

The assumption that there is another, "higher" order of knowledge (*vidya*) illuminating man's essential connection with the world, a knowledge that leads him to liberation and "beyond nature" and which is radically different from our ordinary, sensory, and sensuous knowledge (*a vidya*) is, of course, the *leitmotif* of Hindu culture and speculative philosophy—an object of both fascinated acceptance and derisive rejection. I am, however, not concerned with the "truth" of this assumption. In any case, such matters are inseparable from an individual's vision of reality, legitimized not by "evidence" but by its being shared by a cultural consolidation. Here I am more concerned with the very real consequences that this belief in the possibility of knowing "ultimate reality" has for the picture of ideal adult and the Hindu notions of the goals of adulthood.

Consistent with the prescribed shift of mental interest from "outside" to "inside," the different Yoga schools have developed different paths toward the common goal of liberation. In Karma Yoga there is neither a physical withdrawal nor an overt break with the adult's previous activities and life style. What is demanded of the individual in the second stage of adulthood is a conscious and remitting effort toward disinterested action, toward cultivating detachment from the fruits of work. Raja Yoga, through such practices as *pratyahara, dharana, dhyana,* and *samadhi,* concentrates on the transformation of the individual's habitual modes of experience. Jnana Yoga frontally assaults the portals of *vidya* through the techniques of *sravanam, manana,* and meditation on the five great sayings (*mahavakyas*) of the Upanishads. Bhakti Yoga, eschewing the sedate piety enjoined for the neophyte, increasingly demands a different kind of devotion (*para bhakti* as contrasted to the earlier *apara bhakti*), comprising of the feelings of utter helplessness and complete dependence on the godhead. And at the end of all these paths stands the liberated man, the *jeevanmukta*.

From the foregoing discussion we see that the Hindu conception of the ideal adult can only be understood within a two-stage "theory" of adulthood. The first stage marks a completion in the process of individual socialization in which instinctual activity is tamed and transformed into mature loving and caring relationships. The second stage of adulthood, on the other hand, requires a process of desocialization—an emotional withdrawal and renunciation of libidinal ties. The focus in this stage shifts to a radically different process that is aimed at transforming individual narcissism (with its roots in the primary narcissism of the infant) into its maturest form—the "cosmic narcissism" of the liberated man. Whereas the first process is preparation for life, the second process is a preparation for death. As we saw earlier, in the Hindu view death is the only legitimate concern of the later stage of adulthood. Indifferent to humanist ideals and incompatible with the humanistic framework that has strongly influenced the development of psychoanalysis, the second process is often pejoratively called mystical and its aims labeled as pathological and regressive.

The chasm between the Yogic and the psychoanalytic views on the final goals of adulthood is, however, not unbridgeable. There is a bridge in Heinz Kohut's concepts of mature narcissism, cosmic narcissism, and postulation of separate developmental lines for object ties and narcissistic development [21]. Even closer in spirit (especially to Raja Yoga) is Bion's work. Bion goes beyond the medical model of psychoanalysis and sees the pursuit of 0—his sign for ultimate reality represented by such terms as absolute truth the godhead, the infinite, as the aim of psychoanalytic endeavour. Consequently, he can talk of a stage "unencumbered by memory, desire and understanding," can distinguish between a sensuous and psychic reality (akin to the Hindu distinction between *avidya* and *vidya*), and can write. "The suspension of memory, desire, understanding, and sense impressions may seem to be impossible without a complete denial of reality; a criticism that applies to what is ordinarily meant by reality does not indicate undesirability for the purpose of achieving contact with psychic reality, namely, the evolved characteristics of 0" [22].

A fundamental reason for the divergence in the two images of adulthood lies in the visions of reality that govern psychoanalysis and the Hindu tradition.

The psychoanalytic vision of reality is primarily influenced by a mixture of the tragic and the ironic. It is tragic insofar as it sees human experience pervaded by ambiguities, uncertainties, and absurdities, where man has little choice but to bear the burden of unanswerable questions, inescapable conflicts, and incomprehensible afflictions of fate. Life in this vision is a linear movement in which the past cannot be undone; many wishes remain fated to be unfulfilled and desires ungratified. Fittingly enough, Oedipus, Hamlet, and Lear are its heroes. The psychoanalytic vision is however also ironic insofar as it brings a self-depreciating and detached perspective to bear on the tragic: the momentous aspects of tragedy are negated, and so many gods are discovered to have clay feet. It tends to foster a reflective adaptation and deliberative acceptance. The tragic vision and its ironic amelioration are aptly condensed in Freud's offer to the sufferer to exchange his unbearable neurotic misery for ordinary human unhappiness. On the other hand, the Yogic (or more broadly, the Hindu) vision of reality is a combination of the tragic and the romantic. Man is still buffeted by fate's vagaries, and tragedy is still the warp and woof of life. But instead of ironic acceptance, the Hindu vision offers a romantic quest. The new journey is a search, and the seeker, if he withstands all the perils of the road, will be rewarded by an exaltation beyond his normal human experience. The heroes of this vision are not the Oedipuses and the Hamlets but the Nachiketas and the Meeras.

These different visions of reality, as stressed earlier, combine both the subjective and the objective. Their aim is to impose a meaning on human experience and not the discovery of any absolute truth. Inevitably, they set up ideals of psychological maturity and adulthood that may converge in some respects yet deviate in others. It is the great merit of the holistic approach to the life cycle that it makes us aware of the relativity of all such images governing contemporary life cycles. In addition, it makes us sensitive to the importance of these encompassing images for man's sense of orientation in life and to the disturbances in psychic household that arise when the ancient images begin to shatter under the impact of rapid social change.

Notes and References

1. For a detailed discussion of human development in India, see Sudhir Kakar, *The Inner World: A Psychoanalytic Study of Hindu Childhood and Society,* Oxford University Press, Delhi, 1978.
2. Kakar, S. The human life cycle: The traditional Hindu view and the psychology of Erik Erikson, *Philos. East West,* 18 (1968), 5. See also, Erik H. Erikson, Report to Vikram: Further perspectives on the life cycle. In *Identity and Adulthood in India,* Sudhir Kakar, Ed. Oxford University Press, Delhi, in press.
3. Schaeffer, R. The psychoanalytic vision of reality, *Int. J. Psychoanal.,* 51 (1970), 279–297.
4. For a summary and discussion of the psychoanalytical goals see Robert S. Wallerstein, The goals of psychoanalysis: A survey of analytic viewpoints, *J. Amer. Psychoanal. Ass.,* 13 (1965), 748–770. See also Stephen K. Firestein, Termination of psychoanalysis of adults: A review of the literature, *J. Amer. Psychoanal. Ass.,* 22 (1974), 873–894.
5. Balint, M. The final goal of psychoanalytic treatment, *Int. J. Psychoanal.,* 7 (1936), 206–216.
6. Kris, E. On some vicissitudes of insight in psychoanalysis, *Int. J. Psychoanal.,* 37 (1956), 445–455.
7. Wallerstein, *op. cit.,* p. 754.
8. *Ibid.,* p. 759.
9. Reich, W. *The Sexual Revolution.* Pocket Books, New York, 1975.
10. Erikson, E. H. *Childhood and Society.* Norton, New York, 1963, p. 266.
11. Erikson, E. H. Human strength and the cycle of generations. In *Insight and Responsibility,* Norton, New York, 1969.
12. Erikson, E. H. *Childhood and Society, op. cit.,* p. 265.
13. Pandey, Raj. B. *Hindu Samskaras.* Motilal Banarsidas, Delhi, 1966, p. 227.
14. *Gobhila Gryha Sutra* II.2.16 in Pandey, *op. cit.,* p. 227.
15. *Paraskara Gryha Sutra,* I.11.5, in Pandey, *op. cit.,* p. 228.
16. *Ibid.,* 1.8.8, of Pandey, p. 227.
17. Buhler, G. (tr.). *The Laws of Manu.* In *Sacred Books of the East,* Vol. 25, M. Miller, Ed. Clarendon Press, Oxford, 1886, pp. 214–215.
18. Vivekananda, Swami. *The Yogas and Other Works* (S. Nikhilanada, tr.), Ramakrishna—Vivekananda Counter, New York, 1953, p. 467.
19. Kakar, *The Inner World,* Chapter II.
20. Vivekananda, *op. cit.,* p. 432.
21. See Heinz Kohut, *The Analysis of the Self.* International University Press, New York, 1971.
22. Bion, W. R. *Attention and Interpretation.* Tavistock Publications, London, 1970, p. 43.
23. For a detailed discussion see Schaeffer, *op. cit.*

From the Traditional to the Modern: Some Observations on Changes in Indian Child-Rearing and Parental Attitudes, with Special Reference to Identity Formation

D. M. Bassa, M.B., D.P.M., M.R.C.Psych. (India)

Introduction and Data

There is a dearth of meaningful material in the area of changes in child-rearing attitudes and practices in relation to child development. The observations in this chapter are based on 20 years of experience in a community health center in a Bombay slum where traditional values prevail, plus a 15-year detailed sequential follow-up of over 100 children from birth; on individual, group, and family long-term therapy carried out in a teaching hospital; and on experience in a children's orthopedic hospital and child guidance clinic.

Considering the size of the country and its population, generalizations about Indian behavior, unless adequately qualified and seen in depth, are likely to be erroneous and misleading. Yet, for purposes of discussion and study, categorization is necessary. Socioeconomic conditions, child-rearing and personality development, and interpersonal

333

relationships differ from group to group, depending on whether the feudal, the preindustrial, the industrial, or the postindustrial type of community predominates. Nevertheless, certain common threads can be seen running through them all. The extended family is an almost universal feature, certainly in the emotional if not the physical sense, and the emotional climate generated by this has certain regular characteristics. Traits like unqualified loving, compassion, magnanimity, restitution, making amends, forbearance, "sparing" loved objects from one's aggression and demands, sharing, accommodativeness, tolerance of physical and even emotional deprivation, politeness, deference, avoiding confrontation to the point of the sidetracking of major issues and restraint in sex are so ego-syntonic and so highly valued by the individual, the extended family, and the group that reaction formations, including pathological degrees of self-abregation, self-denegration, and masochism may be difficult to recognize.

The commonest reactions to stress in this type of setting seem to be containments, apathy, withdrawal (physical or emotional), the resort to magical practices in attempts to appease supernatural agencies, depression, psychosomatic and hypochondriacal disorders, and regression to dependency (physical and emotional) on one's loved figures, who are only too accepting till one can recoup. Financial or other material help is often asked for and only too willingly given, even to the point of depriving oneself. The joint family, then, is very much like a friendly and indulgent mutual insurance society or a welfare state, such as Britain, where dependency is encouraged and fostered with assurances of care from cradle to grave. Children and old people are highly valued, but adolescents must behave themselves and keep under control their omnipotence, rebelliousness, and sexual drive. Minor rebellion and peccadilloes may be overlooked and even connived in, but anything more threatening is put down with a firm hand, accompanied by direct or underhand concessions.

Parents wear themselves out in the service of their children, young and old, unmarried and married, in order to ensure that they themselves will be cared for in old age. Parents and relatives take it for granted that they should manage for their siblings, children, nephews, and nieces such matters as a choice of spouse or career, with all their attendant problems, to the extent, sometimes, of regulating their interpersonal affairs and even the frequency of sexual intercourse. The younger ones, out of their own sense of inadequacy and dependency (rationalized as obedience and respect), are only too content to agree, connive, or submit, albeit with some degree of spoken but mostly unspoken disagreement on a low, grumbling note, which may or may not be heeded, depending on the elders' own anxieties and sense of security. Where such disagreements are ignored, the immature young person may sabotage career or marriage or both.

CASE STUDY

Rukimini, 18 years old, the only educated member in the family of an affluent sweetmeat merchant, would have liked to continue her education, but when at the end of high school a proposal arrived, she could not turn it down, out of a sense of loyalty to her father. A week after marriage she developed dyspareunia, vomiting, and abdominal pain. Her husband in the village 400 miles away, also a student, did not mind her continuing her studies not indeed returning to the parental home in Bombay repeatedly after spending only a few days with him, ostensibly for treatment and she was about to be diagnosed as a case of abdominal tuberculosis when, fortunately, the psychiatrist was called in.

The adolescent in India, in contrast to his Western counterpart, seems better able to contain his sexual and other pressures in the hope that in their superior wisdom the elders are bound to ensure their satisfaction at the right time. (Even though this means postponement of emancipation, individuation and identity formation, to some extent.) Self-fulfillment is thus to be sought for and found within the family, not in a frantic search for love outside it. In contrast, the Western child seems increasingly to belong to a faceless community from the age of 1½ to 2 years, starting with the nursery, the play group, and the kindergarten, and setting in motion the process of alienation that comes to a head at adolescence and leads to the pursuit of gratifying object extrafamilially—a process facilitated by the environment.

A naive and helpless trust in elders gives to Indian behavior a peculiar, charming, childlike quality, liable to "exploitation" by authority figures both inside and outside the family. An additional feature is the Indian capacity to bear doubt and confusion and to tolerate the gray area between fantasy and reality without undue anxiety.

Child Rearing

Overprotected throughout, the child is shielded from reality, even though he participates in and witnesses all the adult activities in the family from morning to night, helping and being asked to help in every possible chore from baby minding to stirring the curry. This sets the stage for a spurious independence and pseudomaturity in which one becomes grown up in the doing and feeling of things, but only under deference. In the early days, at least, the child is not confronted with reasonably consistent and firm limits, discipline and habit training (apart from toilet training) being delayed and suddenly and summarily enforced when he has become or threatens to become a little petty tyrant. At this point he is treated to a bewildering combination of blandishments and threats that becomes increasingly harsher until the child submits and conforms (often with his spirit broken). In psychoanalytic terms, the pleasure principle predominates much later than is usual in Western cultures, and reality is introduced more precipitately. The effect is to lay the foundation for high ego ideal, but severe superego formations are not well integrated into an ego that is too weak to withstand their pressures. This results almost inevitably in an overuse of projective and splitting mechanisms. Thus, hand in hand with lackadaisical and permissive behavior go high expectations of the self and high expectations of others. Guilt, depression, and alienation are avoided or rather submerged within this welter of inconsistency, tolerance, and acceptance of the letter of the law. Is Indian culture, then, a guilt culture, a shame culture, or a sham culture? Perhaps all three, like most cultures. Guilt is perhaps greater than in the West and more defended against. The basis is laid for pregenital fixations and regressions and polymorphous perverse activities (except kissing) to persist into adult life.

Infancy

The infant is adulated and overprotected by the mother and other caretakers (including servants and older siblings), and infant-type care is prolonged beyond the first year through "on demand" breast (or bottle) feeding, the late introductions of solids, excessive body contact and carrying, and sleeping with the mother or other caretakers.[1] Thus with multiple caretaking, with having his needs met abundantly, though not always wisely or consistently, and with being treated like an animate plaything that is sometimes coddled, sometimes coaxed, and sometimes teased and tantalized, it is not surprising that the end result is a curious admixture of unbound trustfulness, to the point of gullibility, mingled with sudden and unexpected reactions of mistrust. With all these fixating factors, regressions are common, and passage to separation, individuation, and autonomy of succeeding stages is rendered difficult. Parental behavior can be understood as a recapturing of the lost narcissism, omnipotence, and symptoms of infancy through identification with their infant.

The relative infrequency of child abuse epitomizes the contrast between Indian and Western child rearing. The incidence of baby battering seems to be low, partly because it is not overblown by the media, partly because the Indian mother seems more tolerant and masochistic, but especially because mother and child are shielded from each others' aggression and provocativeness by others who intervene, divert, bribe, or comfort as the seduction demands. The lone Western mother lacks such comprehensive support systems that help to dilute and attenuate the basic conflicts and struggles.

The Toddler Period

In the sample quoted earlier, 80 percent of the toilet training had started before the 6th month and had been completed for day and night by the 17th month, on an average. This precocious toilet achievement against the background of postponement of all other aspects of training makes the issue of consistency a critical one in the development of the Indian child. Autonomy rarely comes smoothly. At some arbitrary date—when the mother becomes pregnant, or a grandmother dies, or an aunt or servant leaves the home—then quite suddenly carrying, feeding, and dressing may stop, and independence is thrust upon the child. Thus negativism and the battle of wills

---

[1] In one sample of 25 slum children, 18 were still at the breast at 15 months. The average age of weaning from breast or bottle was 17.3 months. Full switch over to solids had not taken place at 20 months and was delayed in some until 30 months. Experience with most other children except perhaps those from very westernized families was similar.

comes much later than with the Westernized child, when he can put up greater resistance and so provokes harsher measures from his parents.

Quite apart from whether they can be afforded, toys do not play a very important role in the life of the toddler, since he is involved in body play with elders, including his mother. Aggression is not sublimated into play, nor are his fantasies elaborated in play, but there may be much biting and pinching of his mother's (failing) breast, invoking some counteraggression from her. As a consequence, most children enter the next stage with unintegrated impulses and unresolved problems relating to dependency, sense of achievement, self-esteem, self-assertiveness, individuation, control, and sublimation of aggression.

The Preschool Period

The presence of many loving and disciplining agents means that the "family romance" is not as intense as in the West, quite apart from the fact that the boy's love for his mother is shared and his fear of his father spread among other children. At this stage the child may be sleeping with an aunt or grandmother (whom he may call mother, with his own mother being addressed by her first name), and his main source of fear may be an uncle responsible for disciplining him. The dilution of the "family romance" may well be one of the most important determinants in the apparent stability of the Indian marriage, in that it makes jealousy and rejection easier to tolerate.

Adolescence

As he enters adolescence, the average teenager is by and large conforming and obedient and continues so throughout this period (except when he enters his peer group). His life is very much arranged for him, and he follows the family line, achieving a spurious self-identity entailing very little struggle. In his fleeting identifications and pseudoidentity he has something in common with an emerging trend in the West, but because of opposite factors: too little rebelliousness and too little integration of new influences as opposed to too much rebelliousness and haphazard integration.

In a questionnaire study submitted to students there was a paucity of manifest erotic dreams. In females especially the dreams were highly romanticized and dealt with love, marriage, home, and children. In clinical practice the young Indian male frequently presents with concern over nocturnal emission, equated with loss of virility. Sexual excitement is perceived as heat that has to be eliminated and sex as something dirty. This seems to create a dilemma so that nocturnal emission and masturbation are followed by much guilt. This correlates with what seems to be a low level of sexual activity and the ideal of "sparing" the opposite partner, even though verbal sexual abuse is extremely common at lower social levels. Since sexual gratification ideally is permissible only after marriage, sexual drives are inhibited, along with experimentation in general, innovativeness, creativity, and integration of new values. Many young men deny ever having had nocturnal emissions or masturbated, and this is often confirmed on follow-up. Yet they claim to have fairly successful marriages. A common form of sexual neurosis presents with leakage of semen at odd times, fatigue, pains in the bones, a low threshold for excitement, and constant weak erections.

The child brings into adolescence a weak ego, a severe superego, and high ego-ideals that now become oppressive without any hope of even partial fulfillment except in the most abstract fantasies such as service to the poor—a highly valued ideal. The weak ego is not resourceful enough to create opportunities or take advantage of whatever opportunities the environment provides. Even where parents are liberal and provide ample opportunities, progress is seen as by favor of authority figures. Hence the exaggerated importance given to teachers.

Sexual experimentation is limited because mingling of the sexes, except in a small, highly Westernized minority, is frowned on, and takes the form of crushes, sometimes very subtly manifested, on the elders in the extended family. The defenses against open acceptance of this are naturally very strong, and it takes considerable time and tact before educated young women will accept a questionnaire statement such as "The Indian teenager can take any liberties with his older brother's wife except take her to bed." This is understandable because teenage girls have similar crushes on uncles and brothers-in-law. A constant refrain of teenage infidelity in Indian poetry (written, no doubt, by uncles and uncle surrogates) could be triggered by the sudden cooling off of teenage nieces. This process of experimentation in the joint family, facilitated by the many loved ones available earlier during the oedipal period, helps in the integration of feelings but keeps at bay any tendency to physical gratification, the postponement of which is conditioned by a variety of factors already mentioned, but especially by hope.

If it is correct to say that in Western teenagers there is a tendency to actualize and concretize fantasies, sexual acting out being only one aspect of this process, then it could be said that in Indian teenagers this process is inhibited by defenses against activity in general, with these reinforced by idealism, vague altruism, and other reaction formations.

Conclusion

If one were a mental health counselor and believed that counselling would bring about deep changes in people, one might tell Indian mothers to love their babies less, to discipline their toddlers earlier and more consistently, and to join with their husbands in reducing their adolescents' guilts. One might tell Westernized mothers to love their babies more, to discipline their toddlers later and a little

Table 1. Traditional versus Modern Indian Life

	Traditional	*Modern*
Status	Agrarian, urban slum; $30 a month income	Upper middle class; $300 a month income
Education	Illiterate; dropouts from grade school	Both parents university educated
Homes	Makeshift, without plumbing but immaculately clean inside, especially in the kitchen	Modern homes with plumbing and other facilities
Family	Joint, extended	Nominally nuclear
Marriage	Arranged	Arranged

Table 1. (*Continued*)

	Traditional	*Modern*
Main mothering persons	Mother, grandmother, aunts, siblings	Ayah, mother, grandmother
Delivery	At home by traditional midwife; modern hospital in city	At home by traditional midwife; modern hospital in city
Antenatal	Dependency needs met by family	Maybe so
Rooming-in	Automatic, with little anxiety, at grandmother's; anxiety-relieving	At hospital; not often anxiety-relieving
Breast	12–24 months; close relationship to mother	2–3 months; given up because of "no milk"; bottle 1–2 years
Supplement	Nominal, at 6–15 months	Modern cereals at 4–6 months
"Weaning"	Carried out by total family; onto slops	By mother onto solids
Sleeps	With mother or grandmother until 4–5 years	With mother 1–2 months; then in a cot
Body contact	Much; especially with carrying	Mainly with ayah
Toilet training	Introduced early by grandmother at 3–4 months; achieved by 8–18 months; no diapers	Introduced by mother on potty at 6–12 months; achieved by 12–24 months
Cardinal crisis	Intense	Somewhat less so
Main disciplining agent	Grandmother, mother, aunts, uncles	Ayah, mother
Self-feed	From about 2–4 years	About the same
Self-dress	From about 2–4 years	About the same
Self-bath	From about 2–4 years	About the same
Toys	Hardly any	Mostly for show and decoration
Education	From 5–6 years to 10–12; rote memory passively acquired; no self-discovery	From 3–4 years to 20–25 years; somewhat similar experience
Occupation	Agricultural, unskilled	Professional
Outlook and orientation	Feudal	Industrial and postindustrial on the surface

less arduously, and to join with their husbands in putting up with their adolescents' aggression and moderating their own counter-aggression, at the same time attempting to induce in them a greater sense of responsibility for what they do and ways for making restitution—something that deep down the adolescent longs to do. One might also tell Western fathers, since women must work, that there can be few ways to be more supportive than to prevail on governments to legislate for 2 years' paid maternity leave. To Indians enamored of Western practices, to anthropologists seeking to incorporate piecemeal child-rearing practices of primitive and preindustrial societies, and to Western youth in search of the perfect society in developing countries, one might say, "The grass could be greener on your side, or you could make it so."

1. Indian children seem to be in three developmental stages at one and the same time as a result of maternal anxiety and intrusiveness delaying separation and prolonging dependence. The absence of playthings accentuates this, transforming the mother (breast) into a transitional object.
2. All the classical developmental crises are bypassed in the Indian child (separation-individuation, oedipal, adolescent), leaving only a *cardinal crisis* between dependency and nonconformity. In the traditional family this results in dependency and conformity; in the modern family, owing to premature separation, there is a surface harmony but underlying resentment, opposition, and ambivalence.
3. Because of the peripheral role of the Indian father and because child rearing is predominantly done by women, the Indian boy is at the mercy of his oedipal impulses in addition to lacking strong masculine models of identification. He grows up to become soft, weak, impractical, idealistic, guilt-ridden, and depression-prone like his father. There is a marked dilution of the "family romance."
4. Because of the prolongation of the preoedipal phase, there is an oralization and analization of oedipal strivings so that sex becomes dirty. The early toilet training conduces to a severe superego and obsessional trends.
5. The only continuity in the life of the Indian child is guilt reinforced by shame at the end of the cardinal crisis.

Mother India does not easily let go of her children. She safeguards her youth against violent change by keeping them dependent and conforming.

Appendix

The main differences between the two ends of the continuum of behavior are shown schematically in Table 1.

Changes in Indian Village Societies and Their Impact on Child Development: A Personal Perspective

G. M. Carstairs, M.D. (Britain)

My involvement with India began 61 years ago, when I was born in Mussoorie during the height of the hot weather. The first 8 years of my life were spent in Rajasthan in a mission compound on the fringe of a large military cantonment, part of the now vanished British Raj whose memory still lingers on—perhaps nowhere more strongly than in those Indianized and yet determinedly conservative institutions: the club and the officers' mess. In those days British children were brought up by Ayahs, and in later childhood (if their parents could afford it) by nannies imported from home, and they were usually segregated from Indian children. However, this custom did not prevail in the mission compound. Throughout my early years my playmates were nearly all Indians, the children of Indian Christians or Hindus or Moslems, high caste or low caste—it did not seem to make any difference in our games of marbles or goolie-danda or kabbadi or kite flying, which changed with the seasons. Our common language was Hindustani, which I must have spoken more often than English up to the time when I was taken back to Scotland to begin my schooling. Many years were to pass before I returned as an anthropologist to Rajasthan to share the life of villagers, but when I did so, it felt like coming home. The sounds and idioms of Hindustani came rushing back, like long-forgotten memories, and a thousand sights, smells, and everyday customs were things remembered rather than things encountered for the first time.

Of course, there were also many things that I had to learn. It was a new experience for me to live immersed in the traditions and beliefs of Hindu villagers, day after day, month after month, and season after season. The fact that I was a doctor, prepared to offer my services—limited though they were—to anyone who cared to consult me helped to bring me into contact with the intimacies of family life. Indeed, this happened on the very first night of my 6 months' stay in the small hamlet of Sujarupa, which was my introduction to fieldwork. After some preliminary reconnaissance by bicycle I had decided on this village because it was small, homogeneous in caste, and cordial in its welcome; so I duly arrived on camelback, with my tent, one for my cook, and all our gear and pitched camp a hundred yards from the main entrance to the village. That night my tent was crowded with more than a score of men and children making music and singing *bhajans*. The concert was suddenly interrupted by the appearance of a young farmer, Hira Singh, who begged me to come to the rescue of his wife, who was possessed by a devil and in grave danger of her life. It was with great trepidation that I took my hurricane lantern and my stethoscope and followed him through the dark to his house from which, as we approached, we could hear loud wails and moans. These cries became louder when we entered the house and found a young woman rocking on the ground in apparent agony; they reached a crescendo when I proposed to examine her physically. However, there was no lack of family members to reassure or scold or threaten her, and soon she quietened down sufficiently to allow me to discover that she was in the throes of childbirth. I noted with relief that it was a normal headfirst presentation and that the fetal heart rate was vigorous and steady.

I told the husband that his wife was possessed by a healthy little devil, who would be with us very soon; sure enough the husband made another appearance before midnight at our resumed singsong, bringing news of the birth of his first child, a boy. Like husbands everywhere, now that the crisis was over he wanted to assure us all that of course he had known all along that this was no devil's work— but women are so foolish and so easily frightened that they make a drama out of nothing.

This incident, whose full import I did not realize until much later, gave a most auspicious start to my 6 months' stay in Sujarupa. Quite soon I was invited into the guest room beside the entrance to the village, and then offered a small stone and mud-walled dwelling, a former goat shed, which became my home for the rest of my stay. This was in the heart of the village, only a few feet away from the shrine built by its founders, the brothers Suja and Rupa who had sunk the first well and begun to clear the jungle about 80 years ago.

As the months went on and I found myself gradually coming to understand more about the villagers' world, there were three inter-related aspects I found particularly important: first, their perception of life as precarious, full of uncertainty, and potential dangers so that it was necessary to consult the omens before undertaking any important decision or task; second, the all pervasiveness of supernatural beings and agencies, some of them protective, like the snake gods who guarded the fields, but mostly capricious, powerful, and frightening; and third, the helplessness of the isolated individual. In this mysterious, often threatening environment it was essential to have allies, helpers, advisers, and the most important source of such help was one's family. To defy the all-pervasive gods, local godlings, evil spirits, ghosts, witches, and sorcerers was unthinkable; even to try to be self-sufficient in counteracting such forces was seen as overweening temerity that must lead in the end to disaster. Several of my Indian psychiatrist colleagues have drawn attention to the fact that dependence on parents and parent surrogates is viewed very differently in India than in the West. In the latter culture great emphasis is placed on self-reliance and on action that masters the material environment, and a prelude to such action is seen as the cultivation of freedom from dependence on others, no matter how well intentioned their support may be. In India, no less emphasis is placed on living *in harmony* with the natural, social, and supernatural environment, rather than trying to dominate it; here, material accomplishment is not despised but is seen as likely to succeed only if it accords with the will of the gods and of one's caste fellows. Most major achievements are the result of communal undertakings in which leadership and authority are more important than individual effort.

The ultimate value, "man's chief end," as the Scottish catechism puts it, consists not in piety nor in practical attainment but in self-mastery reached through withdrawal from the illusory world of the senses into the realm of psychic experiences, made accessible through the practice of meditation. In order to make progress in this direction one must have a benevolent guide, or guru. The guru is usually a male figure who has renounced his sexuality and thereby divested himself of the threatening aspects of a father, but in fact, he can be better conceptualized as a blend of the nurturing and supportive aspects of the mother together with the knowledge and guidance of an idealized father. Many months later, while living among a more sophisticated though still rural community of high-caste Hindus, I became aware of the high level of tension between adolescent sons and their fathers. It was axiomatic that sons loved their fathers, but observation showed that their attitude was dutiful, constrained, and charged with fear—in striking contrast with the easy exchange of affection and even teasing between a grandchild and his grandfather. Constraint and inhibition of feeling especially sexual or even tender feelings toward one of the opposite sex were the leading characteristics of proper behavior. At times it seemed to me, as it has done to other Western observers such as Lois and Gardner Murphy, that a Hindu's adolescence and early manhood is a protracted battle against sensuality, in which guilt feelings are constantly being aroused. In many men's life histories personal tranquility is only attained when they have reached the stage of renouncing carnal desires altogether, and it is particularly at this stage in life that veneration of the guru, the nonthreatening father, the always supporting mother, reaches its fullest height.

There is, of course, in every society a constant dialectic struggle between "life as it is" and "life as it ought to be." The anthropologist is continually being told about the latter, while he looks about him and notes the former being lived all around him. While living in the midst of traditional high-caste Hindus, I often had the sensation of being transported back into the repressive conventions of our own Victorian society, complete with its neuroses and demonstrations of hysteria.

Today, the West represents a much more permissive society than the one our parents and grandparents grew up in. One after another, taboos have been broken; feelings previously denied or suppressed have been given free expression. Social reformers of a generation ago believed that this greater freedom of self-expression would have a salutory effect on the personality, liberating the next generation from guilt and anxiety. It does seem to be true that young people in our society have fewer "hang-ups" about sex than had our generation, but there seem to be just as many who undergo spells of anxiety and depression during their later adolescence. Only the provocative factors have changed: the essential crises of achieving personal identity as a man or as a woman still involve some of our young people in agonies of self-doubt. One manifestation of the new zeal for self-expression is the rather strident assertiveness of student homosexuals in the men's and women's "gay rights" movement; for some the presence of these alternative modes of resolving their identity crises can lead to a premature abandonment of the inner struggle as they throw in their lot with one or other of these minority groups.

But these are the concerns of young people—and their parents—in the West. In India the villages have been changing comparatively rapidly since independence: roads, buses, and the ubiquitous transistor radio have all made villagers more aware than their ancestors ever were before of changes taking place in the other world of the big cities. Those villagers who have lived and worked in the cities bring back new ideas and new expectations, and help to bring about change.

Not all the influences of the city are quite what one would expect. For example, even 25 years ago young men used to leave the villages I lived in to work as far afield as in Ahmedabad or Bombay, but this was not necessarily a liberating experience. In those cities they tended to live together with caste fellows from the same area, if not from the same village, and more than one of them told me that these temporary exiles, surrounded by strangers, tended to comply with the niceties of caste observances more strictly than they ever did at home and to insist that their younger kinsmen did the same.

In the South Indian village called Kota, where Dr. Kapur and I carried out a survey of psychiatric symptoms, we noted that a rather significant change was coming about in the way of life of two of the communities we studied, the farming Bants and the Moger fishermen. Both of these castes had practiced matrilineal inheritance for countless generations; after marriage the wife remained in her mother's group of huts where her husband was something of an interloper, held on sufferance. Their children looked to the mother's brother for guidance and instruction, just as they looked to their mother's mother for their share of the family inheritance. Since independence, however, the government had been trying to legislate matriliny out of existence. At the time of our survey, in 1972, about half the married couples from these two groups had made the changeover, as could be seen by the fact that the wives were now living in their husband's territory, at some remove from their mother's huts. Among the women who had made this change, there was a significantly higher prevalence of psychiatric symptoms as compared with the other women who still remained in their home territory, surrounded by their own close kin. Unfortunately, our survey did not include young children; it would have been interesting to see whether those who were now growing up in a setting their mothers appeared to find stressful also showed more symptoms than did children brought up in the old way.

There is, however, yet another tributary of new experiences and pressures for change, in the persons of men and women who have come back home to their village after having lived abroad for some years. In India we call such people "England returned" or "America returned."

There is an interesting contrast between the North American and the British experience of Indian immigrants. As a general rule, North America admits only rather well-educated Indians, doctors, skilled technicians, businessmen, and the like. In Britain there has also been quite an influx of the less educated and the less highly skilled, who have been absorbed into semiskilled occupations. The mode of life of these two groups is quite different. The former have a much better command of English and for the most part lose little time in adopting the mores of their British or American middle-class neighbors. Their children grow up speaking English with the accents of their new country, in which they feel quite at home. In contrast, working-class immigrants in Britain tend to cluster together in quite large communities in the industrial cities. There they recreate small

Indian townships, with bazaars and cinemas showing Indian films. Their womenfolk often speak very little English, but instead converse in their native Hindi, Punjabi, or Gujerati with neighbors from their own language area. Their children live between two worlds, between the Western environment of school and work and the strong Indian orientation of their family and community.

Many middle-class immigrants quite consciously identify with their country of adoption; but working-class Indians very often have the ambition to earn enough money to enable them to return home and end their days in their village of origin. Their children are usually curious to see their motherland, but having done so by no means all of them want to live there, and yet they do not feel entirely at home in the West.

Contrasts are evident in the relation between parents and children in the two groups of immigrants. The middle-class families usually live alone, separated from their close relatives; whereas the working class tend to reconstitute at least a semblance of the extended family and a number of members of their local community. Indian children immigrants from working-class homes have distinguished themselves both from West Indian youngsters and from their British classmates; the young Asians tend to be more studious, more respectful of their parents, and more law-abiding. It is only in later adolescence that they become aware of the fact that their lives are much more circumscribed than those of their class fellows. One of the commonest causes of family disharmony arises when adolescent girls find that their West Indian or English friends are beginning to date boys, conduct their mothers and fathers find quite unacceptable, so that they start to plan a suitable betrothal for their girls—and this in turn can give rise to fresh quarrels, and even to girls' running away from home.

Middle-class immigrants, in contrast, tend to live in predominantly Western communities and make their friends there. Some of them have acquired an English or American spouse—in which case they have usually adopted the West as their permanent home and expect their children to do so as well. Their ties with their culture of origin become progressively weaker, so that when a relative freshly arrived from India comes to visit them they are reminded of the degree to which they have been distanced from their origins. The children who were born or reared in the West are even more cut off from the old culture; they may feel curious about it, but then do not feel part of it—and yet I have known instances of young Indians who had their entire schooling, right through university, in the West and yet have chosen to make their adult careers in India, but these are exceptional cases.

It is possible that the most profound culturally "distancing" factor is simply this: the language in which a mother talks to her children when they are first beginning to speak. Among the families of working-class immigrants this is usually their native tongue, if not a local dialect; among the middle class it is often English. A number of psychoanalysts, including the late Dr. Eduardo Krapf, former Chief of Mental Health of WHO, Geneva, have written about the conduct of analytic therapy with bilingual or multilingual patients. Dr. Krapf treated many such patients when he practiced in Buenos Aires. Most of these patients spoke Spanish, English, or German, but many were of mixed parentage, and he noticed that when the analysis began to touch on deep, infantile material the patient would revert to his mother's original tongue. Even if it were one he or she no longer spoke fluently, its early-learned phrases still carried a profound, elemental emotional significance.

In my own personal analysis I was interested to find that in very early memories interactions with my mother predominated, in spite of the fact that at least as much of my waking life must have been spent with my Hindi-speaking ayah, Soni Bai. (Incidentally, that analysis revealed a psychological hazard of upbringing in a missionary family which has not been mentioned in the psychoanalytic literature. I had spent some time reliving my rivalry, my triumphs, and my guilt in relation to a slightly older brother, who underwent severe sibling rivalry where I was concerned—only to find that I, in turn, experienced sibling rivalry toward the "Baby Jesus" on whom my mother appeared to lavish even more care and attention than she did on me.) It may be, of course, that if my analyst had been a Hindi speaker, I might have recalled some emotionally charged Hindi baby-talk; as it was, the earliest Hindi I could remember was when my parents took me for a visit home, when I was 4. My ayah traveled with us as far as Bombay, and as she waved goodbye from the pier I said to my mother: "Soni Bai kya pedal chal rahi hai?"—("Is Soni Bai coming on foot then?").

It is characteristic of Western families to be largely isolated, and this intensifies the relationship between an infant and its mother—and it also renders the infant more vulnerable to the effects of inadequate mothering. In the Indian extended family the primacy of the mother-child bond is still apparent, but it is not a monopoly; there are usually several mother surrogates who offer the infant a variety of experiences of mothering—but when the child is frightened or unhappy none of these is so comforting as his real mother. The experience of British children who grew up with an ayah as well as a mother may have had effects of which their parents were unaware; their relationship with the ayah may well have awakened sensibilities other than those they learned from their own mothers. How else was it that when I returned to Rajasthan, 26 years after having left there as a child, I felt immediately, inexplicably at home. It was as if at a very early age I had become emotionally attuned to two worlds, that of a Scottish Presbyterian household and that of the mysterious, god-haunted Hindi world, in all its inexhaustible variety outside the mission compound.

It may seem that I have wandered rather far from my original intention, which was to contrast the stresses of rapid social change in Indian villages and cities among the lowly educated and the Westernized middle classes and among families from each of these backgrounds who have become immigrants in the West. The common element I recognize in each of these contexts, although more markedly in some than in others, is a weakening of formerly unquestioned, powerful, and relatively unchanging cultural values: these were expressed in traditional society in religious observance and in formal rules governing one's behavior toward family members, caste fellows, and other people in one's community. All these have greatly changed in a single lifetime—and not only in India.

Nine years ago I heard Margaret Mead deliver a remarkable lecture at a Mental Health Congress in London, in which she recalled the tensions that used to develop between American immigrants from Europe, who clung to their old ways of life, and their second-generation children who grew up as young Americans. Had they remained in Europe, the elders would have guided their young people, imparting the age-old traditions of their inherited culture, but in America the situation was reversed. The children were better informed about the American way of life and often had to teach their parents. Today, said Dr. Mead, societies are changing so rapidly that all of us who are parents find ourselves in somewhat the same position as those first-generation immigrants. Without having crossed any ocean we discover that our own culture has become in many ways changed, new, unfamiliar, but our children who have grown up with the changes seem more at home in the modern world than we do. We are all immigrants from an Old World that has already largely disappeared.

The need to adapt to this unprecedentedly worldwide phenomenon of change is felt in Indian towns and villages only a little less strongly than in immigrant communities. It can confidently be expected that many people, among the old as well as among the young, will suffer emotionally as a result of the interruption of old continuities. Such casualties of personal experience will need, as they have always needed, the help of "support figures" within the circle of their close relationships. In traditional societies they were always there, if not within the extended family, then somewhere in its cultural projections, in gods, priests, or gurus. In modern societies, whether those of the village or of the city, of the place of one's birth or among distant, unfamiliar surroundings, the need on the part of young people passing through a maturational crisis to find support figures is no less pressing than before but if traditional sources of support are no longer to be found, tomorrow's communities will have to create new ones, or else their growing children will suffer that most demoralizing of all experiences: to need help and to find none.

A Note on the Down-trodden Hindu Wife: Myth or Reality?

The role of women, like so many aspects of that diverse culture, appears to vary widely in different parts of India and in different communities. They are seldom, if ever, given so ostentatiously subordinate a role as generally seems to be the case in the Muslim countries, particularly in traditional Arab states; yet to Western eyes they seem to be treated in many ways as the obedient slaves of their male lords and masters. This subservient role is idealized in religious teaching and is particularly emphasized in those regions where the Rajput warrior-princes used to hold sway. Their community, even more than those of the other twice-born castes, used to regard a wife's meaningful existence as having come to an end when her husband died. All over Northern India, but especially in Rajasthan, one finds memorials to dutiful wives who have enhanced their family's honor by committing *suttee,* immolating themselves on their husbands' funeral pyres. Significantly, on these tragic though proud monuments, the date of the event and the name of the husband—but not that of his wife—are engraved upon the stone.

In Rajasthan women of the major high-caste groups observe *purdah,* none more strictly than the wives of former princes or princelings, and vestiges of this seclusion of the womenfolk are observed even among women of the artisan or farming communities. For example, village women will draw their headcloth well down over their faces when in the presence of a strange man. When a young bride comes to live in her husband's village, she must observe this custom in the presence of all his elder male relatives and village neighbors; only when she is much older and the mother of sons will she be fully accepted as "one of the family" and allowed to show her face more freely, and even then decorum reasserts itself on formal occasions. Life in the girl's parental village is much more relaxed, because there nearly everyone is a close kinsman in whose presence she need not veil her face. Hence the expression "gaon men chori, parccon men lori," which means "at home one is always the little girl, elsewhere one has to act the bride."

Small wonder that a girl has mixed feelings when she leaves her mother's house on the third day of her wedding ceremony to join her bridegroom and his all-male escort in the long walk to her new home. It is expected of a bride to wail on this occasion, to express her grief at parting from her mother. My friend Dakhu, a 16-year-old bride in the Rajasthan village where I lived for some 6 months certainly wailed to good effect: we could still hear her when the wedding party was three-quarters of a mile down the road. When she came back a few weeks later I asked her if she had been putting it on, but she denied this vigorously: "And I tell you, brother Morris, every morning when I see that hill over there called Acram Ahat in the far distance I weep again because it reminds me of home."

She was just commencing her long apprenticeship to the role of a young wife, first to rise in the morning then all day and every day exerting herself to please her mother-in-law, her husband, and eventually her children. It is true that there is no more venerated figure in Hindu legend than the totally self-sacrificing mothers, but let no one deceive themselves that this role is easily acquired. There is one festival of the year called Holi, in which women are given licence to assert themselves openly and shamelessly, making fun of strange men and singing bawdy songs. Here we see an example of a saturnalia, an occasion for a licenced return of the repressed. Another such occasion came to my attention during another village wedding, this time of one of our young men. I joined all the other men in the party, who went to the bride's village for 2 nights of feasting, but I returned a day earlier, joining the solitary old man who was left to guard the womenfolk. That night I heard and saw our village women perform songs and dances that I witnessed at no other time. They were unusually cheerful and excited, with a sort of hectic gaiety. This was especially the case when they performed an action song, standing in a ring taking turns to cradle and nurse a rag doll that was passed from one to another and then, as the song grew faster, it was thrown with increasing violence across the center of the ring, and finally, amid shouts of laughter was flung out of the ring altogether. They enjoyed this so much that it was given two encores.

Here, surely, was an expression of pent-up repressed hostility toward their infant tyrants and against their own infinitely tolerant, submissive role. Some years later a female medical student from Edinburgh visited this village, at my suggestion, and told me that the women gathered in a place apart to regale her with special "women's songs," and these included a reenactment of their rag-doll singing mime. It is often said that within the privacy of their own domestic hearth, Hindu women can assert themselves well enough, but that cannot happen so long as the mother-in-law is head of the household. When it does come about, it is a delayed reward—or revenge—for years of submission as the *lori,* or young bride, of her husband's mother's domain.

The Modernization Process (and Its Pains) in the Indian Adolescent Female as Observed in the Therapeutic Situation

Alan Roland, Ph.D. (U.S.A.)*

It should be kept in mind that the following results of a therapeutic inquiry—an 8-month psychoanalytically oriented research project—are preliminary and tentative and thus mainly a stimulus to further investigation. The project itself can be regarded as a kind of corollary of the social science research that is exploring various aspects of change in modern India. This particular effort is aimed at ascertaining this process of modernization at a level below that of surface consciousness and is mainly based on therapeutic, counseling, and supervising experiences coupled with discussions with various mental health personnel and social scientists.

The approach is based on the current social anthropological perspective that tradition and modernity may be complexly interwoven rather than being intrinsically opposed, as had been originally considered. The focus of interest, therefore, is to understand to what extent the new psychosocial developments are being integrated smoothly into the emerging identity or resulting in inner conflict.

* Senior Research Fellow, American Institute of Indian Studies.

One must distinguish here between modernizing factors that are intrinsically Indian in scope and those that are Westernizing ones imported from abroad and stemming from antithetical value orientations and social patterns. The problems of assimilation may be radically more different and more difficult in the two cases.

There are further limitations to the possibility of any psychological generalizations that can be made because of the confounding and complicating factors of caste, class, and region. The subjects under discussion are drawn from the middle and upper-middle classes in urban centers such as Dehli and Bombay, where they have had English medium instruction throughout their schooling and at times considerable exposure to Western ideas. Some come from families with more modern or Western values and others from more traditional ones. The sample, nevertheless, can in no way be regarded as representative.

Some Methodical Problems

Western psychotherapy, grounded for the most part in psychoanalysis, has met with considerable opposition in India because of its rational and reductive approach to religious and spiritual development, usually interpreted in the context of early parent-child experiences. Many of India's leaders of psychiatry are profoundly involved in the Indian spiritual tradition, in meditation, and in a pressing need to reassert the presence of a basic Indian identity over and against Westernizing values antagonistic to Indian culture. This, of course, has also been the response of Indian leaders from Vivekananda to Ghandi over the last 100 to 150 years.

A second type of resistance to the acceptance of the analytic method originates in the emphasis, or in Indian terms, the overemphasis that Western therapists *theoretically* place on the curative nature of cognitive processes, such as interpretation, as contrasted with the importance of the real relationship. As has been duly noted by several authors, the Indian patient often relates to a therapist as to a family elder or guru and expects real involvement from him. Thus some Indian therapists trained in the West but basically identified with Indian rather than Western culture have commented that the classical psychoanalytic mode of relationship, or rather relative nonrelationship, is unsuitable for most Indian patients. One has the impression that it is the more Westernized psychoanalyst who attempts to maintain the classical type of psychoanalytic relationship. For these psychiatric leaders the Indian sociocultural values of closely involved familial relationships, based on mutual interdependence and consideration and great sensitivity to the other's feelings and possible narcissistic hurt, are quite at odds with the psychoanalytic viewpoint.

Closely related to this last issue are a cluster of other values involving psychoanalytic emphasis on the patient's self-expression, self-reliance, independence, and individuation in social situations—all contemporary Western values, and even basic assumptions of individual development. In those instances in which the individual is embedded in the matrix of traditionally well-defined family relationships and the sense of self is identified with the family and its traditions, free and spontaneous self-expressiveness could be regarded as threatening, hurtful, and disrespectful. The goal of well-being is not to separate from the family but to function well within it.

The issue of individuation is a subtle one, not easy for the Westerner to fully comprehend or even to describe. Although there is undoubtedly a great deal of individuality in the Indian personality, individuation of the self is not a prominent feature and appears to be in opposition to the major thrust of traditional Indian psychological development that stresses dependability rather than individuation. The emphasis in the Indian psyche is not on the "I" or the "I" and the "you," as in the West, but rather on the "we" and the "we" and the "they." Individuation is most encouraged in the spiritual realm, where the individual's inclinations, temperament, and stage of development are taken into account, and where the individual is generally free to practice as he or she wants. In certain modernized, urbanized environments there seems to be somewhat greater individuation, in a social sense, than in the traditional environment, as well as individuals with a rich blend of individuation in both a Western and traditional sense, and there is no doubt that changes are gradually taking place.

There is one further set of resistances that an analytically oriented therapist meets with in treating the Indian patient that is also related to the culture. First, there is often a strong reluctance to discuss matters private to the family and its regulation. There is a reluctance to express thoughts that are inimical to other members or seen as harmful to their honor. This in no way implies that the Indian patient is out of touch with his feelings and impulses; in fact, one gets the impression that beneath the reluctance to communicate and the greater presence of secrets there is perhaps an even greater awareness of feelings, fantasies, and impulses as compared with a Western patient.

A second common resistance is passivity and a need to be told what to do. This can be met more than half way by the Indian therapist accustomed in family and work relationships to be constantly guiding others. Unfortunately, when this occurs, the passivity tends to get reinforced. Finally, there is at times an expectation and apprehension that the therapist will act as an extension of the family to get the patient into line, especially if the patient is involved in self-assertion against the family. This fear may become intensified if family members demand to meet with the therapist and lead to the patient becoming overtly cooperative but passively resistant to the treatment.

Changes Resulting From Westernization and Modernization in the Indian Adolescent Female

The project involved a sample of girls who were receiving counseling at various colleges in Bombay. Almost all of them were the first females in their families to attend college. By and large, they came from traditional, middle-class families, from Hindu, Moslem, Christian, and Parsee communities, and from various parts of the country—Bombay, Sind, Gujerat, Goa, Punjab, Bengal, and South India. All had attended English medium schools; all live in unitary families (because of housing conditions in Bombay), but all had extended family relationships.

The manifest reason for their being sent to college was that this would not only enhance their prospects for marriage to a college-educated boy (considered highly desirable for economic and status reasons) but also would increase their chance for gainful employment following marriage. For the first time they were occupying the same educational milieu as boys, could dress as they pleased, and in general were in a much more unstructured environment that allowed greater freedom in the choice of courses and activities. Yet, at the same time, they all expected to have their marriages arranged and maintained a respectable distance from the male students.

There was one striking problem that came up with the 18 and 19-year-olds that could almost be labeled a "stranger reaction." They displayed an extreme uneasiness and lack of confidence with students they did not know, either male or female, and developed "ideas of reference" although not of clinical intensity. For example, they imagined they were being stared at, criticized, and talked about behind their backs. On first glance, this looked like typical adolescent "paranoia" familiar to Western observers, but here it seemed to have additional cultural roots. The reaction was further complicated by the fact that they themselves, much against their own reason, developed similar attitudes to others, thus setting up what Cameron termed a pseudoparanoid community with everyone suspecting everyone else. Dynamically it was clear that in criticizing another, one was being critical of a forbidden part of oneself and thus maintaining a measure of moral self-respect.

Interestingly enough, the girls did not perceive the parents in their unitary families as being unduly critical of them. On the contrary, they felt them to be loving and considerate, if not always understanding about the exigencies of college life. They reported that they were quite free at home and under no compulsions. What did emerge, however, was a pervasive climate of parental attitudes that conveyed implicitly or obliquely the necessity for a girl to be extremely careful in her dress, in her behavior, and in her relationships with boys *in public* because of what people might think and say; of the effect this would have on the reputation of both the girl and her family, thus endangering her marriageability. References would be made to neighbor's daughters and the consequences of their misbehavior. In this way strangers begin to represent a subtle menace to be watched with wariness and caution.

In previous generations the girls from traditional families would generally have had their marriages arranged earlier and without prior exposure to the unshattered stimulations of college life, but the modernization movement brought with it a bombardment of novel experiences and contacts, particularly heterosexual ones. There is evidence to suggest that sensuality tends to be more controlled than repressed in the Indian personality, so that the college experience may generate defensive internalized parental attitudes toward the stranger conducing to a "stranger anxiety." Everyone outside the family is a stranger and therefore a potential threat. As a result, the adolescent becomes as circumspect as possible, to the point of extreme modesty inhibition, except among family members and close personal friends. The freer the college atmosphere, the more likely is it for the parental attitudes to take the form of projective identification and bring about a mutual mistrustfulness.

Some of the girls were gradually able to talk about conflicts with their mothers at home and the ways in which they handled them. The commonest technique used was by containment of anger, with withdrawal from contact and a retreat into silence until control over their feelings was regained. They seemed unable to convey directly to the mother their sense of injury, however hurt they might feel. Instead, they preferred to commute it in some nonverbal fashion such as declining to eat while insisting that they felt perfectly all right. The mother might sometimes take cognizance of these nonverbal cues and inquire further about the situation, but more usually it was the daughter's task to make excuses, apologies, and amends if things were to be patched up. She might do this by silently helping around the kitchen or with the housework without broaching the issue of the conflict. Some of the girls would acknowledge displacement of anger onto younger siblings, or cousins if they lived in a joint family. Several reported occasions of inexplicable depression that would last for awhile and then just as inexplicably clear up. These various mechanisms, ranging from conscious containment to depressive reactions appeared to be the main traditional mechanisms for handling mother-daughter conflicts. In the few cases in which the daughter summoned up enough courage to confront the mother, she had the conviction that there was no other way open to her to mend the relationship—either the mother was too rejecting or too easily hurt. Sensitivity to being hurt as well as to hurting others are prominent themes in the counseling of these college girls, and this applies to female patients as well. It may be a characteristic feature of the Indian psyche in general.

CASE ILLUSTRATION

A concluding example of the effects of modernization will read in parts like a psychoanalytic case in Western society, though some of the reactions are particularly Indian. It concerns a girl in her middle 20s from a South Indian, Christian, middle-class family. She is the fourth of five children, all of whom had entered the religious life. Characteristic of this particularly Christian community, there is a great emphasis on education to advance the status in life. The patient was clearly the least-favored child of her mother, who regarded others as brighter and more religious. Her unusual intuitive gifts and lively personality were not appreciated. She spent a very unhappy, lonely childhood, became something of a problem in school, and was always very shy. However, her father, while not being overly close to his children, seemed to be more emotionally stable than the mother, and served as an important model of competency and intelligence.

She went on to college and postgraduate work, doing reasonably well, and more importantly, found that she was responded to in a very different way than from her mother. This increased her confidence, gained her friends, and eventually found her a husband—someone, who, common in the Christian community, was quite suitable for her. She now has a highly responsible position as a teacher and counselor in a good school and is much appreciated in her work.

In therapy she had been helped to express a variety of feelings that relieved various somatic complaints. It has been reported that this bottling up of feelings is a fairly typical defense in Indian women. When she came into treatment she had been recently married and was living with her husband's family in a joint family setup. It made her uncomfortable and guilty whenever she and her husband went out socially and left her sister-in-law and mother-in-law at home. The same guilty reaction also came up in relation to unmarried girlfriends as well. Upon careful investigation, it turned out to be a case of projective identification, in which she felt empathetic for an old, unhappy, lonely self, which she projected onto others. This interpretation felt very right to her and enabled her to live her current life in a much happier way, without being obsessively concerned with hurting her in-laws or friends. She then brought up the problem of her inability in postgraduate work to share with others her excellent counseling work with maladjusted children. By means of dreams and other material, displacements from the mother onto other older work-figures were traced, ranging from feelings that no one would listen to her to the other extreme of becoming upset if spoken to with anger. Throughout treatment, it was clear that she was very aware of her feelings, particularly of her anger, but dealt with them through containment and withdrawal, cutting off communication, and at times losing all sense of sympathy.

In this case, the modernizing opportunities available through college and postgraduate education, together with later professional work, enabled this girl to have many experiences and responses unobtainable at home. Being Christian, she could also choose a husband to her own liking. Thus through education, employment, friends, husband, and therapy, she was able to find a very different and satisfying kind of life for herself. Without these modernizing influences, it would not have been possible for her to differentiate herself and her self-image from the matrix of the traditional family.

References

1. Neki, J. S. Psychotherapy in India. Presidential Address, Indian Psychiatric Society, 29th Annual Conference, Calcutta, January 1977.
2. Pande, S. K. The mystique of Western psychotherapy: An Eastern interpretation. *J. Nerv. Ment. Dis.*, 146, 425–432.
3. Singer, Milton. *A Great Tradition Modernizes*. Praeger, New York, 1972.
4. Surya, N. C., and Jayaram, S. S. Some basic considerations of psychotherapy in the Indian setting. *Indian J. Psychiatry*, 1964, pp. 153–156.
5. Cameron

Changes in the Family and the Process of Socialization in India

M. S. Gore, Ph.D. (India)

The effort here is to approach the theme of the Study Group—Children and Parents in a Changing World—from the vantage point of a sociologist. Since this sociologist is an Indian, he focuses more specifically on the Indian situation. Here again, because of his specialized interest, what he has to say is more likely to be related to the urban, middle-class family than any other group. This presentation deals mainly with the social and familial changes in India as they affect—or are likely to affect—the process of socialization within the family.

The Theoretical Framework

In sociology the term "social change" is used to refer to changes in the institutionalized patterns of living characteristic of a society. Individuals in a society may also experience other changes related to age- and sex-determined or occupational roles, but such changes, at the level of individuals or groups, would normally be regarded as a part of the dynamics of that society and are provided for through social mechanisms that facilitate adjustment to such changes. However, since even the major social changes, that is, changes in the major institutional structures of society, may also begin only as changes experienced by individuals in their own lives and not necessarily as institutional changes identifiable as such, the distinction between social change and social dynamics is not easy to make in relation to concrete situations. It is an analytical distinction, one that is often made after the change has become too marked to be missed. The institutional structures involved may be in the area of kinship, education, religion, government, the economy, and the like. When one speaks of changes in the institutionalized patterns of behavior, one also refers by implication to changes in the realm of values, in the subjective perceptions of individuals, their aspirations, motives, and so on.

Two major approaches are currently prevalent in the study of social phenomena—including the phenomenon of social change. These approaches are often labeled as the structural-functional and the Marxist or material-dialectical approaches. In an analytical sense the two are not mutually exclusive insofar as the Marxist approach is also an approach that is based on an identification of social structures and a study of the functions subserved by them in a given society at a given point of time. However, in their emphases, in the kinds of literature that they have given rise to, and in the historical roles that they have played, the two approaches have been very different. The scope of this chapter is limited to a consideration of social and familial change as it affects the process of socialization. The conceptual framework used for analysis is that provided by the structural-functional approach.

Traditional Indian Family

The traditional Indian family has been described in sociological literature as the joint family. The jointness of this unit lay in the composition of the household which often consisted of an aged couple, their adult sons and wives, and young children belonging to the older parents as well as the young couples. However, the jointness also applied to a commonly owned property, a common purse, a common kitchen, and the mutuality of obligations that bound the members together. This joint family had to face three important problems:

1. The distribution of tasks between adults.
2. The establishment and legitimation of a definite line of authority.

3. The assimilation of the married women who came from other households into the joint family corporation.

These problems were tackled by laying down the fact that authority in the joint family rests in a formal sense with the eldest male member, though in actuality he might share it with or delegate it to different persons in different spheres. The age and sex basis of higher status and authority was generally supported by the norms of a tradition-bound society that generally accepted these norms in other spheres of life as well. The lack of occupational differentiation within the family—which was ensured partly by the limited occupational diversification of an agrarian society and by the institution of a joint inheritance of familial property—minimized the differences that might otherwise have arisen in the outlook and income of the adult males. The potential disruptive influence that the women might have exercised was minimized by the norms of early marriage, intracaste marriage, and arranged marriage. The women thus entered the new homes while they were still young; they came from homes that were not culturally very different, and they came without any prior exclusive claims on their husbands. The culture of the family segregated and subordinated the female. Further, the significance of the conjugal tie was itself subject to limitation—often perhaps unsuccessfully—by subordinating it (in terms of its moral claims on the male) to the filial and the fraternal ties and the obligations they engendered.

The traditional joint family fulfilled varied functions in the rural context. Like all families it was involved in:

1. The procreation and socialization of the young.
2. The intrafamilial management of tension and the regulation of affect.
3. The production and consumption of the economic unit.
4. The provision of social security for the contingencies of old age, widowhood, orphanhood, disability, and the like.

The ability of the joint family to subserve these functions depended on the particular social context in which it functioned—the context of a largely agrarian, occupationally undifferentiated, traditional society in which age and experience were respected, the status of women was subordinated to that of men, and the major cultural theme was one of ensuring continuity—continuity of the family, of the caste, of religion, of past knowledge—rather than a theme of innovation and change.

The Traditional Socialization Model

The process and the content of socialization in the joint family differed from what was sought for or achieved in a modern nuclear family unit, and they were more directly supportive of the society in which they flourished. One of the family's major characteristics was the presence of several adults of both sexes and a conglomerate of children in the household. A child had to relate itself to many adults, all of whom represented sources of authority and gratification to varying degrees.

The child's mother had a special emotional and interdependent relationship with the child that was recognized and allowed, particularly when the child was still at the breast. In a large household the young mother often found that her relationship to her child was psychologically the closest and most meaningful—closer, sometimes, than even her relationship to her husband. The "lonely" mother's emotional need for the child and the significance of a son as a guarantor of her status in the joint household made her want to keep her son emotionally close and dependent on her, even in later life. Her need coincided with the younger child's own need for a dyadic relationship within the large joint household. However, once the early stage of physical dependence was over, the child had many potential mother surrogates.

On the other hand, the affective role of the father was considerably circumscribed by social and cultural norms. In addition to the fact that he was not as constantly at home as the mother, the father was also restrained culturally from taking special notice of his own children or from playing with them, since propriety demanded that he relate equally to the other children in the household and custom demanded that he assume an authoritative rather than affective role.

The smallest children spent most of their time in the women's section of the house, whereas those 5 years and older were mainly with age cohorts of siblings and cousins. The older group were as likely to be chastised or reproved by any of the elders in the family; the major source of gratification for each child, however, came from one particular woman, mother or mother surrogate.

The content of socialization—or the verbally communicated message—would emphasize for the child the need to accept the authority of elders in the family, the importance of accepting obligations for all its members, the significance of tradition and of conformity to it, and obedience to the norms of caste and religion. Culturally, the great epics emphasized the virtues of filial love and duty, of equal sharing among brothers, of respect for elders, and of idealization of the mother.

The joint family household was a patriarchal household. It was one in which the line of authority was always clear, but the exercise of authority was often shared and modified by consultation. Children brought up in the household were loved and sometimes spoiled, but they were expected to abide by the authority of the family. In the initial phase of upbringing there was great freedom in letting them be, but this soon gave way to discipline and obedience. Children should be seen but not heard in the presence of their elders. There was generally no effort made to exclude them from adult company, so that they were often able to listen to discussions between adults from which they presumably drew their own conclusions. It was the duty of the adults to protect the children, ensure their well-being, and prevent them from consorting with undesirables. The child's physical needs were always given priority—particularly by mothers—over their elders' needs.

The child in the joint family had a lot of company, but the process of upbringing did not emphasize the individuality of the child. His recognition as an individual with exclusive claims for affection, guidance, and attention came usually from the mother or mother surrogate, but for the rest of the family he was just one of the children. This sense of being one of the group was often dominant. Discipline was varied and included corporal punishment administered without guilt on the part of the adult. Other kinds of punishment included the withholding of sweets, exclusion from company, denial of food for short periods, and confinement, in extreme cases. Severe physical abuse was not common.

Some of the older themes in child rearing included the following:

children must be cared for and caressed; they must be obedient and dutiful; and they must be groomed to follow parental examples and aspirations.

The Pressure for Change

The traditional family is still in existence. Irrespective of the household composition, the familial relationships continue to follow the patterns created by the joint family. In the urban areas, however, certain changes affecting the familial goals have appeared and have tended to modify the family life style and the modes of upbringing. The change is still marginal in some ways but important in its potentialities.

The urban social context—particularly the present-day urban context—is different in some significant ways. The relatively undifferentiated occupational structure of the rural areas is not characteristic of the city. Occupational differentiation is a feature not only of urban society as a whole but also of the family, so that sons do not follow automatically in the father's footsteps. This is especially true of the educated, white-collar groups, but even in the working class, although fathers and sons may belong to the category of skilled or unskilled labor, their employers and their emoluments are often very different. Difference in income, occupation, and education are not conducive to joint family living, particularly when a common purse is maintained by the family. Even living in a joint household and eating from a common kitchen may present problems—especially after the death of the two parents.

Apart from occupational differentiation, there have been changes in the age of marriage of the urban middle class. This has gone up largely because a young boy, whose future economic standing depends on his education and ability rather than on his father's landed wealth, is no longer considered "eligible." The rise in the age of marriage has meant that the girls have to be kept occupied during the years prior to marriage in the parental home. Education, first to the school level and now to the college level, provides the substitute occupation. The later age of marriage and education prior to marriage in the case of girls raise problems for the joint family. Girls who now enter married life at the age of 20+ and after 4 years of college are not as easy or as willing to be molded to the pattern of the new family and its particular requirements. Besides, over the past 40 or 50 years every young girl who enters her hubsand's family as a daughter-in-law or sister-in-law has tended to be more educated than the other older women in the family. The younger but more educated daughter-in-law may find it difficult to accept an authority pattern based on age and seniority.

Apart from these situational changes and pressures, new ideas have also exerted their influence. The concepts of equality and rationality have affected the family as they have affected other institutions. The concept of equality has been argued in favor of women. It has opened up opportunities in education and occupation for them; it has led to a modification of the family law both in relation to property and inheritance; it has given them political rights; and it has enabled them to organize themselves as an articulate, though not necessarily militant, group.

The concept of rationality challenges the legitimacy of tradition as a basis for action. In the joint family in which family tradition was often the basis for allocation of family resources, the introduction of rationality as a norm opens up the scope for discussion, difference, and disagreement. This affects the socialization process, particularly in the case of the adolescent and postadolescent youth.

New ideas have also flowed in as a part of the Western, liberal approach to child upbringing and education—ideas that have resulted from the work of Freud and of creative educators like Froebel, Montessori, and Dewey.

Familial Change

The new social context and the new ideas are mutually supportive, and they both make it difficult for the family to continue to function as it traditionally did. The following observations indicate some of the directions of change. They apply primarily to urban, educated, middle-class families, since these are the ones most directly affected by the new changes.

Although there are no conclusive, nationwide data, there is some indication that in the urban areas the proportion of truncated joint families—families from which some of the adult males with their wives and children have moved out—has increased. This may happen not as a result of formal division but as a result of nuclear units moving out either for reasons of inadequacy of housing or for reasons of nonavailability of jobs in the original place of residence. Sometimes these reasons may be genuine, and sometimes they may be culturally acceptable legitimations of an action undertaken for other reasons. Such truncation does not give rise to neat nuclear units. One nuclear unit may leave the household, and what is left behind may still be a joint household made up of two brothers and their dependents or one brother and the parents or some such combination. Although urban households are smaller in size, they are not strictly nuclear in the European or American usage of the term.

Another form of adjustment to the new situation may be for brothers to live under the same roof but have separate kitchens. This pattern is probably more common in smaller towns where the family originally lived in an ancestral home.

However, whether they live jointly or severally in different households, the mutuality of obligations may still continue to bind the brothers, at least for one generation. It will be common for them to accept responsibilities for the education and the like of their nephews and nieces, to help one another in difficulties, to function for one another as sources of temporary credit, to visit for relatively long periods during vacations, or to ask a female relative to come and stay with them to tide over a temporary crisis when the woman of the house is unwell.

Nevertheless, even where the joint household continues, there is usually one distinct change: the primacy of the conjugal tie in comparison with the filial or fraternal tie is no longer seriously challenged. Furthermore, the quality of husband-wife relationship has changed in some ways. The husband and wife spend more time together by themselves and exchange ideas. Even today, however, marriages are largely arranged by parents and other elders, and the pattern of marriage following a period of courtship is not common. What sociologists have identified as the "romantic complex of love" is not the factor that brings a young boy and young girl together, nor does it play a central role in their postmarital relationship. The mutual expectations are still largely traditional.

Finally, there is also greater equality and communication between adult males—whether they live separately or in the same household.

The traditional joint family was often characterized by a measure of reserve between adult brothers or even between father and son. This reserve may have been due to the clear status differentiation between them or, at times, it may have served the purpose of clothing covert hostility.

The Changing Socialization Process

The pattern of socializing the young is also changing in certain ways. Parents in urban homes are much more concerned about their children and their future than was common in the rural home. This has been necessitated by the differential occupational pattern and the need to make an early choice about the educational stream to be pursued. If the household is a joint one, the children may still not receive a highly individualized treatment on the part of the elders in the family, but decisions about children have become much more directly the responsibility of their parents than of the elders in the family as a whole. The degree to which this has happened varies a great deal from family to family.

In the urban middle-class family there is greater consciousness, even greater self-consciousness, on the part of parents about the importance of their parental role and how it might affect the children. If highly educated, they have begun to experience the problems of choosing between the autocratic, democratic, and permissive approaches to child upbringing. The problems of adolescence, which were not discernible above the surface in the rural family, have now begun to be identified. The situation of a child defying the parent or an elder was very unusual in the joint family, and if the child did seem defiant, the parent or another elder would punish the child immediately, without hesitation or sense of guilt. The educated parent today often seems to be caught between his natural inclination and the dictates of "good parenthood."

The difficulties of the parent-child relationship become more noticeable during the postadolescent and early youth stages of the child's life. The young person has enough education to question the basis or justification of the do's and don'ts prescribed by the parents, and he may set no value on the experience of the elder generation or their fears on his behalf. In many middle-class homes the conflict of wills may not become critical or explosive, but in some it does. In either case the conflict is not well-balanced. The young person is, of course, economically dependent, but at the emotional level the modern parent appears to need the acceptance and approval of his offspring more than the other way round.

Among the new themes in child rearing are the following: children should be given maximum opportunity for developing their potential; parents should not impose their occupational or other preferences on their children; children should be told the reason why they may or may not do particular things. The newness is not in the themes but in the emphasis.

Conclusions

The picture of familial change and change in the socialization processes is not very clear. The difficulties are both because there are not enough studies on the subject as because the picture is highly varied. The rural joint family of the higher caste is different from the rural joint family of the lower caste in the types of compulsions it generates. The educated, middle-class, joint family in the small town is different from the rural land-based or business-based joint family. The small-town nuclear household is different from the big-city professional person's nuclear household. Some of the differences arise out of household composition, some from the nature of the urban context, some from the type of education and mass media exposure that they imply, and some depend on whether the nuclear family living is a first-generation or a second-generation experience. Further, religion is an important variant. Parsees and some of the urban Christian families no longer share in the culture of the joint family at all.

The limitations of these observations on family life and family change should, therefore, be borne in mind. What has been called the traditional joint family may still be the contemporary family in a rural setting—especially if it is a higher-caste, land-based family. The changing urban family is likely to undergo more change, depending on the education level of the family members, their occupations, and the ethos of the urban community in which they live.

Our knowledge is currently too inadequate to say whether there is a clear continuum of change. My suggestion that there is one is at best a hypothesis.

Situations and Settings: A Search for an Optimal Environment

Christopher C. Benninger, Ph.D. (India)

Until very recently architects and planners based their concepts and ideas on utopian notions of perfection. Their values evolved along a clear path of history from the classic harmony of Greek and Roman proportion to the grand spaces and structures of the Renaissance to the Reformist sense of order, hygiene, and equality in the late 19th century, and through a period of rebellion against the classics in favor of a response to modern and industrial function. During all this time they were a profession concerned primarily with things and only secondarily with the users—people. When they did consider people it was in the sense of the industrial designer fitting his product to a user's performance standards, rather than in the sense that they were creating environments that would be part of a total context of human development. When these principles were extended from individual buildings to mass urban plans, or when they had to work in communities whose resources were small, the gaps in their understanding were laid bare.

It is from the architecture of scarcity that new attitudes have developed and new understandings have been sought. These new concerns have led architects to accept the hypothesis that every human environment represents a balanced design of social, economic, and physical constraints that must be understood before new limits are set through design and plans. A three-way relationship between the physical, the social, and the economic aspects of environment can be represented as follows:

SITUATIONS generate REQUIREMENTS/ABILITIES generate SETTINGS

This infers that a set of requirements project an intent for settings, and certain abilities generate a possibility for settings. Priorities act as a structuring device between the needs of any household and its ability to pay for their fulfilment. In more affluent societies the relationship is less tight as the means are greater.

Let us look at a simple requirement/ability model which includes changes corresponding to the development of a family that is a recent migrant to an Indian city. What kind of settings correspond to their inherent needs and means and what kind of official (public), entrepreneurial (private) and community (popular) responses result? Figure 1 traces through time the changes in a family's *situation*. The situation that generates requirements and abilities is in turn a product of the restraints and opportunities of the society.

The trajectories show the shift in needs for three different elements in the family's situation. These are accessibility, security, and status. These elements of the family's situation overlap considerably with three elements of all settings: location, tenure, and level of development of shelter, respectively. It is location that provides physical accessibility, tenure that gives legal claim to a residence, and the level of development of shelter that adds to the status of the family.

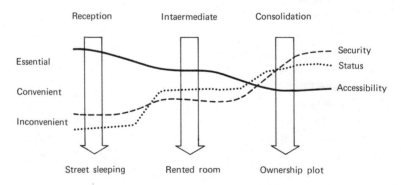

Figure 1. Requirement/ability model.

Because there is a match between situations and settings in every phase of the family's development I call this the optimal model of habitat mobility [1]. The model is described below in terms of its situations and settings.

Reception

In the first phase the household is composed of a single member who is a recent migrant to the city with no job, skill, or social group. He buys leftover food from the market and picks up casual work on a daily wage basis. He would find a high level of shelter, with its high regular rent, an inconvenience. As an independent bachelor his status needs are low. As such, any status gained from a good room would be of little use. He would also find the legal ties of monthly rent inconvenient, as his income is not regular, and he has more pressing needs than shelter. Besides, he is not concerned about the security of the tenure he would gain as a tenant. But to him the accessibility he gains from location is essential. He has to be on the spot when anyone comes in search of a laborer for the day. His source of cheap food is also at the wholesale market nearby. The setting that matches his situation is street sleeping, posing as a second-class passenger sleeping in the railway station, or, if he is lucky, staying free with a relative. The match between his situation and his setting makes an extremely responsive environment. Though it may look better, a rented room in a lodge costing half his income would be a poor setting causing frustration and inconvenience!

Intermediate

In the second phase of his family development he marries a girl from his village through arrangement of his father and brings her to the city, where a child soon is born. Through regular contacts he now has steady work. With added income he has collected some belongings: a radio, some cooking utencils, blankets, and clothing. With these possessions and a wife he needs a secure place to live. Security through tenure is very convenient. Accessibility is still important, but less so than in the first phase. With a "friends' circle," collected after a few years in the city, and with a wider group of relatives from his wife's side he requires some status. All these conditions can be fulfilled by renting a room in the city center. This may be in an old subdivided house, a chawl[1] or in a hutment. This gives a partial picture of the resolution of needs within means in the intermediate phase of family development.

Consolidation

After several years in the city and several new additions in the family, our migrants are in a position to know what their potential in the city is. The head of the family has a regular job for which he has developed some skills. In addition, other members of the family are working either part-time or casually. It is known to the family that income may drop off due to illness and with old age. The romantic hopes that were brought to the city have evolved into a clear set of real possibilities. The family would like to consolidate whatever gains it has made in the city. Whatever investment is being made in housing in the form of rent would be better spent on their own house. Status is more important now that daughters are approaching marriageable age, and the "city-bred" sons of the house want better things. A bicycle and more stable employment have reduced the need for accessibility in a city that is better understood and more "visable" to the family. With old age in sight the family feels the need for a more stable residence. It would like a claim to dwelling regardless of whether money is available for rent. For this security, the family would like its own home where it can even generate extra income through rentals or a small workshop in the back yard. All these situational priorities elicit requirements that are satisfied by squatting on vacant land and pressuring the authorities for legal recognition of tenure. Moving to an open site and building one's own shelter that can be upgraded over the years is the best setting for this situation. It offers an opportunity to invest in something for the future and to build a decent house piece by piece, as and when economic conditions permit, thus increasing status. It also grants more independence in decision making. By living in a setting

---

[1] A *chawl* is a multistoried dwelling structure in which each apartment is composed of one or two rooms, accessible from a common stair and balconies across one face. W.C.'s, water taps and baths are common. Before their construction was made illegal they were built by industries for their workers.

with community mates, one optimizes his condition further, having neighbors with common needs and friends from whom to take help in times of crises. This then represents a match between an appropriate setting and the family's situation in the consolidation phase of development.

Unfortunately, this optimal model of movement from one matched situation and setting to another is rare. The findings in Latin America of John F. C. Turner [2] and William Mangin [3], which support this model as a theory of urbanization, result from richer societies with less-developed systems of public control. The legislative structure that controls the development of Indian cities makes settings so expensive through unrealistic standards that it is impossible for the average man to consolidate into viable urban settings [4]. The rent-control acts have made it uneconomical for either the private or the public sector to build rental housing within the means of the average man. Thus, legally framed, official schemes produce settings that are beyond reach of the vast majority of households. These factors tend to direct investment toward high income ownership housing [5].

Figure 2 is a sketch of the income distribution in Ahmedabad. Multiples of level of subsistence are shown vertically, and the percentage of households in each multiple is drawn on the horizontal. Lines are drawn to indicate schemes available to households earning at that level and who are capable of spending 15 to 20 percent of

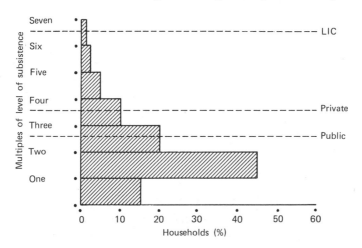

Figure 2. Income distribution in Ahmedabad.

Situations and Settings

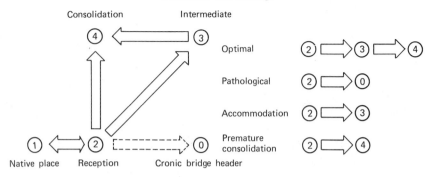

Figure 3. Change models.

their income on housing. It can be seen that many are neglected and must therefore provide their own housing. They do this through their own efforts in the popular sector.

Faced with the dilemma of having no choices in the formal system, urban households resort to illegal methods of finding settings . . . they squat. It is presently estimated that 33 percent of the households in the city of Ahmedabad live in such illegal settlements and that these settlements are growing three times as fast as the rate of the population as a whole [6]. The inferences of this ad hoc approach to city building and casual view of human development are many. We are creating a low-security society in which investments in the future are risky. This results, in turn, in alienation from the society that provides no place for a large number of its members. Instead of the optimal model outlined above, several alternative models are evolving that attempt to relate situations to settings with the minimum tension. They are illustrated in Figure 3 in terms of their flow from situation to situation and setting to setting. Each circle represents a basic setting that has been described. The direction and timing of movement between different settings places households in different models.

Pathological Model

When a migrant cannot integrate with the city socially, economically, and physically, a pathological situation arises. The migrant becomes a chronic "newcomer" unable to change or to improve his condition. Unlike the genuine newcomer or the seasonal visitor with whom he shares the street, he has his family and his belongings with him. The situation is often due to psychological, physical, or other handicaps. The family makes its living by begging or through some marginal business.

Accommodation Model

In the optimal model the family easily moved into a rented dwelling. In the present urban context this move is very difficult. Since the tenant is guaranteed possession of his quarters at the same rent year after year, it is uneconomical for him to leave. The value of the rent depreciates to a point where the owner cannot afford to maintain the structure. Under these conditions rental housing is not a viable investment. Some new units are created by subdividing older houses, but there is a growing shortage. The difficulty of finding dwelling and the depreciating rent encourage households to remain in rented rooms. As the family grows its needs for more space, for status, and for more choice grows, and the match between the intermediate phase and the rented room is broken. Security, reasonable locations, and a paucity of alternatives encourage the persistence of this poor match.

Premature Model

With an end to the construction of chawls and the saturation of rented dwellings, new families have little choice but to squat in a hutment early in their development. This occurs before they can make a good choice of location or before they can conceptualize the long-term growth of their settlement. Since no plans exist for these settlements in the public sector, the families often fall prey to middlemen, who themselves have squatted or rented the property from the owner. These parties then sublet the land in small plots for a huge profit.

These are some of the more predominant models. There are others wherein the migrant fails and returns to the village, and still more where the boy is born in the city and builds his family around the setting inherited from his father. In an economy of scarcity this is very common.

In the vast majority of cases there is not a good match between the situations and the settings. The family just has to accept whatever setting it gets. Given the strength of their culture and the slow growth of their economy, there is little hope for changes in their situations. Settings, however, could be more responsive and bring better environment.

An Optimal Environment?

Given the above, what would an optimal environment consist of? Obviously, there is no such static reality. An optimal environment would be one in which a number of settings would be matched to situations prevalent in the society through which families move during their development. It may be possible to characterize those settings and to compare them with the existing set of possibilities to deduct positive policies for change.

In the foregoing discussion several settings were identified. Each setting is distinguished from the others by the intensity at which a particular set of qualities is operant. The quality of accessibility, for example, can drop off in intensity as the family moves progressively to new settings and a more stable urban existence. Other qualities also are expressed at different intensities in different settings. A good setting, if it is to respond to situations, should contain particular qualities that are required in the situation. These qualities, when expressed in a material sense in a setting, could be called manifestations of the qualities. If we identify and describe those qualities, we will have good programmatic information with which we can evaluate existing settings and design new ones. Figure 4 identifies three generic settings and the implications of qualities operant in them. The indications in the figure (−, 0, +) infer whether the quality and its manifestation have a negative and unwanted effect in the setting, a neutral and accepted effect on the setting, or a positive and possibly necessary effect on the setting. At the top of the diagram *situations* are listed. At the bottom *settings* are listed. On the left-hand side *qualities* are listed, and on the right-hand side *manifestations* of the qualities are noted. Qualities and manifestations and situations and settings are characterized according to their relationship to each other. Manifestations, then, are the realizations of qualities

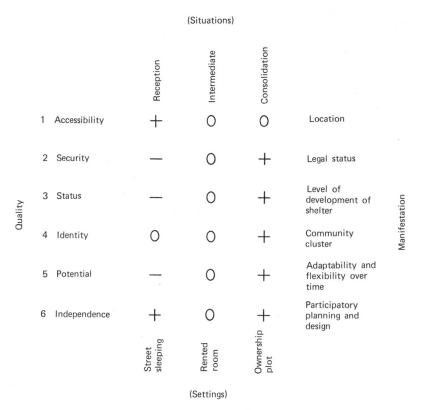

Figure 4. Manifestations of qualities.

through physical, organizational, and institutional reality. In a healthy, optimal environment settings are also the physical, organizational, and institutional realities of situations. Some of the qualities which as elements persist through all the situations are discussed below.

Depending on the phase of development of the family and its resultant situation, qualities that seem on a cursory view to be universally positive have a negative effect. Someone may wonder how potential, for example, could be negative in any circumstance. The answer is that these qualities here are not taken as general abstractions but as given material reality, and therefore they have associated costs. It is with regard to priorities that structure the situation and ability to pay that structures choices that a quality can be negative when its acquisition rules out the ability to acquire more critical qualities, such as accessibility. Again, the principle that situations generate requirements and abilities which generates settings rules. These qualities are discussed in more detail below, and the child as a participant in the environmental process is noted.

Accessibility

In addition to the physical manifestations of accessibility there are also social and economic barriers and channels to opportunity and self-realization. Access to skills that open up employment opportunities must also be considered. Access to information about jobs, life styles, processes, and markets all contribute to the opportunities and barriers an environment contains. In India we have identified a family type distinct from the Western nuclear family and from the traditional Hindu extended family. Like a nuclear family it is small, its growth dependent on the number of children. Like the extended family it shares a common purse. But unlike both there are no breadwinners. All the members work to support the family, and no one income would be sufficient for survival [7]. Because of this financial relationship, which in turn is very dependent on the intricate social ties of the individual family members, I have called this family type the symbiotic household. If the location is good for only one worker, it destroys the economic basis of the family. In this type it is also common for the work hours to be broken up into small segments rather to be in a continuous sequence, as in a factory or office. A child may go to a house in the morning to clean floors and in the evening to wash utensils and take out garbage. A poor location, distant from the job-intensive areas of the city, reduces the role and contribution the child makes in the symbiotic household. At the same time he is losing his chance for a nonformal education that may be essential preparation for his adult life. In the planned, isolated community he may go to school and learn to read and write, but these are not the skills he will need, nor does it answer the immediate questions that arise in the family of which he is a part. Poor accessibility may rob the child of irreplaceable informal experiences that are essential to his development.

Security

We have discussed security in terms of one's claim on his dwelling place and in terms of one's right to inhabit a particular place. Other forms of security such as persistent good health, a continuing job, and a strong relationship with friends and family add to the sense of stability. Although these may be illusive, a stable claim to the place one lives is not. A family that is forced to move periodically loses the social and economic contacts which only time can make. At the same time the individual viability is hampered. For the child who experiences forced removal from his sources of income and familiar network, the loss may be irreparable. He may lose confidence in his ability to be.

Independence

Here the term is meant as the amount of control one has over one's own environment. It indicates he has a number of choices open to him in terms of the context of his setting. Operationally, it may mean a family can choose the timings of the investments they make in their homes or what kinds of materials and finishes they want within their means. Self-help through site and services schemes gives this kind flexibility and choice. If properly planned such schemes will provide open plots large enough to allow growth over time [8]. Each family member participates in the constructive process of discussing what to build next, organizing the materials toward a common goal and actually building their house together. For the child, the raising of a house is a hopeful and positive sign. If he can participate in the work he gets the feeling of importance and a sense of participation in a future that is real and meaningful. He also sees through the actions of his parents that they are not silent bystanders to the fate of the world, but that they have plans, concerns, and abilities to bring solutions. In so building their own house the parents provide a model that says, "you can change the world." This is a very important message in modern-day India. Another aspect of independence is decision making at the community level. This raises the question of to what extent the family and community can make decisions involving hundreds of households. New microlevel institutions have arisen as a response to the corporate planners who make decisions paternalistically on paper from within their air-conditioned offices. The canned solutions are rejected; the community refuses to be pushed from one place to another; it creates a forum for debate and discussion and begins to make decisions for itself. The child, witnessing his parents in open debate and discussion, gains respect for the social concerns in which the dialogues are cloaked. He sees his family involved in bigger questions than its own survival, and he is aware that his parents and he himself are citizens who have responsibility to causes and human dilemma. In different phases independence means different things. It has perhaps least importance when the young man settles into the position of a householder and the family is young. But when he enters the city and as the family matures, independence is essential.

Identity

Caste, religion, and provential group still provide a strong sense of belonging to a man who may otherwise be lost in a city full of change and seeming chaos. Peer-group relations, occupation, and dress will also help bring identity to a family in the city. Living with one's caste and village mates in a community provides a link to the past and to the roots of one's existence. This can be accomplished by providing community groups the opportunity to live in close physical proximity. Size is also an important consideration. The massive schemes official planners create tend to "ghettoize" the inhabitants, creating a stigma around being poor. The single, repetitive house, stamped out in thousands, is a symbol of the low value society puts on the inhabitants. This projects on the child the idea of his unimportance and helplessness in a massive, faceless society.

Status

The argument has developed along the theory that the better one's house, the higher one's family status. Other sources of status can be one's occupation, income, and social position. But these chance opportunities are limited in the Indian society. Especially for the adolescent members of the family, with strong peer group ties, the level of development of shelter is an important source of status, and more so for the eligible bride for whom the house will be the symbol of the family's importance. This is not just the hypersensitivity of the inexperienced young. In looking for a groom for their daughter a family is looking for a good house as well. Youngsters who have been born in the city know the importance of their house as a measure of status and its importance to their future.

Potential

Settings have different levels of potential, and potential has its corresponding costs. Thus in the reception stage living in a high-potential setting would inconveniently drain resources that are needed for survival. At the intermediate stage potential is not essential and may even involve more initial investment than would be easily available at the time. A high-potential setting needed at consolidation would include the possibility of investing as resources allow and as need demands. A flexible and adaptable setting, perhaps in the form of a growing house on a small plot, would fulfil this. The importance to children of a "future" has been noted above. Having an ability to act in the future, even though present resources may not allow it, is a kind of savings. Its value grows with time, and when other inputs become available it can be cashed in. The small, "finished" house leaves no thought for the future or room for imagination. For children and young persons this may unnecessarily close mental doors.

Good and Bad Settings

Thus a setting that may look good to one family from the viewpoint of its situation may be bad for another family in its situation. As middle-class professional planners, architects, and social workers, we tend to forget this and to judge environments as static things from our own values, which often place high emphasis on neatness, appearance, cleanliness, and order. The last few years has been a global period of debate and discussion about environment. But the time element of environment, with its forward and backward links, has been missing. Settings have been confused with environment for this reason, and again, using ethnocentric measures we have placed our professional, Western and middle-class yardsticks against these settlements and condemned them. There is, though, light at the end of the tunnel. Though we still lack a great deal of information, we are more correctly trying to optimize the relations between situations and settings, qualities and manifestations. More emphasis is being put on the processes of life than on perfect models. This spirit is growing in a number of disciplines, and the sharing of concepts between diverse professionals is becoming a common phenomena. Perhaps through this interaction we can attain a truly ideal model of environment, but within our new terms of reference.

References

1. Benninger, C. C. Models of habitat mobility in transitional economies, *Ekistics,* February (1970).
2. Turner, J. F. C. and Goetze, R. Environmental security and housing input, *Carnegie Rev.,* October (1966).
3. Mangin, William. Squatter settlements, *Sci. Amer.,* October (1967).
4. Benninger, C. C., Rules and regulations, *Human Settlements,* (a Report for the United Nations). Mysore University, Institute for Development Studies, 1975.
5. Paul, S. Housing policy: A case of subsidising the rich?, *Urban and Rural Planning Thought,* January, 1973.
6. Government of India, Special report on Ahmedabad, *Census of India,* 1961.
7. Marris, P. *Family and Social Change in an African City,* Northwestern University Press, Evanston, 1962.
8. Benninger, C. C., Design criteria for developing contexts, *Ekistics,* March 1972.

General Discussion

A. Potamianou, Ph.D. (Greece)

Dr. Gore has helped us to understand changes in family life and structure, at the same time, he has also cautioned us in evaluating such changes. Although he stressed the fact that the joint family system was becoming looser (at least in some of the urban areas, and especially in the middle-class families), he went on to emphasize that the extended family continues to maintain its ties without a serious challenge. Although the changes he found were marginal in size, their potentiality had to be considered respectfully. The data that he gave us, coming, as it did, from a sociologist, has opened up a number of intriguing questions that need to be further investigated by the dynamically oriented clinician.

One cannot, however, agree with his contention that when one speaks of change in the institutionalized patterns of behavior, there is a reference, by implication, to concurrent changes in the realm of values, aspirations, motives, and subjective perceptions, firstly, because an individual may block out, consciously or unconsciously, perceptions that seem dangerous or threatening to him and second, because research data are available indicating that people can adapt their outer behavior to the models proposed (through group pressure or the influence of the mass media) and still not change their ideals, expectations, and inner representations.

Dr. Gore has also observed that Indian children were expected to abide by the authority of the family and that they responded to this edict submissively. Could it be that their submissive feelings, disallowed within the family, were not completely submerged but manifested themselves in other groups under different forms? Freud, for example, remarked on the ambivalent feelings toward teachers that were frequently displacements from parental figures and pointed out that this often interfered with the child's learning. There is no question that the child is at high risk for learning disabilities if he transfers mainly negative feelings from his home to his school. One can ask oneself if this displacement mechanism, observed in the underachieving youngster, is similar to what happens on a general scale in India. Furthermore, in view of the fact that Dr. Gore has observed that youth nowadays are being permitted to say "no" to their elders and to question their "do's" and "don'ts," one wonders how this younger generation will react to the new freedom and how this will be reflected in the system of internal representations.

I was also interested in his comment that, until recently, the relationship of the Indian woman to her child was more meaningful and closer than to her husband but that this situation, too, was in the process of change because shifts in the living arrangements of the joint family gave the spouses more time together to develop a closer relationship. This affect will inevitably have an influence on the inner child-object representations of the women. We clearly need to study in close detail the transformations from beginning to end that take place in all these situations of change so that we can understand the process better. Such transformations, however, are not always easy to understand from the outside and may often seem paradoxical. McClelland, for instance, has pointed out that technical innovations, such as providing fishermen with nylon fishing nets, sometimes had an opposite result from the one expected. The fishermen, instead of becoming more active and achievement oriented, often abandoned work as soon as they gained quicker and easier money.

It would seem that the family, both as an external reality and as an internal representation, serves the individual member as a screening device for the defensive, antidepressive, and adaptive functions of the ego, because what the individual cannot sustain, the family group often can. This was what Freud spoke of in his *Group Analysis and The Analysis of the Ego*. This poses the difficult question as to how far one should encourage the disillusion of this protective family shield, even if its external and internal representations seem at times to stand in the way of social development.

Having said all this, one should remember that change cannot be stopped and that the younger people in India, as elsewhere, will always be more on the side of change. For them, the powerful ode of the Indian poet Sitarania must be very appealing:

> These people. . . .
>
> Who can hinder now their onward march? Who can set limits to their illimitable hopes?
>
> They will measure the immeasurable winds. . . .

With regard to Roland's paper on identity conflicts in Indian life, I expect that all of us would agree on the principle that child-rearing patterns, family structure, and family expectations strongly influence identity formation. However, the diversification of the sociocultural subgroups of India's rapidly changing society, the information that we have had from Gore pertaining to the loosening of the joint family system (although the extended family still maintains its hold on the individual), the discouragement of caste solidarity, and finally, the inevitable erosion of religious archetypes (because of population mobility and the dissemination of mass media information) all make it extremely difficult to assess the intrapsychic economic value for the individual and for the group of the conflicts induced by these changes. In Greece the current tendency is in the direction of a negative identity formation, and I wonder if this is true for this country.

We have to face the fact that the old child-rearing practices are no longer rewarding in the context of personality development. And we still do not know to what extent the changes in family structure and function will generate autonomy or produce stresses of such intensity or duration that they seriously impair the psychological homeostasis of both individuals and groups. The effects may be subterranean. Wittkower and Warner, at a meeting of the International College of Psychosomatic Medicine in 1964, reported a high rate of gastroduodenal ulceration in Hindus as compared with Moslems and Christians. They hypothesized that this stemmed from the recession of the caste system into a new status that was previously unknown in India's tightly organized social hierarchy. They also reported a high rate of coronary heart disease in the Singapore Indian population vis-a-vis the Chinese and Malayans. We must ask ourselves, therefore, whether these modifications in the life patterns of the Indian people are more detrimental than beneficial.

I have a final comment on the allegedly nurturing, warm, and protective Indian mother. I have found that one can learn interesting things about what is really happening in a culture by looking at the products of its art. For example, one can see the differences between the ideals, the living experiences, and the expectations between the 5th and 6th century in Ancient Greece by looking at the statues. Here, in India, I was struck by two facts: first, in examining the children's art one rarely sees elements of their real environment included in the design, almost as if the children were turning away from their surroundings; and second, in Indian sculptures one often sees the mother giving the breast to the child, but the expression on the mother's face indicates that she is not "with" the child. If this is a reflection of something that the artists themselves have really experienced, then the turning away of the children could correspond to the turning away of the mother. This might also be the explanation of why the Hindus cling to relationships as if it was impossible for them to sever the umbilical cord, why they turn to a guru to substitute for the nurturing mother, and why they resort to experiences that sustain fusional fantasies as in yoga or meditation. All this may originate in an absence of "holding" in Winnicott's sense of the word. Perhaps one should reexamine the perception of the Indian child's primary relationships in the light of the hypothesis that what has been observed by both sociologists and psychologists concerning the Indian mother could in reality be a coverage for extremely ambivalent feelings toward her children in that the latter may bring narcissistic satisfactions in terms of status but may also constitute a heavy burden for mothers already overwhelmed by difficult living conditions.

E. Hoch (India)

Having worked in India for the last 21 years in different areas and settings, I have been impressed by the great diversity of situations and patterns of change. For instance, there is a marked contrast between the sophisticated setting here at the B. M. Institute in Ahmedabad and my present field of activity in Kashmir, where a high percentage of the population is illiterate and where the cultural patterns are those of the Moslem community. The sociocultural role of women in the Hindu family does not hold good among the Moslems for whom divorce is very easily obtained. The place of women is very insecure as marriage, in their words, is "very cheap," both in the concluding and resolving. Consequently, there is quite a lot of depressive illness among women. Contrary to the experience here and in Western countries, the child patients that I have seen were all girls suffering from such "silent" disorders as anorexia and depression, and they were brought by mothers who themselves showed signs of depression.

In studying change in a country like India, one has to distinguish three sectors of the population: the first is still "traditional" in the true sense of the word and relatively unchanged: the third is one in which change has already taken place, and one can roughly call it "modern"; between these two there is a "transitional" sector that should really form the main target for any studies of change, since it involves a great confusion in attitudes and behavior. In the longitudinal study carried out at the B. M. Institute we found that a third of the children lived in consistently traditional joint families, another third in modern nuclear families with highly educated working mothers, and a final third were children of fairly highly educated mothers unable to utilize their education and having to submit to the dominance of an old-fashioned mother-in-law. It was in this last group that child-rearing practices appeared to be least effective and where the rating or regression on the number of problems among the children was highest. An interesting aspect is that sometimes, as a result of change, the first and third sectors greatly differ from each other. In the area of family planning, for instance, the need is not felt in the traditional sector. Infant mortality is still high, and a large number of births is necessary to make up for the losses. In the most modern sector, emancipated couples already plan their families because they themselves feel the need. The middle sector is one in which the need can be stimulated and which is presently becoming ready for the message. On the other hand, as a result of change, the first and third sectors may come to resemble each other. We found, for example, that the most modern mothers were again resorting to patterns similar to the traditional freedom from constraint in infant rearing, while in the middle sector one could discern tendencies toward greater strictness. Similar tendencies can be observed with reward to certain fashions and clothing and hairstyle ("the more things change, the more they remain the same"). One has, therefore, to be careful to distinguish between the "still" and the "again," between the "not yet" and the "no longer."

In India the great problem exists in the enormous backlog of still undeveloped sectors of population. This means that "change" in any area continues almost indefinitely and, furthermore, that part of the most advanced population has already undergone a great deal of change so that the process of "catching up" leads to a variegation of patterns. The train of progress for change is a long one; by the time the engine has arrived at its terminus, the end carriages may still be a long way down the track. Dr. Ramlal Parikh's comment about the importance of starting "change" from below, from the "grass roots," and not imposing it from the top struck a similar cord in my thinking. From my observations, some of the recent developments in India have led to an increased strengthening and differentiation of already "developed" areas, while little effort has been spent on bringing up the most backward sectors. This has merely widened the gap. I would also agree with him that it is a whole way of life that has to be changed; all too often, the changes that we see are only superficial and compartmentalized. This is a hazard imposed by the traditional structure of Hindu society; it was not up to the individual to develop his full potential but only to function within the strict prescribed limits of his caste. The Bhagavad Gita explicitly states that in order to reach spiritual salvation, it is better for a man to remain faithful to the duties of the caste into which he has been born, no matter how long this may be, than to strive for a station in life for which he has no prerogative. Aspirations thus were limited and development often onesided. As things stand at present, social mobility is theoretically feasible in every direction, but one frequently gets the impression that people who have been previously restricted are now unable to sustain a higher level of operation. Among young people, such as students, complaints of poor concentration and excessive "wet dreams" ("leakage syndrome") are becoming increasingly common. One can observe this again in connection with another aspect of the old Hindu social order where, in addition to the horizontal stratification of castes ("varna"), there is also a vertical division into "ashrama" or stages of the life cycle. The first of these stages is that of the "brahmachari," a concept that is all too often misunderstood as signifying only a need for sexual continence, whereas it has a more inclusive meaning of "containing," of holding in and saving up one's potential for a worthwhile aim in the future. Nowadays there is not much evidence of this "containment"; on the contrary, there is an emerging pattern of immediate dissipation that might be regarded as an influence of western "consumer society."

An interesting feature in psychiatric practice is the presence of manic phases in very young patients and in people who in no way resemble the classical pyknic type, which makes me suspect that a cultural element may be involved. I have termed this the "cultural decompression syndrome," analogous to caisson or diver's disease, resulting from being transferred too rapidly from a high underwater pressure chamber to the ordinary atmosphere. I would see it as another illustration of the poor capacity to "contain."

Some of the presentations have referred to the early start of schooling in India. One gets the impression that the need for engaging in formal learning at too young an age cuts off the development of fantasy and creativity. One is often surprised to find how limited are the interests of even academically educated people, who often have very little to say outside their specialized professional field. Perhaps this may also account for the fact that Indian patients, when put on the analytic couch, are more likely to fall asleep than engage in "free association."

Some of the lack of depth in the changes that have occurred may be due to the fact that the "modernisms" have been imposed ready-made. I think that there is a world of difference, for example, between the use of electricity in a country that has contributed to its discovery and gradual evolution and its importation into a country that has not passed through the many stages of its development, where the people might very well consider it as "magical." One can have illiterate electricians and motor-car drivers but, as compared with Western mechanics, the integration of what they are using into their total world image is not the same. This is one aspect of what I have described as "primitive autism" or the tendency to regard people and objects only from the point of view of what one can get out of them and not in their total context of meanings. This is perhaps the most prominent in nomads. Change has brought with it the "modern automatism" of technology, which again implies a similar spirit of exploitation. The former can easily be converted into the latter, but what is left out, or skipped, is the stage of being able to "care" for someone and something, to see a person or thing in all his or its potentials and connections of meaning, and to be willing to promote its optimum development in all respects and not only in those that happen to be useful to oneself. This is something that cannot be taught by mere "technical aid," but needs human examples of "care."

One final remark about child-rearing practices in India: in our longitudinal study, obsessive-compulsive patterns tended to appear when the child has to learn to clean himself with water after defecation. This involves touching what previously was not supposed to be touched and sets up almost a model for a compulsive situation. We also found that aggressive ratings were highest in those children whose toilet training was started earliest and most rigorously, and that those who started earliest often finished latest. The mothers from nuclear families also seemed more able to improve their child-rearing methods from one child to the next than mothers from joint families in which the mothers-in-law dictated the practice.

S. Lebovici (France)

In relation to Dr. Carstairs' paper, I would like to offer a French viewpoint on the "syndrome of emigration." In Paris one can find classrooms where 50 percent of the children are from emigrant families and have failed to adapt, after repeated trials, to the normal educational environment. In this respect Portuguese families have very special difficulties. The children often have to teach their mothers French, although the native language is spoken at home and all the mothering is done in that tongue. All these create specific difficulties in the growing up of these children. I would say that they are both expectable and understandable. However, I would take issue with Margaret Mead in her assertion that the "syndrome of emigration" is a universal one in the sense that all parents become emigrants in a rapidly developing and changing society. In my opinion, the feeling that the parents have that the world is changing too rapidly stems from their wish to avoid their conflicts with their children. Any process of training and transmitting values is fraught with conflict, and because parents shy away from this and leave the children to cope for themselves, they tend to generate a "culture of shame" rather than a culture of guilt that originates from conflict. The children are ashamed for lack of internal standards. Their superego has not been mobilized, and so they react by overidealizing society and thus setting up external standards for themselves. In growing up, every child has to kill off his parents and teachers as part of his internal conflict in order to build a sane and efficient self that is capable of functioning autonomously.

Psychoanalysis has made use of Indian philosophical concepts, as is evident in the work of Freud, Jung, and Fromm. The process of individuation and identity formation, given such a prominent role in the presentations by Roland and Bassa, is a more recent product of Freudian (more specifically Eriksonian and Mahlerian) psychoanalytic development. Even psychoanalysts who practice a family approach are often engaged in tracing the sources of identity in the interparental and the parent-parental relationships.

It should be theoretically possible to establish a bridge between psychoanalysis and Indian philosophy, making use of the concept of the self in its equation with the continuity of the living experience; the latter concept is not very dissimilar from that of narcissism as employed by Winnicott.

A final word about the sex ratio in clinic samples: our own experience has seen a change from 25 years ago when over 70 percent of referrals were boys; more recently, it is falling below 60 percent. Why are girls appearing more frequently in our practice? Is her position in the family and her importance to the family becoming more secure and significant? The answer is uncertain because of two seemingly contradictory factors: female children are cognitively ahead of their male counterparts right into adolescence, and behaviorally they tend to externalize this and therefore to be less visible clinically. On the other hand, current studies are indicating that girls are being reacted against by mothers and boys, a factor that could increase the incidence and prevalence of emotional disorders in girls. If this latter factor has been historically constant, one might be able to attribute the change in the sex ratio to the cultural change.

C. Chiland (France)

I think that we should be cautious in accepting all the implications of Roland's presentation, because it is important to remember that psychoanalysis is not only a mode of treatment and investigation, but it is also a very comprehensive and systematic theory. Therefore, if analytic treatment appears difficult to put into practice with Indian patients, this in no way means that the theory loses its value as a tool for understanding what is taking place (or not taking place) in the patient. Furthermore, if one has a narrow conception of the Oedipus complex, one can very easily challenge its universality, but if the Oedipus complex is viewed as originating in basic differences between the sexes and the generations and a very necessary confrontation for the child in the construction of its sexual identity, then one can say with some confidence that Indians, like everyone else, do have an Oedipus complex. India has its own pathologies (as, for example, those dealing with the attainment of the hermaphroditic ideal) that would indicate that the Oedipus complex is everywhere latent in this culture. The dissolution of the boundaries of the self is an end that has been pursued by the Lindoric philosophy: Atman is Brahma. This is also what one finds, less clearly, in the Christian mystical experience.

D. de Levita (Holland)

Dr. Carstairs' paper impressed me in two ways: first, its almost lyrical quality and second, its modesty. The author combines in himself the analytic incisiveness of a psychiatrist and the inquiring mind of a social anthropologist—a rare combination. The seemingly simple vignettes gain in profundity as one reflects on them. Life in the Irish-Presbyterian mission appeared to have two contradictory sides to it: there was the home with its somewhat superior and exclusive Christian attitudes, and then there was the playground with its assortment of children from every class, caste, and creed. The child, however, is not aware of these differences and interacts spontaneously and unself-consciously with his peer group. We find very much the same thing in our clinical work with upper and middle-class patients: the parents set the social boundaries and insist that their children do not mix with those from the lower classes because of the "bad habits" that they might pick up; whereas their children feel isolated and hungry for peer relationships. Parental values, which make no sense to the child's cognitions and emotions, are imposed on him and not generated by him. In Indian society today there appears to be a definite trend toward upward mobility which often means that values, prevailing at the new levels, are taken in without being integrated so that an internal dissonance results.

Carstairs also draws our attention in a way in which the Indian villager perceives his own life as somewhat vulnerable, subject to all kinds of influences that lie beyond his control. He needs constantly to appease these powers by ritual expiation and sacrifice. I might add that this type of primitive, animistic theology can manifest itself unexpectedly at the highest levels of Western culture, showing that we are all "brothers under the skin." A political humorist in Holland recently explained to a visitor that the bureaucrats governed the country. When he was asked who made the decisions regarding the implementation of policy, the answer was, "The higher ups, that is, the astrologers!"

Another anthropological viewpoint with clinical implications sees the individual Indian trying to live in harmony with the natural, the supernatural, and the social environment and needing a support system to accomplish this, which is where the guru makes his appearance. Professor Carstairs looks on the guru as a blend of the nurturing and supporting aspects of the mother and the knowledge and guidance of an idealized father. Many of the patients in treatment seem to need to make a guru out of their therapist in order to be able to harmonize their internal and external worlds.

I was especially fascinated by the fact that he found evidence of adolescent turmoil even in the Indian rural areas, suggesting that it is not simply an artifact of the Western world. By providing young people at this stage with a moratorium (Erikson), the turmoil can be avoided, but the adolescents pay a price for this as our clinical experience informs us. Besides, moratoria are not easily available in our particular culture, and may be a specific product of urban life. In the rural areas the adolescent drifts into adult roles, conflict or no conflict.

I have a personal comment to make about the emigration syndrome. When I was living in London I came upon many educated and sophisticated Dutch people who had never entered an English home. On exploring this further, I came to the conclusion that the immigrants were attempting to avoid acculturation. It seems that to be able to live comfortably in an alien culture without losing one's own identity requires considerable maturity, and the more usual way of dealing with the insecurity of the alien status is to establish one's own native community within the larger community and immerse oneself in it.

Manoj Shah (India)

One has constantly to bear in mind the fact that India is a country of 600 million people with only 600 psychiatrists, so that there is an enormous logistical problem in the delivery of mental health services. What one can do under such circumstances becomes severely limited. We also have to remember that India is a country that is changing, and that change may either strengthen the ego or weaken it. That it does the former more frequently than the latter would seem evident from the fact that the sick are only a small minority, relatively speaking. If change is introduced gradually in small doses, there is every reason to hope that larger numbers will be able to cope. The concept of psychological immunity to change, developed by Dr. Anthony, would seem important to consider in this context. Our Health Ministry has evolved a plan for training villagers in health care, beginning with courses in nutrition and hygiene. In an era of increasing change, when the Indian people are often anxious and bewildered by the exposure to novel experiences, it seems easier to introduce changes in health care gradually, following this up with changes in mental health care as reflected in child-rearing practices. Using local people, who already have a place in the community, makes the work of assimilation easier, and the interest may be later consolidated through the mass media. In physical health as in mental health, our greatest hope lies in primary prevention.

W. Rickards (Australia)

I have attempted to relate the general gist of the presentations and the discussions to our situation in Australia where the population is exploding and developments are extremely rapid. Increased upward social mobility forms an important part of all this, so that lower-class families are in the process of acculturating to the aspirations and values of the upper classes. The children who have been carried along with their parents into this new subculture are finding it difficult to adjust to the new expectations and are very soon on the road to becoming failures. This often devastating problem, with its impact on the mental health of the child, is being handled more and more by educational authorities and less and less by child psychiatrists, whose helpfulness in this respect is clearly not yet recognized. The problem, however, lies not only with the new children and the new families (and in the context of Margaret Mead's remarks, all upwardly mobile individuals are in her sense emigrants) but is aggravated by the school's failure to meet the problem with new understanding and new curricula. A shortage of teachers makes for additional aggravation. The children, presenting with boredom, underachievement, and a restless hunger for exciting or soothing distractions, are at risk. The way ahead seems blocked to them because of the lack of job opportunities at this stage. As a consequence of this flux of change, homes are increasingly in jeopardy, and families are too "broken" to be able to interest themselves in such matters as school progress. The good and bad aspects of change seem inextricably bound together. Anthony has implied the importance of "good enough change," and it seems to be clear that to bring this about we need good enough parents with good enough children. It is my impression, shared by, I believe, workers across the world, that although adolescence appears to be a period of normative crisis, it is the early adolescent (12–14 years) that appears to be the most vulnerable. There seems to be two ways of coming to terms with the enormity of change: a small proportion become rebellious and make sporadic attempts to disrupt the conventional environment around them, but the greater number either become alienated, emotionally disturbed, or conforming and intellectually numb. The parents, who often look as if they were in the latter part of their own adolescence, can do little to help with the dilemmas that wrack the immature psyches of their offspring. From what we have heard, as compared with the Australian adolescent, the young Indian is less individuated but more dependable in the context of the extended family. We should, however, be cautious of adding our quota of stereotypes to the picture, although Anthony has shown how the stereotypic reactions of the parents and their stereotypic portrayals of the adolescent add to the burden of pressures imposed on the young people. We need to take these multiple determinants into account when assessing the impact of change from the clinical point of view.

Kiyoshi Makita, M.D. (Japan)

The two presentations of Anthony and Solnit mesh together like a beautifully woven Indian carpet with both horizontal and vertical threads. The first provided a broad overview, while the second added the necessary depth. Both laid emphasis on the interplay of inferred internal and observable external change. Although it is an important move in psychiatry to explore transcultural differences as evident in surface phenomena, it is equally important to detect the basic similarities underlying the outer manifestations and to understand both within the same encompassing theory that would be valid across cultures. In brief, the examination of cultural differences must proceed hand in hand with the search for universals and unification. In this process our current theories and our present techniques of observation might both prove inadequate to the task of reducing (in Meyerson's terms) "diversity to identity."

The question of what "change" really is does not elicit a ready answer, especially in its psychiatric connotation. Anthony's suggestion, derived from Toffler, that "change is life itself" crystallized something for me. The multifaceted nature of change, covering the biological, the psychological, the sociocultural, and the historical, does seem to make it coterminous with life. One would also agree with him that what is of the essence is the amount and rate of change; other aspects are more culture-bound and variable in effect. Also relatively immune from cultural variability are the intrapsychic changes that occur in all individuals, irrespective of ethnic and social differences.

Anthony's paper impressed me on two grounds: his mention of the biological substratum of change and his classification of "change syndromes," most of which would be applicable to the Japanese people. As an eclectic, I welcomed the inclusion of brain morphology within the same spectrum as the psychodynamic, although to some it may seem a far cry from the neuron to the intrapsychic! We need both, at least for the present and foreseeable future.

Since Japan is a monoracial and monocultural country, we do not experience the change syndromes resulting from immigration and acculturation, and foreigners who want to live in Japan are very limited in number. Japanese children who accompany their parents on business or scientific visits to foreign countries for periods occasionally suffer in their school adjustment on returning to Japan, but this may well be related in individual vulnerability. However, even in as small a country as ours, there are cultural differences among prefectures, and the cultural shock syndrome could well apply to our domestic subcultural conflicts.

What interests me the most is the "future shock" syndrome. Although Toffler described it as "the most important disease entity of tomorrow," with us in Japan it already is one of the most important ailments of *today*. We see many cases from our university, college, and senior high school population. The rate of change, as broadcast through the media, is shocking for these youngsters searching for some solidity and sureness. Yesterday's prime minister is today's criminal, past generals of the army are involved in directing murder, and successful businessmen have been publicly exposed as fraudulent exploiters. Japan, too, has had its Watergate. For the youth there would appear to be no reliable models for identification in this state of flux, and so identity problems become even more exaggerated. Is it surprising that motivation toward success is diminished when success is linked so catastrophically to failure! In part, these reactions stem from the failure of the parents to adjust themselves to rapid social change and to modify their enthusiasm and ambitiousness to have their children attend university. At present, 50 percent of high school students are college bound. The wish for higher education is admirable in principle, but in practice it creates a glut in the upper echelons of employment leading to misery-provoking discrepancies between the level of learning and the job level. And the parents sacrifice themselves to accomplish this. Understandably, the point of crisis in the child's progress is soon reached and results in what I would call the "failure syndrome" not included in Anthony's nosology. After two or three failures, the youngsters are exhausted physically and emotionally, lose their ideals, and become pleasure driven. School for them is little better than a social club. Competition of any kind is avoided.

I would agree with the principles of prevention contained in Anthony's presentation, although in a psychiatrically less-advanced country like Japan, it would be difficult to realize. We have difficulties with the idea of interdisciplinary collaboration, since sectionalism is still rampant and rigidly maintained; but even that can change when change is the order of the day!

S. Lebovici (France)

Despite the excellence of the papers and the richness of the discussion, my first impression was of a submersion in an ocean. However, on observing a session of Indian dancing I at once grasped what our colleagues from this country meant when they spoke of the harmony of mind and body as an ideal to be pursued. In this subcontinent with its rich and ancient history and culture, change is very much in the air because of the twin processes of Westernization and urbanization. Following our site visits, I had a feeling of estrangement (*unheimlich*) from viewing, at close quarters, the spectacle of poverty and misery. But even in the midst of this saddening human condition there were oases of relief—the sight of young mothers with their babies, little girls mothering their even smaller siblings, tranquil old men apparently at peace with themselves and their dismal surroundings. It was with some effort that I could turn my attention from such experiences to the clinical and therapeutic concerns of our own field. Solnit reminded us at this meeting of the continuity of relationship between bodily approaches at one extreme and highly sophisticated interpretative approaches at the other end, and Coelho advised us to drop our preconceptions and attempt to understand the richness that lies behind specifically Indian approaches—meditation, yoga, and the like. We did our best in this latter respect, but our lack of knowledge of Indian philosophy was a decided shortcoming. Furthermore, we came with a confused experience of it in Europe: some of the most eminent people are practitioners of the Indian approach but so also are a host of marginal individuals—hippies, drug addicts, and alienated young men and women, many of whom are attracted to what is advertized in popular magazines as "Indian psychotherapy." In the face of all this pseudotherapy, we need real information from our respected colleagues who practice in this mode. As a psychoanalyst I must try to assess the value of this approach from within my own frame of reference, allowing for the bias this entails. Lourie spoke of the importance of pain and discomfort during early life that could stem from both internal and external sources. For the baby, a major difficulty is in discharging emotions adequately at a time when the full elaboration of feeling is impossible. I am in favor of the new discipline of infant ethology, but I am quite convinced that even the most precise observation is useless without an understanding and interpretation of what is being observed; otherwise it is no more than an actuarial exercise. Our own observations focus on the mother-infant "eye-to-eye dialogue" and on the creative anticipations of the mother. The patterns of mothering that become manifest also reveal danger signals for the future well-being of the baby, for example, a mother who feeds her baby with a bottle while casually reading a magazine at the same time. Nor should we overlook the baby's given name in such interchanges, since it may tell us what part the child plays in the mother's fantasies, as for example, when it is given the name of a much loved father or of a brother who died: the future of the child may be determined by the unconscious meaning that he has for the mother. One should not, therefore, overlook internal factors in our understanding of infant behavior. I also think that there has been some misunderstanding of psychoanalytic theory that needs correction.[1] For instance, the Oedipus complex, as the nucleus of this theory, must be understood not as a symbolic and anecdotal account of a love affair between a boy and his mother but as a consequence of the neonatal condition that directs the human neonate of necessity to find and to recreate an object to gratify his hallucinating wishes. The same is true for the libido concept, in which the sexual energy of eros can be displaced, transformed, or sublimated in the form of tender feelings. For many reasons it seems to me too difficult to elaborate on links between psychoanalytic psychology and the Indian conception of the psyche. What we can do is to build clinical bridges between Western and Indian clinical experiences. For example, the psychotherapy of illiterate people as described by Hoch is not dissimilar to what we in the West try to do with so-called "multiple-problem families" who are also inaccessible to the interpretative approach and with whom one also needs to get some immediate effect at the first contact to avoid a rupture of the therapeutic relationships. Lourie also drew our attention to the maternal care furnished these days in the West by fathers. No doubt this does have some practical value for the family, but we also need to remember the importance of differentiating the father-mother images for the children and that in the preoedipal stage the father may take the place of the bad mother and provoke a stranger response. It is also true that the Western father is also becoming anonymous to his children, often lacking in any sustained interest in them. The children in turn know very little about him and his work and ignore him, as pointed out by Mitscher-

---

[1] Dr. Serge Lebovici is the immediate Past President of the International Association of Psychoanalysis.

lich. In all our deliberations we have to bear in mind the vital equation:

$$\text{change} = \text{transition} = \text{conflict}$$

For "good enough change," to use Anthony's expression, one needs at least two or three generations to learn how to cope with the conflicts involved, how to preserve some measure of constancy and how to achieve a necessarily new and different identity.

Some Reflections on1 the Changing World in India

Reginald S. Lourie, M.D. (U.S.A.)

We have learned so much in Ahmedabad that we should share with others that I began grandly to think that we could write *the* message of Ahmedabad to the Melbourne Congress. However, as I look at the threads of ideas we have collected in this city, I became much more humble in the spirit of the economic life of Ahmedabad, and it then seemed more useful to think like a textile worker and weave together at least some of the threads with those which this International Study Group brought from Dakar, Bled, and Jerusalem, as well as those that we brought from our own countries along with those made available to us so productively by our Indian colleagues.

To begin with, we brought from Jerusalem as one thread a somewhat oversimplified classification of the capacity of children and families to change. First, there is a segment of the population that can accept and fit in with change. Here I would include the delinquents, because even though they are violating society's morals, at least they are individuals who have the energy and capacity to do or at least try to do something to adjust to both internal and external conditions. Second, there is a group of individuals who follow along the leads provided by those in the first group. And finally, there are those who cannot fit in with change and must either be helped or carried along or else they lag behind, locked into old patterns.

James Anthony and Albert Solnit have taken these headlines and given them depth and brought the most up-to-date information on child development as well as their own experience in defining what vulnerabilities there are in the evolving human organism that can interfere with the capacity to deal with change. These brilliant essays come back to the biological makeup of the individual and the early developmental experience as major factors that determine which capacities to change would emerge. There is a still further basic refinement I would suggest as a factor in the constitutional structure of the individual growing out of our current studies of children, namely, the integrative capacities of the child or, if you will, the synthetic functions of the ego. My own experience and continuing interests in this area of function began in a study carried out in the early days of World War II on the selection of pilots. We found that a significant group of normally functioning subjects gave scattered or disorganized responses under experimental stress in contrast to an equal number at the opposite end of the spectrum —individuals who appeared to organize better under stress and/or anxiety. Later, in our work with children, we found once again that the ones who organized better and developed satisfactorily under adverse or changing conditions were the ones who needed only crumbs of good experience to develop normal autonomous ego functions. Those, on the other hand, who disorganized under stress and lapsed into helplessness (and sometimes hopelessness, as when they have difficulty in collecting their thoughts), required a much longer period of dependency. If not recognized early, there also ensued not infrequently a preoccupation with keeping everything the same in addition to a variety of avoidance mechanisms for dealing with the sources of anxiety or stress. Depending on the degree and ease of disorganization, these individuals had difficulty in dealing not only with large but also with small changes. The fact that they were more commonly males made one wonder if centuries ago this group was already recognized in India and that the glorification of the Mother-goddess and the drive to be near her, considered together with the breast symbols scattered so liberally through the temples, were all manifestations of dependent males provoked by ironic stress; this, of course, is merely an intriguing speculation.

The most common pattern of change that the very young child

must face is adjustment to a double standard. This is followed by triple and quadruple standards as they become older and have to function outside the protecting family. Dr. Bassa describes this with the infant facing the inadequate or unavailable breast. One example of the concept of the double standard is the 2-year-old who is proud of having dry pants but then is encouraged, albeit with understandable reluctance on his part, to go into the water with his bathing trunks. One saw the toddlers at Ramdeo Pir Ni Taki Community Center solving the problem of having to deal with a double standard by walking around without pants! This brings me back to Dr. Bassa's description of the successful toilet training beginning in the first months of life and completed well before 1 year of age. It takes me back almost 40 years when I was a very young child development researcher in Myrtle McGraw's laboratory at the time that she found that the child did not have voluntary control of the lower segments of the body until myelinization had reached the lower motor neurons, as indicated by the fact that he was able to stand and begin to walk. It was not until then that voluntary control over the bowel and bladder sphincters was possible. Therefore, one must ask, in connection with this early toilet training of the Indian child, who is the one who is trained? Is it the child or the mother? And is this another aspect of the Indian child's prolonged dependency.

Change is always a disruption that brings pain. If it is constructive change, it upsets the status quo at the same time that it opens new horizons. Adam and Eve may have found this out unhappily, at the time of their banishment from Eden when their precipitate leaving resulted in Adam (or was it Eve?) organizing better under stress and initiating what was the science of agriculture in biblical terms! We heard about Vasana being reconstituted after a disaster in Indian history and mythology. In more modern times de Toqueville pointed out how much pain and subjugation humans were able to tolerate and live with uncomplainingly until their conditions improved. Only then did loud complaints and hurts come to the surface. We heard this type of complaining in a mild way at the community center that we visited. Now that each house had a washroom, there were complaints that never existed before that the washroom needed doors. In more violent ways, the aggression which we heard being repressed in the Indian child's extended family (with the exceptions described by Dr. Hoch) can emerge like a lanced abscess, as is evident in the violence reported in Indian and Western newspapers. Dr. Gore and Dr. Carstairs described how the aggression belonging to sibling rivalry is directed outward from the family toward other groups. In addition to the examples they gave, I recently read about an Indian village that depended for sustenance on the sale of grapes to a winery. Some villagers learned how to make wine which they sold, and the village prospered. The women in the village, who had been bare breasted, were now able to buy clothes that covered their breasts. In a neighboring poor village, the women also began to cover their breasts, whereupon the women in the first village became indignant and violently opposed their poorer neighbors' upward mobility! Is this the same process that goes on in families, when the 2-year-old pushes the 1-year-old who is trying to learn how to walk, and says, "Get down, you're a baby, you can't do that." In other words, sibling rivalry can be displaced from the family as individuals develop broader horizons.

This takes me back to when, in development, the fundamental patterns of thinking are established. We must always be cognizant of the powerful influence of the repetition compulsion. For reasons we do not yet know, the first new experience, particularly if repeated, becomes permanently impressed, even if it is later put out of conscious awareness. Thus in the earliest years what is beautiful and what is ugly is established in the individual's mind. I do not know how this principle works in India, although Morris Carstairs gave us some examples of it, but in the Western world this is why the fat boys and girls, and the skinny boys and girls, and the ugly men and women, by advertising standards, all get married. It also gets down to the senses of taste and smell as factors in the ability to accept change. This is why I wonder if the SEWA project is not starting too late with children well past the earliest years. Is this why the young graduate of the program set up his home back in the slums when he married, even though he had a washroom in it? This is why the Catholic church says, "Give us the child for its first seven years," and why I was so pleased to hear that the B. M. Institute now has a program for babies 0 to 2 years of age.

I would like to make just a brief comment on the use of education as the basis of change in the context of teaching children to avoid alcoholism. In the 1880s laws were passed by 45 of the states in the United States requiring that the evils of alcohol be taught to children at every grade level from the first grade on, and a set of textbooks in the curriculum has been used to this end. From the increasing prevalence of alcoholism in the United States, one must certainly wonder about the efficacy of this educational approach to correcting problems of impulse control.

The mention of the young man's marriage reminds me of a pattern of change that seems to be taking place in India away from arranged marriages, which goes one step away from the traditional patterns. We found in the classified sections of the Sunday newspaper inquiries for marriage partners with descriptions of the applicants' physical, professional, and financial situations as well as descriptions of family backgrounds. It dramatically emphasized to us that India is in a state of change in many different ways, but it also bore out Professor Gore's observation that slow change is the best, because this may well represent the first step away from the arranged marriages.

The use of education in changing patterns of living and expectations from relationships really begins in the early years of life. Anna Freud pointed out how if one wants a smiling baby, one lets the baby know how much its smile is appreciated. In the slum, we see education for survival as having the highest priority. When this is primary, it takes precedence over all the other instincts. The early imprinting along these lines can block out other paths for learning. The 5- or 6-year-old child who we have seen assuming care and feeding of the baby has learned impressive skills, but is it at the expense of fostering curiosity in other forms of learning? Does it put a premium on concreteness of thinking in other forms of learning and would these two factors prove handicaps to the child's ability to adjust to formal learning in school?

The need for population control appears to be inevitably tied to improvement in health. The underlying drive reported to us in India is the need in poor families to have enough children to take care of the parents in their old age. With the high infant and child mortality in this group of the population there is the additional need to have enough children so that some at least will survive. One can understand why at the last WHO expert committee meeting on child mental health the representatives from the developing countries kept returning to the need to deal with the physical illnesses of children. You must have live children before you can practice child psychiatry. The inference is that any voluntary population control will fail as long as India takes a strong country-wide health program and as long as children continue to represent a life insurance policy for the parents.

Dr. Carstairs' observations on adolescents in first generation immigrant families reminds me that there was no significant delinquency in the Chinese-American youth before World War II while they remained in their extended families, but as soon as these young people became involved in the general community, a high level of delinquency resulted.

Benninger's thoughtful paper illustrates how the education of the planner must include an understanding of human development. The challenge for us is to take his important categories of societal needs, natural phenomena, communication systems, and other networks of supply and add to them the information that we have about the human family and its developmental needs, so that together we can arrive at the goal that Doxiadis calls "Utopia." That is, the creation of cities that takes all this into consideration. As we look across the river in Ahmedabad and observe the growing number of apartment houses, one wonders whether there is a vestigial nesting instinct still at work in men (or perhaps in the minds of architectural planners who insist on building these human versions of beehives!).

There is currently a worldwide controversy about violence on television, giving me a *deja vu* experience. I recall the same worries about comic books and movies years ago; however, if one looks at the themes involved, they seem to be the same ones handed down from generation to generation, ones that originated in our religious texts, which are full of bloodcurdling violence. The only difference appears to be that now the violence is expressed and dealt with in terms of modern forms of destruction, communication, and transportation. One aim of the media is to create the child and his family in the image of a national ideal that serves a cultural value in preserving constancy and continuity within the flux of change. One other virtue that the media might espouse is the maintenance of cultural differences in the face of a fast-contracting world, with its increasingly rapid communication and transportation systems, so that they do not get lost. In dealing with the instincts that underlie violence and its accompanying guilt, there is in India not the psychotherapist but the Guru, so that religion takes care of the unconscious conflicts by mergers with the ultimate, the eternal, with Krishna.

In thinking about such authority, I would like to quote from the still unpublished paper by Zelnick, titled "Psychic Disequilibria and Social Change."

Attachments to authority diminish when major segments of society experience the conditions of felt injustice, and relative deprivation in the distribution of economic and social rewards. When individuals in groups appear to be gaining at the expense of others, attitudes toward authority and the conscious awareness, the idea that authority is unjust or permits inequities, becomes a force that shapes earlier defensive and adaptive structures and leaves the change in individual societies. The ability of alternate sources of authority to compete successfully for allegiances, directed formally elsewhere, depends on how deeply they appeal to the possibility for equity while assuring those disaffected.

The Ahmedabad Discussions on Change: An Indian Viewpoint

B. K. Ramanujam, M.D. (India)

Let me begin with the development of psychological theory in India as a part of the philosophical system. As Venkoba Rao has described it, it has evolved stepwise over a period of centuries from primitive animistic thinking into a highly complex system during the Vedic and post-Vedic periods. This would indicate that even in ancient times there was sufficient flexibility in the Indian mind to discard long-cherished notions and explore newer ones. The important point to bear in mind is that these notions had a relevance to a particular age, meeting some of its epistemological needs and failing to meet others. As long as this is remembered, there is no need to argue over the issue of their being the "ultimate truths." The sages at the time, from all accounts, allowed considerable scope for debate, discussion, and varying interpretations, and it is clear that the same open-mindedness is needed to put both their knowledge as well as our own to the critical tests required in any branch of science. When one hears that to solve present-day problems we have to go back to the past "truths," one cannot help but wonder if this is not another manifestation of the resistance to change. In a peaceful, agrarian milieu, with little to worry about except the seasonal aberrations of the monsoons, there was time to think about the origins of human distress and search for panaceas. As Dr. Anthony has mentioned, the situation today is different because of the acceleration of change that has precipitated a state of "future shock" so that we no longer have the time to contemplate life, since we are being swept along by it. We need to mitigate distress as it occurs. Change is not what we seek but what is imposed on us as an inexorable historical process. Dr. Lourie has commented on the vulnerabilities of the evolving human organism and on the constitutional makeup of individuals that makes them able to organize themselves under stress. Clearly, these capacities and vulnerabilities are biologically and not culturally determined. What the culture does, perhaps, is to imprint certain value systems that can either enhance or retard the capacity for adaptation. In our country, with its teeming millions, such constitutionally based individual differences tend to be overlooked and discounted by the collective viewpoint, so that the cultural factors are brought very much to the forefront in our thinking. Thus in analyzing the conditions of life and change in an agrarian society, our focus would be on the family and not on the individual and his frailties. Every contribution of labor toward a collective goal of reaping a good harvest is important, and under such circumstances the individual is simply a part of the household, with his survival dependent on the survival of the family. Each village being a closed community, all its inhabitants are mutually supportive in meeting the minimal needs of community life. Such interdependence requires a clear-cut delineation of role functions and power structure in order to minimize conflict. At the same time the system has to make allowances for individual aberrations as a collective problem and provide for the containment of these, so that the balance of societal stability is not tilted. The very clear injunctions against certain behaviors and the prescription of expiatory rituals if they do occur are clear indications of a highly sensitive recognition of human weakness.

Within a social system of this kind, authority figures emerge as a further stabilizing factor. The role of the guru is a case in point. Guru is a much misunderstood designation that is often treated as a monolithic concept when, in fact, it is highly variable. There are gurus who are authoritative, gurus who are benevolent, who are quite permissive, gurus very much involved with the community, and gurus who isolate themselves from common humanity and seek their own salvation. Just as in the West one seeks an analyst or therapist with an orientation suitable to one's needs, one does the same in the case of the guru. Similarly, every guru, like every therapist, has his successes irrespective of the system to which he subscribes. All societies have their sages, sometimes professionalized, sometimes not, to advise them on the basic issues of existence—the relationship of self to the world, of the individual to his family, and of parents to the children that they are raising.

This brings me to the discussion of child-rearing practices that show a wide variation, depending on the particular sample being studied, the region from which it comes, the ethnic and caste status and the source of referral, such as school, physician, or clinic. At the B. M. Institute the clinic sample differed significantly in many areas of child care from the school sample. It is also difficult to generalize because the different inquiries lack a common frame of reference and a common scientific language. Furthermore, our expertise in this country is at present very limited. All we can share with one another are the demographic facts and figures.

Despite these limitations, we can still arrive at some understanding, for example, that the mother-child relationship is generally intimate and involved up to a certain point but determined by adult considerations and values; that there is a sudden increase in what is expected of the child as soon as he is old enough to take on minimal responsibility; and that the arrival of siblings on the scene creates conflicts that are externalized, since the values do not encourage an open expression of sibling rivalries. One frequently also observes a precociousness in development due more to the exigencies of circumstances or the need for survival than to a fulfillment of the child's own emotional needs. This can have an impact on creative and learning abilities, as indicated by the high rate of dropouts and learning difficulties in the school population. In this context Dr. Anna Potamianou was surprised to find in the drawings of 9 and 10 year olds in our school that there was no evidence of any impact of their immediate environment, or in other words, that their perceptions of the world they live in were not reflected in their artwork. We have found that many of these children are very concrete in their responses to CAT, and clearly this area needs further study. Aggression and its manifestations are critical to the understanding of the changing Indian personality. In a society that values nonviolence and that teaches the sacrifice of one's own needs for the benefit of the group, the naked expression of aggression on trivial provocation raises the question of how much have controls been internalized and to what extent the Indian people practice what they preach. One has the sneaking suspicion that the acting out of our children and adolescents in a violent manner is unconsciously abetted by the adults, but this is only a suspicion! Are adolescents any different here in India? From our clinical experience and from what we observe all around, it is hard to escape the conclusion that they are indeed. We need, as clinicians, to extend our investigations beyond the clinical walls and to take a closer look at the social scene if we want to know more about the normative development of adolescence. It might tells us, for example, whether the so-called "turmoil" exists as a significant entity in our culture.

About therapeutic strategies there is, I think, less controversy. We follow, as I am sure that you do, the basic therapeutic principle of fitting the modality of treatment to the needs of the patient. The details of a particular intervention vary as much among us as no doubt they vary in Western practice. Coelho has observed that scientists should make their findings available to the people and that the insights should be translated in language that is understandable to the people, but he should know that in this country social scientists have no voice at all as yet in policy making, and this is where we lag behind the Western world. But things are changing, perhaps slowly, but hopefully for the better. Your visit has already catalyzed change at this Institute, and we are very grateful.

Postscript to Dr. Ramanujam's Discussion

Shipstone [5] has pointed out that today's family *everywhere* is a new phenomenon and that new patterns of family life are emerging *everywhere* due to multidimensional changes in the world.

This is more true of India than perhaps of any other country. Chained in tradition with its thousands of years of history, rooted in thousands of years of its culture and religions, social change in India is affecting family life in a very significant way. The Indian family is caught between the "old" and the "new," the "traditional" and the "emerging" patterns of family life. Some changes are providing new freedoms and opportunities, new guarantees for selfhood and for being a person in one's own right; but some other changes are disruptive of family life and security and unsettling to the individual.

The changes taking place in the joint family involves attitudinal changes to family obligations, decision making, the relationship between husband and wife, and the socialization of the children. The nuclear family unit, the changing role, and the upgraded status of employed married women have given rise to new values and attitudes that are not supportive of the traditional code of behavior [4].

The transition from one family structure and style to another is not easy, and there is some ambivalence on the part of family members to the change. The younger ones may complain "of the suffocating atmosphere of the he joint family" [3] but are still not prepared psychologically to break away from it. What they seem to want at the present time is "limited change" [1] or some sort of compromise that would allow fuller scope for the proper and healthy development of the individuality of the young. This is what is basically at stake. At present, the family continues to function like a clan, and modes of address and scales of authority are still more or less regulated, giving the appearance of "personal relationship but not really recognizing the family member as an individual with his or her distinctive features" [2].

References

1. Gore, M. S. *Urbanization and Family Change.* Popular Prakashan, Bombay, 1968, p. 232.
2. Hoch, E. *The Changing Patterns of Family in India.* Christian Institute for the Study of Religion and Society, Bangalore, 1966, p. 92.
3. Kapadia, K. M. *Marriage and Family in India,* 3rd ed. Oxford University Press, Bombay, 1966, pp. 291–292.
4. Ramanujam, B. K. The Indian family in transition: Changing roles and relationships. *Soc. Action,* 22 (1972), 16.
5. Shipstore, E. I. Educating the Indian adolescent: Role of the family, guidance and student services. *Soc. Action,* 22 (1972), 26.

The Changing Indian Scene: An Overview of the Ahmedabad Conference

Peter B. Neubauer, M.D. (U.S.A.)

I would like to begin by quoting the greatest of Ahmedabad's former residents, Mahatma Gandhi, whose Ashram was such a moving and at the same time stimulating experience for all of us to visit: the quintessence of eternal India underlying all the flux of change. He said: "Do not swallow all I have been saying because my facts may be wrong," reminding us of the need to keep an open, skeptical, and challenging mind, especially when the issues are charged with emotion. And the topic of change in India, as everyone has no doubt felt through this entire week, is a very emotional issue. What Gandhiji is telling us is to be sure of our facts, irrespective of who makes them, before jumping to conclusions.

My second introductory point is to warn you ahead of time that my remarks will be biased in the direction of my own interests and that I will be formulating my own personal reaction, selectively, to the presentations and discussions. You do not have to swallow my "facts" unquestioningly, any more than I have to swallow yours! We do not, therefore, need to be apologetic to one another.

My third point of departure is to contrast the Indian profile of the changing scene and its repercussions with our last year's experience in Israel, where change was progressing at a remarkably rapid rate. There we found people from more than 50 countries, with different histories, backgrounds, child-rearing practices, and habits, attempting to come together to build a new future, a new social structure, and a new identity. Israel must have been, or ought to have been, the prototype of the concept of "future shock." The social and emotional problems generated by the process of accelerated acculturation has been great and has taken its expected toll on some of the participants. There were those who were already too damaged prior to immigration to adjust without massive welfare support to the changes imposed on them, and there were also those who were ready to move faster than the conditions allowed. Social experiments, such as the kibbutz movement, represented new, thoughtful, and mature ways of finding answers to the utopian aspirations that continuously haunt the human mind.

The Arab population found itself exposed to this gathering momentum; their medical, educational, and work opportunities suddenly opened up new choices with their attendant advantages and problems. Israel is a future-oriented country, and the power of ideologies (social, religious, and national) as an ingredient of change had to be understood in order to measure the capacity of people to adapt to change, to tolerate frustration, and to make the necessary individual sacrifices that all change exacts.

At the end of our meeting there we found ourselves also in the process of change and needing the conceptions and preconceptions we had brought with us. How did the individuals cope under these special circumstances? What was the response of the inner life as a rapidly changing environment? What were the psychic mechanisms involved, and finally, what was the incidence and significance of the disorders that ensued?

It is in this context that we have to understand the two introductory papers by Doctors Anthony and Solnit. Dr. Anthony sacrificed his gift for practical illumination and his talent for drawing on clinical vignettes in exploring the human conditions in favor of providing us with a classification and nosology of change. Apparently, he did not want us to lose ourselves in a global and amorphous world of change or become too narrow in our approach. He therefore offered us three categories within which to view our topic: the meaning of change, the field of change, and the process of change, to which he added specific areas for the study of change: the neurobiologic, the immunity and vulnerability response, and the clinical syndromes of change. He laid stress on psychosomatic and somatopsychic interactions and the biosocial and sociopsychic patterns. If we were to follow this outline systematically, we would undoubtedly avoid one-sided formulations and premature conclusions. He wanted to make sure that we included responses to abnormal rate of change, whether too fast or too slow, and degree of change, whether too much or too little, and to the kind of change, whether too diverse or too restricted, outside a context of normal adaptive patterns. This is important, because if we take as our topic change as a part of life, in all its manifold forms and complexities, then our field becomes too wide and our investigations insufficiently focused. On the other hand, if we overemphasize the clinical and the pathological, we may underestimate the adaptive maneuvers and the normal variability with its crises, stresses, and symptoms. I return to this point later.

Solnit focused his address on the inner, the psychological maneuvers and experiences and the inner awareness of change. He suggested that the theory of trauma would help us to understand the reactions to sudden change in the context of the hypothesized "stimulus barrier" (the psychic defense system) and the concept of developmental tolerances. There is an obvious bridge between the concept of variations within the norm and developmental tolerances. For the purpose of clinical assessment, these two concepts provide us with the orientation request to judge the effect of change on the individual and also expose the limits of our present knowledge. Solnit then proceeded to examine the impact of acute disasters, such as the Buffalo Creek incident, and the need to differentiate between the adaptive external maneuvers to cope with disaster and the prolonged internal disequilibrium that persists, sometimes indefinitely. Here he introduced—as Anthony did—the relationship of individual vulnerability to the at-risk environment, warning us not to generalize without asking into account the individual life history and predisposition. In his words, each child co-determines or selects *his* environment, and thus one has to determine for each individual his affective environment.

He then went on to suggest that in order to learn more about the process of change, we should look closely at what takes place during development as well as to examine the biological and environmental factors that also appear to be involved. In studying developmental progression, we can learn that there is no even continuum, no easy passage from the old to the new and that organization leads to reorganization and to new structural formations. Each state has its own conflicts and resolutions, to be followed by new tasks. Development is characterized by progressive-regressive swings and symptoms that are age appropriate, or better, change appropriate that can constantly appear and disappear. Observing this fluctuating process, one may gain comfort from it and a better perspective of what may be expected during change.

In thinking of some of the stresses and strains that beset each generation in transition, and of Mead's statement that developmentally we are all immigrants, I was reminded of the adolescent stage, with its disorganization, its upheaval in psychic structure, and the reemergence of the old (and, at the same time, the turning against the old, so that old symptoms reappear in both old and new guises), and amidst all this ferment, its formation of a new ego ideal and a new identity. The environment may interfere with these processes conducing to regressions and fixations or to precocious progressions with its pathologic consequences. One cannot extend the developmental model to include all formal change, but since change is an inherent part of our inner psychic as well as outer experience, it would seem worthwhile to explore systematically the potentialities of the epigenetic model for the study of change. The challenge before us is to differentiate between those crises, stresses, and symptoms that are a part of change from those that interfere with it. This understanding may also help to determine our modes of therapeutic intervention.

As Anthony has pointed out apropos the various presentations, both Western and Eastern, we are all struggling to integrate what sometimes looks like conflicting and incompatible propositions regarding the traditional and modern and have not been so successful in doing so. There appears to be two major trends. On the one hand, there is the Indian tradition, its ancient history and the richness of its spiritual life in which emphasis is placed on living harmoniously with the natural, social, and supernatural environment and on communal rather than on individual understandings and achievements. In the West stress is placed on self-reliance and on actions aimed at mastering the material environment. Thus dependence on parents is viewed very differently in India and in the West. One should respect such differences, seek to understand them, and refrain from assessing them hastily without adequate knowledge, background, and experience. One must have lived for some time (and not 2 weeks!), "Withdrawn from the illusory world of the senses and in the reality of the psychic experience." Most of all, as a transient, one must suspend judgment, always an exacting task, at least for Westerners! Neki added to this discomfort when he stated that any psychotherapeutic system that did not owe its loyalty to the transcendent goals of mental health (which, of course, includes most Western psychotherapeutic procedures), would be ipso facto rather than helpful. His own inclination was to remain within the traditional system and develop an Indian methodology of treatment. With such built-in restrictions, science would become culture bound and not a search for truth, at least in the opinion of this reporter. On the other hand, there is an opposing trend that stemmed from data presented by those Indian colleagues who have either applied modern clinical methods or have presented clinical findings in a framework with which we were familiar. Dr. Gore, for example, applied social science concepts to outline for us the family patterns now prevailing in India, and we were thus able to compare his findings with our own. Ramanujam, in his careful demographic studies reflecting change in our time and the influence of urban life on changes in diagnostic categories, allowed us to compare the differences and similarities of disturbances in both countries. Transcultural psychiatry is only feasible if we can share a common scientific basis and approach.

In a narrower sense, however, we are not and should not be concerned with the issue of whether the traditional should be cherished and maintained or whether new forms of living and new approaches to living are to be preferred, or even of how we can understand each of them. Our topic asks us to focus on change, the assessment of change, and concomitant psychic experience and stresses. At the same time the pull toward the traditional or toward the modern is also a part of the process of change, and in the context of our topic we have many insightful contributions. Perhaps, because it may have been a less-complex task, Benninger addressed himself most clearly to the subject of change. He outlined an optimal model—life as it ought to be—and formulated three steps: a beginning one, locational change and its housing requirement; an intermediate one; and a consolidating step. He added that "unfortunately" this optimal model of movement was rare and therefore proceeded to outline other models, the pathological, the accommodating, the premature consolidating, which are terms that appeal to us because they seem to conjure up developmental analogues.

Chiland presented an important longitudinal study of adolescents in a changing world, in which she described the interaction of changing developmental stages with a changing environment. Her term emphasizes the many-sidedness of the period. The work studies an antedote to the distorted images of the adolescent that are projected and accepted by the mass media. The adolescents investigated had a similarity to the adolescents of many years ago, giving an indication of the rapid shifts in manifest behavior that are taking place. In her study Chiland found a critical period of development around 15 years of age, whereas American studies have located a crisis somewhat earlier, between 12 and 14 years of age. Chiland explored the identity conflict in urban India and attempted in a dynamic approach to disentangle the various factors contributing to it, while Bassa was interested in correlating child-rearing practices, the separation-individuation process, and identity formation.

Gore examined the pressure for change in urban India and the sociological consequences in relation to occupation, age of marriage, the concept of equality, and a rationality that challenged the legitimacy of tradition. He was, like a good scientist, careful to warn us that his interpretations went beyond the facts and even more in the nature of hypotheses for future testing. I must also mention, briefly for want of space, the vivid account given by Carstairs of the contrast between the North American and British experience of Indian immigrants.

Coelho investigated the impact of television and the pressing need to study this extraordinary tool and its influence on the lives of children and their parents. The mass media represent undoubtedly powerful instruments of change. One must not fail to mention the many and enriching contributions that Dr. Hoch made to the general discussion. Her vast experience blended a variety of fields and gave her a bird's eye view of the great diversity of situations and patterns of change in India. She recommended that the "transitional section" as she called it, should form the object of a future study of change, since this was where change was most likely to manifest itself. She found that the polar groups—the traditional and the modern—resembled each other in many ways. In her longitudinal studies she described the effect of early or late toilet training on successful and unsuccessful socialization and the fact that mothers in nuclear families were better able to improve their uprearing methods from one child to the next, whereas the mothers from joint families were tied down to the practices of their mothers-in-law.

I will mention a few additional themes that emerged from the various presentations. One of these can be summarized under the heading of "developmental variations." Almost all the contributors stated that the normal phase progression, as outlined in the psychoanalytic theory of development, are not seen when one studies Indian children or adolescents. Psychoanalytic investigations by Bassa and Roland indicated that the usual separation-individuation process could not be observed, that individuation did not lead to separateness, that the self was an expression of group identity, and that the ego ideal was an expression of group ideals. Furthermore, it was alleged that adolescence as described in the psychoanalytic literature as a period of upheaval and conflict is never seen in India. Adolescence is a quiescent period, and presumably much of it is due to early and continuing interdependency. Thus intrapsychic conflicts and the emergence of the oedipal struggle around the primary objects could not be documented. These findings led to the question of whether cultural and social conditions impose themselves on developmental progression, perhaps subduing otherwise inherent phase organization, or whether the development that we observe in Western society is a product of our social and family structure and whether the role of the individual in our society is expressed in our child-rearing practices. The Indian child from earliest life on is regulated toward dependency; deviations from it are not tolerated. This may bring about a different developmental and characterological structure.

A second theme centered around the psychodynamics of the conjoint family. The contributors described the social system of interdependence, psychological dependency, and dependability that give wide-ranging protection to each member of the family. Any understanding of the function of the individual must be seen in this context: the child from the beginning of life has interacted with many members of the family. The changes that are observable today in the outside world are a function of changes in family patterns: mothers who accept jobs, the move to urban communities with smaller housing units, and the general national interest in reducing the birth rate. Therefore, a strong correlation was made between individual behavioral function or pathology and specific Indian family dynamics and structure.

The vicissitudes of aggression was still another theme that arose in the discussions. Some stated that in Indian religion and culture aggression has to be viewed as something different from the aggression seen in Western society. The search for harmony and unity and the wish for transcendence of physical desires in the Indian child differ from the wish for mastery, independence, and the search for individual expression that characterize European and American children. It was said that one could find expression of assertion but not of aggression in India. Others brought clinical material that indicated that aggression did have a place in everyday living, that there could be violent outbursts if not within the group then against other groups, that there was evidence of ambivalence, and that there were various forms of symptomatology that could only be understood if one regarded them as expressions of the aggressive drive.

In our daily practice we are aware of an array of defensive maneuvers such as isolation, repression, denial, projection, but none of these become operative during the pressure of change when this is adaptive or pathological in nature.

We also need to study the personality in response to change in terms of its flexibility and rigidity, its tolerance to change, or its resistance to it. There may be well-functioning individuals in a traditional setting who are quite unable to tolerate the stress of rapid change, and there may be unstructured individuals who do not fit into a stable system but who do well under circumstances of change. Thus the role assignment and function of individuals in a traditional family may shift during change and bring about a remarkable reshuffling of authority assignment and leadership. There are those who suffer during change and those who feel mobilized and comfortable with it with ease; the former become unsettled and the latter pioneers of new frontiers and leaders of new societies. We may all be immigrants, but some of us will forge ahead while others will stay behind. We need to study the personality characteristics as they correlate with periods of transition.

These vivid references are samples of the richness that pervaded the meeting as a whole, both in its presentations and discussions. If one were able to put them together and examine their implications carefully, one might well arrive at criteria for measuring change and for following the processes of change. At the same time, it was not surprising that we also ran into questions for which we had no answer and that represented the limits to our knowledge. The theme of change was chosen because of its worldwide impact on families and our wish to understand the nature of this impact better as well as its effects, because we are all in the same boat, whether our countries are developed or undeveloped, democratic or communistic, all in the state of transition. We do not know as yet to what extent the manifestations of stress and strain are the inevitable price we pay for innovations, the spur to new development, or the symptoms of aberrant adaptation.

Anna Freud, a few years ago in a lecture, addressed herself to the changing conditions of our patients; where once there were inner conflicts due to repression and evident in neurologic symptoms, there was now the opposite: the acting on impulse, the reaching out for immediate gratification, and the location of problems in the interplay between individual need and environment rather than within the individual. Will this change lead to a new form of balance? Is it a necessary reaction to the past, or is it a reaction to the loss of social and family structure and the absence of trusted ideologies?

We heard much about the significance of the Indian family pattern. The conjoint family provides a natural system of interdependence, the advantage to which is security, protection, and provision, and the price for which is obedience, submergence of individuality, a group ego identity, and conformity to the strict rules. One must respect this particular pattern of the human family and learn to assess the personality traits of dependency or identity formation as it is reflected in it. Nor must we attach the same significance to it that dependency carries in Western families. These are basic anthropological propositions.

What, however, is the meaning of pathology within this kind of family pattern? Which symptoms are sociosyntonic? Which socioalien and which need to be modified? What sort of and what amount of change can the family tolerate without being disrupted? However useful this particular family pattern may be, surely there must be role assignment within it; there must be those who are preferred, those with authority, and those with executive function, and with all this there must be sibling rivalry. Can change bring about greater flexibility without the loss of the protective shield for all the members? As the community steps in to provide services, day care, health, and education, will this strengthen the family as a whole or will the delegation to others weaken it? In Israel Caplan spoke of the variety of support systems provided by the extended family, in the absence of which support must come from the community, from social agencies, and from health and welfare resources. Can there be a balance that brings about a change and is not simply a shift from one dependent state to another? Most importantly, can one support the family from the outside and still leave decision making to it? And can we support the family's reliance on itself and still avoid making it a passive recipient? What we need at this point in history is careful and systematic longitudinal studies of Indian families in change that might answer some of the questions that have been raised.

We have discussed the usefulness of the developmental model for the study of change, but there is another that has not been explored. It is the therapeutic model. The former permits us to see the forward movement of change, the steps and processes of progression; the latter invites us to review the past, to look backward in order to bring about reorganization, to correct past misconceptions and fears, and to free us from those interferences that do not allow us to be what we are. It aims to open up new choices. In the psychoanalytic model of therapy this is not achieved by direction or clarification or guidance. Psychoanalysis also attempts to achieve a harmony between biological demands of psychic life and our notions of what life ought to be as expressed in our consciousness and in the reality of our environment. It aims for a new synthesis, a new integration, and a blending of life-supporting and assertive-aggressive striving. We can learn from our therapeutic work about what interferes with the attainment of this goal, about the resistances to giving up old projective defenses, even if inappropriate for the present, as for the future, and about the tendency toward compulsive repetition in repeating instead of re-membering. We must explore this therapeutic model systematically and see to what degree it helps us to understand not only the adapta-tions to change but also the ways in which therapy helps in the adap-tation to change. Rilka has expressed, in his own profound and prac-tical way, the changes that he expected to achieve: "I believe in all that has never been said before; I wish to free all my spiritual feel-ings, so that what no one even had dared to wish shall come to me without effort." This is much more than any of us could wish for ourselves or our patients, but it speaks of the ideals of change that haunt us all until death when we can no longer change.

Epilogue

E. James Anthony, M.D. (U.S.A.)

To write about change is to continue mankind's debate through the centuries: does it exist or is it illusionary? Do things change or only people? Are we the agents of change, the products of change, or merely the victims of change? De we need to change the conditions of particular lives before we can change the people who live these lives? Why do some of us thrive on change and others succumb to it? Do men require constancy as much as they need change, and is the well-adjusted life a delicate balance between the two? Is change inevitable, and if it is, is it fruitless to be for or against it?

These and many other questions of the same kind have provoked opposite and apparently irreconcilable viewpoints since the dawn of consciousness and the first perceptions of a continuously changing world. Psychologically, nevertheless, the development of a sense of constancy has as much importance as the development of the sense of change and may function as the needed antidote to it. Like most basic phenomena, change is difficult to define in a way that is inclusive of its many sidedness. One might say very simply that change is anything that happens, whether slowly or rapidly, whether in large or small amounts. Theoretically, both dimensions are measurable, although in practice it is not easy to construct appropriate measures. In order to study change one needs to look at it from the outside as an observer. This in itself poses a problem, since the observer himself is generally caught up in the changes he is observing. He is not standing still, however much he may think he is. This means that in making observations on change, we need to include observations on the changing observer.

In this book the contributors have more or less taken up positions *sub specie aeternitatis* and have looked at the child and his family in a changing world as if they were not part of it themselves. This is a license that all scientists allow themselves: it allows them to be objective, uninvolved and relatively impersonal. For these so-called nonparticipant observers, three sets of changes become apparent:

1. Changes that take place within the individual as a function of his growth and development through the life cycle.
2. Changes that occur in the world surrounding the individual and which may include near events, such as changes in the family, in the neighborhood, or in the school, and distant events, such as changes in the country, in the continent, or in the world. The first set of changes may be referred to as personal and the second as impersonal.
3. Interactive effects of changes in the individual and changes in his environment. At times, a period of rapid and great change in the individual, such as at adolescence, may coincide with periods of rapid and great changes in the environment, both personal and impersonal, and as a result the experience of change is maximized. At a certain threshold, which differs for different individuals, the change becomes stressful, and the individual is then said to be at risk. Whether he succumbs to the stresses of change will depend on his resilience or vulnerability. Some individuals can adapt to large amounts of change rapidly delivered, whereas others, more change-sensitive, may find themselves overwhelmed by even minimal changes. The less resilient ones will tend to become change-resistant and will do their best to keep both themselves and their world "just so." Such resistance to change is found everywhere, but it tends to become especially prominent in areas dedicated to traditionalism.

As one travels across the world (as one does through the pages of this book), one is aware not only of change but also of the way in which change itself changes under different conditions and different circumstances. Pascal was especially aware of this when he remarked that "we find hardly anything which does not change its character in changing its climate." In addition to this geography of change, there is also the history of change: every epoch brings its changes with it, both large and small. Various parts of this book have dealt with historical change and the perpetual dialectic of past and present as recorded by historians and as manifested in the daylong, lifelong relations between parents, between parents and their children, and between families and their environment. Changes over the centuries have led to alterations in personal and social life; changes from the outside have permeated the internal structure of the personality that has not only affected the formation of identity but has at times conduced to massive shifts of human consciousness. We therefore need to take clear notice of change not only in daily human intercourse but also in clinical practice. To quote Wilde:

> The only thing that one really knows about human nature is that it changes. Change is the one quality we can predicate on it. The systems that fail are those that rely on the permanency of human nature, and not on its growth and development.

The capacity to change is important for the mental health not only of the individual but also of the world at large. Change has been said to be the great enemy of revolution, meaning that where stagnation is the rule, upheaval is very likely to occur, and the same is true of the individual.

Coelho and Stein [1] have pointed to the stresses that are resulting from an urbanization of the planet. They predict that even though most of the human race is still rooted in a rural way of life, that if present trends continue, by the year 2000 more than two-thirds of the human race will be living and working in towns and cities. This is astonishing in view of the fact that for nearly 10,000 years our habitats were essentially agricultural settlements and that in oddly 200 years the industrial revolution has produced changes of such a magnitude and rate that new coping skills have become necessary to meet the sociotechnical demands of modernization. These two authors have developed a series of hypotheses to interrelate the factors of change, vulnerability and coping:

Hypothesis 1. Individuals experience psychological stress when there is an unexpected or unusual change in their social or physical environment, such as uprooting due to war or natural disaster or forced relocation.

Hypothesis 2. Psychological stress is likely to increase when environmental change occurs at the same time as a severe life crisis that involves the disruption of emotional bonds, as evident, for example, in the higher morbidity rate in grieving widows and divorcees.

Hypothesis 3. Psychological stress (and concomitant health hazards) are likely to increase when environmental changes cluster at critical developmental periods, such as adolescence, menopause, and other transitions in the life cycle.

Hypothesis 4. Mechanisms of coping behavior are developed in response to environmental change and their efficacy depends on several factors: the awareness of the changing situation, the motivation and readiness to respond creatively to challenge, the emotional and social supports available and the institutional provisions of solutions to such crises.

The syndromes of modernization include the stresses of uprooting (with its attendant psychological alienation), the syndrome of overcrowding that results from the disparity between the individual's demand for space and the supply of space, from the noise that brings about feelings of crowdedness and frustrates desires for privacy, peace and quiet, and from the feelings of isolation and loneliness that paradoxically result from high-density living.

Another characteristic change that has a huge significance for the child and his family has to do with the experimentation with new life styles and nontraditional family structures such as communes and counterculture groups. There have also been changes in the communes themselves. The original commune has now decreased its reliance on drugs and increased its competence in agricultural work. Their members still function literally in terms of property and the sharing of financial responsibility. Surrogate parents continue to be available for children whenever necessary. In many ways, the commune seems to function as an extended family group or at times like an Israeli kibbutz in which children are protected and cared for by the group as a whole. This pattern of general caring for children includes teenagers. It must be remembered that the situation is largely an experimental one and therefore subjected to the waywardness of the members and their level of competence. In some communes the members are undoubtedly disturbed and lacking in parenting skills, and the way of life is consequently disorganized; in such settings it is true that the children do seem somewhat lost, poorly differentiated, and pseudomature. It has been said by McConville [5] that "the point at issue with counter-culture groups is not so much the structures themselves but the intensity with which particular ideological viewpoints may be held, which may in turn interfere with parenting or nurturance and with the necessary evolution of the family."

The total kibbutz situation in its ideological background, complex peer systems, day care, and provision of competent "paraparents" in addition to biological parents, does seem to be a more sustaining and holding culture, chiefly because of its longer experience. There is some support for the view that children of the kibbutz are more self-reliant and less dependent on parenting figures than those from "nuclear" families.

These changes in life styles and new patterns of child rearing are having their impact on conventional systems. Child-rearing modes, outlooks, and practices of existing institutions are already manifesting changes that make them less clearly distinguishable from modes in the counterculture. Eiduson and her colleagues [2], in fact, describe a two-pronged movement of change: counterculture people are becoming resocialized into the mainstream, on the one hand, and mainstream institutions are incorporating changes from the counterculture, on the other hand. As they put it: "This kind of change is not uncommon when vital social and psychological phenomena are under longitudinal study. However, unique to this study may be the rapidity of social change in our culture today, a rapidity which may even be hastening changes that normally take place in the young child."

Apart from the changes brought about by countercultural movements, the women's movement was making a major impact at every level of the social order, combating discrimination and suggestions of inferiority wherever they were found. It was part of the mythology related to sex differences that men came to regard themselves as changers who relished novelty, whereas women were seen as change-resistant, reactionary, and traditional in their outlook. This belief was opposed by no less a person than Karl Marx, who said; "Anyone who knows anything of history knows that great social changes are impossible without the feminine ferment. Social progress can be measured exactly by the social position of the fair sex (the ugly ones included)" [6]. Here he is talking about women not as agents but as indicators of change. Developmentalists have pointed out that little boys do seem to be more active and more exploratory than little girls from very early on, but it is difficult to exclude the cultural influence that may well determine and limit the range of feminine behavior in pursuit of some feminine ideal. The drive for equality on the part of women has had many repercussions on the structure and functioning of the family, on the care of children, on the relationship between the spouses, and on the instrumental roles of father and mother. During this period of transition and change, it would not be surprising to find that more children are becoming disturbed by the disequilibrium in the home, but clinicians, who have observed children adapt to all types of novel situations during their upbringing, are generally optimistic that there will be an adjustment to the new order and that after a period of disquiet the families will settle down. It has been emphasized in several presentations in this book that the capacity to change in response to changing conditions, changing environmental demands, and changing modes of family life is one of the qualities to be considered in predicting the future mental health of the individual. Yet, changeability is not a virtue in itself and in its extreme form can represent a pathological state in which the individual is so inconstant as to lack a central core of identity. A capacity to change should not be confused with abnormal changeability.

The reason why environmental change has been relatively overlooked in the past by clinicians may be due to several causes: their tendency to take the environment for granted as part of the givens of clinical practice and to be relatively unaware of maturational and developmental responses evoked by differing social, cultural, and physical environments. Often the clinician is jarred out of such attitudes and expectations only by acute or disastrous environmental changes. The complex character of the connections between internal, interpersonal, and external factors has transformed the nature of change as understood today into a multifactorial event system leading to greater difficulty in evaluating its reliability, validity, and objectivity. Finally, the increased density of the environment and the increased rate of change and of change agents are in need of study. Life for the child and his parents in today's world is not only understood in a more complicated way—it really is more complicated. In the past the individual and environment were connected in a much more direct way. For example, the Sioux Indians, a century ago, related to the environment through the buffalo [9]:

It is said that when the buffalo died, the Sioux died, ethnically and spiritually. The buffalo's body had provided not only food and material for clothing, covering and shelter, but such utilities as bags and boats, string for bows and for sewing, cups and spoons. Medicine and ornaments were made of buffalo parts; his droppings, sun dried, served as fuel in the winter. Societies and seasons, ceremonies and dances, mythology and children's play extolled his name and image.

There is a "buffalo" in the lives of most families that keeps them together, gives meaning to their lives, and allows them to create a family history that is continuous and coherent. The "buffalo" may become a victim of change, and the family, in a sense, dies along with it unless it can create a new symbol, a new mythology to preserve and sustain its members.

One of the major problems that confronts us today is the lack of preparation for change on the part of the younger generation, and the onus for this must be laid on the shoulders of their elders. The young, therefore, go out unprepared and are consequently bewildered and mystified by the kaleidoscope of the changing world that confronts them. Helen Keller [4], shut in behind her missing senses and groping toward an outside world with which she could have only a fragmentary experience, had yet the wisest comment to make on this serious problem, and we can do little better than be guided by this blind and deaf woman into a better future. What she said was:

Serious harm, I am afraid, has been wrought to our generation by fostering the idea that they would live secure in a permanent order of things. They have expected stability and have found none within themselves or in their universe. Before it is too late they must learn and teach others *that only by brave acceptance of change* and all-time crisis-ethics can they rise to the heights of superlative responsibility.

Bibliography

1. Coelho, G. V. and Stein, J. J. Coping with stresses of an urban planet: Impacts of uprooting and overcrowding. *Habitat,* 3/4 (1977), 379–390.
2. Cohen, J. and Eiduson, B. T. Changing patterns of child rearing in alternative life styles. In *Child Development and Psychopathology,* A. Davids, Ed. New York, Wiley, 1976.
3. Erikson, E. H. Observations on Sioux education. *J. Psych.,* 7 (1939), 101–156.
4. Keller, H. *The Open Door.* New York, Doubleday, 1957.
5. McConville, B. J. *Nontraditional Families and Their Impact on the Child.* Presented at the Regional Study Group meeting of the I.A.C.P.A.P. at Quebec, 1977.
6. Marx, K. *Letters.* 1868.

Index

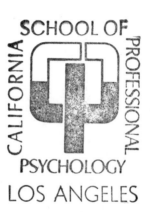

CALIFORNIA SCHOOL OF PROFESSIONAL PSYCHOLOGY

LOS ANGELES